Principles of Perioperative Safety and Efficiency

Jamal J. Hoballah • Haytham M. A. Kaafarani
Georgios Tsoulfas
Editors

Principles of Perioperative Safety and Efficiency

Springer

Editors
Jamal J. Hoballah
Surgery
American University of Beirut
Medical Center
Beirut, Lebanon

Haytham M. A. Kaafarani
Surgery
Massachusetts General Hospital
Boston, MA, USA

Georgios Tsoulfas
Transplantation Surgery
Aristotle University School of Medicine
Thessaloniki, Greece

ISBN 978-3-031-41088-8 ISBN 978-3-031-41089-5 (eBook)
https://doi.org/10.1007/978-3-031-41089-5

This Springer imprint is published by the registered company Springer Nature Switzerland AG
The registered company address is: Gewerbestrasse 11, 6330 Cham, Switzerland

We dedicate this textbook to our patients, to whom we pledge every day to provide with the safest and highest quality care that we can.

Foreword

It gives me great pleasure to write this foreword to *Principles of Perioperative Safety and Efficiency*, as this text represents many different elements of the surgical experience. This is a tremendous example of the remarkable success of the Dr. Pon Fund International Chapter Opportunity program, which is named for Pon Satitpunwaycha, MD, FACS, whose generous donation through the American College of Surgeons (ACS) International Relations Committee has sponsored educational courses by ACS chapters around the world. The textbook is based on the "Principles of Perioperative Safety and Efficiency" course, which was offered in July 2018 in Beirut, Lebanon, by the Lebanese ACS Chapter, supported by a Dr. Pon Fund award. The enthusiastic participation in that course highlighted the need to address, safeguard, and promote principles of perioperative safety and efficiency. The entire perioperative process impacts successful surgical outcomes.

Despite various national and global safety initiatives, perioperative adverse events remain alarmingly high, and this is especially notable in hospitals in low- and middle-income countries, which may lack the resources to address the factors leading to untoward events. This textbook aims to teach healthcare providers the fundamental standards of perioperative safety and efficiency. This text is appropriate not only for surgeons, but also for anesthesiologists, residents of many specialties, medical students, nurses, hospital administrators, and other members of the healthcare team. Many will derive benefit from multiple chapters, including those focused on informed consent in the digital era, cost containment, checklists, medication errors, management of challenging patients, surgical site infections, handling of specimens, error reporting, and data-driven safety and quality measurements.

In my role at the ACS, I continue to focus on our 110-year-old motto, "To Heal All with Skill and Trust." The principles espoused in this text are central to our mission. I am pleased at the collaborative approach taken by surgeons around the world to advance ACS initiatives and improve the care of all our patients.

Finally, I would like to extend my congratulations to Jamal J. Hoballah, MD, MBA, FACS; Haytham M. A. Kaafarani, MD, MPH, FACS; and Georgios Tsoulfas, MD, PhD, FACS for their efforts in the coordination and collaboration necessary to convene these extraordinary surgeon authors. Moreover, I thank each of them for their commitment to the International Relations Committee of the ACS, each having served in leadership roles.

I am confident that this text will be a valuable resource to surgeons and health-care workers in all practice settings.

American College of Surgeons
Chicago, IL, USA

Patricia L. Turner

Preface

> "You must know, my pupils, that operative surgery is divided into two parts: one where the operation is performed safely, and one, on the other hand, where lethal complications arise."
> Albucasis, 1000 AD, On Surgery & Surgical Instruments

Surgery is a high-hazard field. Despite all the technological advances, perioperative mortality and morbidity rates remain high. Despite decades of the patient safety movement, wrong-site surgery still happens. Despite awareness, surgical fires and intraoperative deaths still occur. The journey toward zero preventable harm to surgical patients is long but worthwhile.

It is with great pride that we bring you the first perioperative safety textbook. The textbook is comprehensive, covering multiple areas of safety and quality of the surgical patient, from preoperative to intraoperative and postoperative care. In this textbook, experts in surgical, medical, and anesthesia safety have come together to bring you the latest in safety science and the latest evidence in high-reliability science and have applied it to surgery in order to ensure surgical patients always receive the highest quality and safest care possible.

We hope this textbook serves as a valuable reference to the millions of nurses, physicians, administrators, and healthcare providers who have dedicated their lives to safeguarding surgical patients worldwide.

Beirut, Lebanon — Jamal J. Hoballah
Thessaloniki, Greece — Georgios Tsoulfas
Boston, USA — Haytham M. A. Kaafarani

Contents

Contributors

Jyotsna Agarwal Department of Anesthesiology and Pain Medicine, Hamdard Institute of Medical Sciences and Research, New Delhi, India

Abdulelah Alhawsawi Novo Genomics, Riyadh, Saudi Arabia

Thomas A. Aloia Oncology Services, Maternal Health and Perinatal Medicine, Ascension, Houston, TX, USA

Marie T. Aouad Department of Anesthesiology, American University of Beirut Medical Center, Beirut, Lebanon

Michel Attieh Department of Anatomical Pathology and Laboratory Medicine, American University of Beirut Medical Center, Beirut, Lebanon

Chakib Maurice Ayoub Department of Anesthesiology, Duke University school of Medicine, Durham, NC, USA

Tala Ballouz Department of Internal Medicine, Division of Infectious Diseases, American University of Beirut, Beirut, Lebanon

Fouad Boulos Department of Pathology and Immunology, Washington University in St. Louis, St. Louis, MO, USA

Davy Cheng Schulich School of Medicine & Dentistry, Western University, London, ON, Canada

Meena Nathan Cherian Global Health New Challenge, Geneva Foundation for Medical Education and Research, Versoix, Switzerland

Chrysanthos D. Christou Center for Research and Innovation in Solid Organ Transplantation, Department of Transplantation Surgery, Aristotle University School of Medicine, Thessaloniki, Greece

Julia R. Coleman Department of Surgery, University of Colorado–Denver, Aurora, CO, USA

Jeffrey B. Cooper Department of Anesthesia, Critical Care, & Pain Medicine, Massachusetts General Hospital, Boston, MA, USA

Department of Anesthesia, Harvard Medical School, Boston, MA, USA

Center for Medical Simulation, Boston, MA, USA

Justin B. Dimick Frederick A. Coller Distinguished Professor and Chair Department of Surgery, Michigan Medicine, University of Michigan, Ann Arbor, MI, USA

Roman Dudaryk Department of Anesthesiology, University of Miami, Miami, FL, USA

Ryder Trauma Center, Jackson Memorial Hospital, Miami, FL, USA

Sarada Eleswarpu Department of Anesthesiology, Duke University school of Medicine, Durham, NC, USA

Majed El Hechi Department of Surgery, Massachusetts General Hospital, Boston, MA, USA

Adrian W. Gelb Department of Anesthesia and Perioperative Care, University of California San Francisco, San Francisco, CA, USA

Alex Haynes Department of Surgery and Perioperative Care, University of Texas Austin, Austin, TX, USA

Rana M. Higgins Department of Surgery, Medical College of Wisconsin, Milwaukee, WI, USA

Jamal J. Hoballah Department of Surgery, American University of Beirut Medical Center, Beirut, Lebanon

Ryan Howard Department of Surgery, University of Michigan, Ann Arbor, MI, USA

Kamal M. F. Itani Department of Surgery, Veterans Affairs Boston Healthcare System, West Roxbury, MA, USA

Department of Surgery, Boston University, Boston, USA

Harvard Medical School, Boston, MA, USA

Haytham M. A. Kaafarani Department of Surgery, Division of Trauma, Emergency Surgery and Surgical Critical Care, Massachusetts General Hospital, Boston, MA, USA

Cynthia Karam American University of Beirut Medical Center, Beirut, Lebanon

Petra Khoury Health and Care Department, International Federation of Red Cross Red Crescent, Geneva, Switzerland

Gentian Kristo Department of Surgery, Veterans Affairs Boston Healthcare System, West Roxbury, MA, USA

Harvard Medical School, Boston, MA, USA

Wilton C. Levine, M.D. Department of Anesthesia, Critical Care and Pain Medicine, Massachusetts General Hospital, Boston, MA, USA

M. Sofia Macedo Center for National Health Insurance, Ar Rabi, Riyadh, Saudi Arabia

Wissam Maroun American University of Beirut Medical Center, Beirut, Lebanon

Janet Martin Department of Anesthesia & Perioperative Medicine, Epidemiology & Biostatistics, London Health Sciences Centre, London, ON, Canada

Charbel F. Matar Department of Internal Medicine, University of Connecticut, Farmington, CT, USA

Lydia R. Maurer Department of Surgery, Massachusetts General Hospital, Boston, MA, USA

George Molina Brigham and Women's Hospital, Boston, MA, USA

Elizabeth Mort Department of Medicine, Massachusetts General Hospital, Boston, MA, USA

Marc A. de Moya Division of Trauma and Acute Care Surgery, Medical College of Wisconsin, Milwaukee, WI, USA

Nathan D. Neilsen Section of Transfusion Medicine and Therapeutic Pathology, Division of Pulmonary, Critical Care, and Sleep Medicine, University of New Mexico School of Medicine, Albuquerque, NM, USA

Timothy E. Newhook Department of Surgical Oncology, Division of Surgery, MD Anderson Cancer Center, Houston, TX, USA

Raymond R. Price Center for Global Surgery, University of Utah, Salt Lake City, UT, USA

Marwan M. Refaat Department of Internal Medicine/ Division of Cardiology, American University of Beirut, Faculty of Medicine and Medical Center (AUBMC), Beirut, Lebanon

Department of Biochemistry and Molecular Genetics, American University of Beirut Faculty of Medicine, Beirut, Lebanon

Scott E. Regenbogen Department of Surgery, University of Michigan, Ann Arbor, MI, USA

Samantha J. Rivard Department of Surgery, University of Michigan, Ann Arbor, MI, USA

Marwan Sarkis Rizk Department of Anesthesiology, American University of Beirut, Beirut, Lebanon

Nesrine A. Rizk Department of Internal Medicine, Division of Infectious Diseases, American University of Beirut, Beirut, Lebanon

Mohammad Sabra Department of Internal Medicine/Division of Cardiology, Henry Ford Health, Detroit, MI, USA

Carine Sakr Department of Employee Health, American University of Beirut Medical Center, Beirut, Lebanon

Richard Schulick University of Colorado Department of Surgery, Aurora, CO, USA

University of Colorado Cancer Center, Aurora, CO, USA

University of Colorado Anschutz Medical Campus, Aurora, CO, USA

Jamie L. Sparling Department of Anesthesia, Critical Care, & Pain Medicine, Massachusetts General Hospital, Boston, MA, USA

Department of Anesthesia, Harvard Medical School, Boston, MA, USA

Ali Taher Division of Hematology and Oncology, Department of Internal Medicine, American University of Beirut Medical Center, Beirut, Lebanon

Yasmine Tameze, M.D. Department of Anesthesia, Critical Care and Pain Medicine, Massachusetts General Hospital, Boston, MA, USA

Georgios Tsoulfas Department of Transplantation Surgery, Center for Research and Innovation in Solid Organ Transplantation, Aristotle University School of Medicine, Thessaloniki, Greece

Center for Research and Innovation in Solid Organ Transplantation, Department of Transplantation Surgery, Aristotle University School of Medicine, Thessaloniki, Greece

Patricia L. Turner American College of Surgeons, Chicago, IL, USA

Ulfat Usta Pharmacy Department, Aman Hospital, Doha, Qatar

Mohammad Rachad Wehbe Division of Vascular Surgery, Department of Surgery, University of Rochester, Rochester, NY, USA

Daniel Dante Yeh Denver Health Medical Center, Denver, CO, USA

Abbreviations

AAMC	Association of American Medical Colleges
ABA	American Board of Anesthesiology
ABC	Assessment of blood consumption [score]
ABMS	American Board of Medical Specialties
ACC	American College of Cardiology
ACCP	American College of Chest Physicians
ACE	Angiotensin-converting enzyme
ACEi	Angiotensin-converting enzyme inhibitors
ACGME	Accreditation Council for Graduate Medical Education
ACS	American College of Surgeons
ACS NSQIP	American College of Surgeons National Surgical Quality Improvement Program®
ACS/SIS	American College of Surgeons and the Surgical Infection Society
ADD(s)	Automated dispensing device(s)
ADE(s)	Adverse drug event(s)
AEIs	Accredited Education Institutes
AEs	Adverse events
AGS	American Geriatrics Society
AHA	American Heart Association
AHRQ	Agency for Healthcare Research and Quality
AHTR(s)	Acute hemolytic transfusion reaction(s)
AI	Artificial intelligence
AIDS	Acquired immunodeficiency syndrome
AIMS	Anesthesia Information Management Systems
ALT	Alanine transaminase
AMR	Antimicrobial resistance
AMT	Anesthesia medication template
anti-HBc	Hepatitis B core antibodies
anti-HBs	Hepatitis B surface antibodies
AORN	Association of periOperative Registered Nurses
APSF	Anesthesia Patient Safety Foundation
aPTT	Activated partial thromboplastin time [test]
ARB	Angiotensin receptor blockers
ARM	Anesthetic-related mortality

ASA	American Society of Anesthesiologists
ASCO	American Society for Clinical Oncology
ASH	American Society of Hematology
ASHP	American Society of Health-System Pharmacists
ASPE	Association of Standardized Patient Educators
ASPF	Anesthesia Patient Safety Foundation
ASPiH	Association for Simulated Practice in Healthcare
ATC	Acute traumatic coagulopathy
ATLS	Advanced Trauma Life Support [course]
AV	Atrioventricular
BBP(s)	Blood-borne pathogen(s)
BID	Twice a day [dose]
BMI	Body mass index
BPMH	Best Possible Medication History
CABG	Coronary artery bypass grafting
CAP	College of American Pathologists
CAT	Critical administration threshold
CAT	Competency assessment tool
CBC	Complete blood count
CDC	Centers for Disease Control and Prevention
CDIs	*Clostridium difficile* infections
CDS	Clinical decision support
CHSE	Certified Healthcare Simulator Educator
CICV	Cannot intubate, cannot ventilate
CIED(s)	Cardiac implantable electronic device(s)
CISB	Critical incident stress debriefing
CMS	Centers for Medicare and Medicaid Services
CoC	Commission on Cancer
COT	Committee on Trauma
CPAP	Continuous positive airway pressure
CPC	Committee on Perioperative Care
CPOE	Computerized physician order entry [system(s)]
CRM	Crew resource management
CRM	Crisis resource management
CRT	Cardiac resynchronization therapy
CS	Clinical skills
CSPS	Council on Surgical and Perioperative Safety
CUSP	Comprehensive unit-based safety program
CVR	Chest X-ray
CXR	Chest radiograph
DAC	Difficult airway cart
DAM	Difficult airway management
DASH	Debriefing Assessment for Simulation in Healthcare [program]
DI	Difficult intubation
DMV	Difficult mask ventilation

DRGs	Diagnosis-related groups
DTI	Difficult tracheal intubation
dVSS	daVinci skills simulator
DVT	Deep vein thrombosis
EACTS	European Association for Cardio-Thoracic Surgery
EAS	European Atherosclerosis Society
EBL	Estimated blood loss
ECG	Electrocardiogram
ECRI	Emergency Care Research Institute
ECU	Electrocautery units
EE	Exposed employee
EFL	Expiratory flow limitation
EMI	Electromagnetic interference
EMT	Emergency medical team
EPA	Environmental Protection Agency
ER	Emergency room
ERAS	Enhanced recovery after surgery
ES	Erector spinae
ESA	European Society of Anesthesiology
ESA	Emergency surgical airway
ESC	European Society of Cardiology
ESU	Electrosurgery unit
FAA	Federal Aviation Administration
FDA	Food and Drug Administration
FeO_2	Fraction of expired oxygen
FES	Fundamentals of endoscopic surgery
FFP	Fresh frozen plasma
FiO_2	Fraction of inspired oxygen
FLS	Fundamentals of laparoscopic surgery
FMEA	Failure mode and effect analysis
FSTD	Flight simulation training devices
FUSE	Fundamental Use of Surgical Energy™
GA	General anesthesia
GCS	Graduated compression stockings
GDFT	Goal-directed fluid therapy
GTT	Global Trigger Tool
HAIs	Healthcare-associated infections/hospital-acquired infections
HbeAG	Hepatitis B e antigen
HBIG	Hepatitis B immunoglobulin
HbsAG	Hepatitis B surface antigen
HBV	Hepatitis B virus
HCUP	Healthcare Cost and Utilization Project
HCV	Hepatitis C virus
HCW	Healthcare workers
HERAM	Health Resources Availability Monitoring System

HFE	Human factors engineering
HFMEA	Healthcare failure mode and effect analysis
HFS	Hip fracture surgery
HICs	High-income countries
HIPAA	Health Insurance Portability and Accountability Act
HIT	Heparin-induced thrombocytopenia
HIV	Human immunodeficiency virus
HR	Heart rate
HRS	Heart Rhythm Society
iAEs	Intraoperative adverse events
ICD	Implantable cardioverter defibrillator
ICD-9-CM	International Classification of Diseases, Ninth Revision, Clinical Modification
ICRC	International Committee of the Red Cross
ICU	Intensive care unit
IFU	Instructions for use
IHI	Institute for Healthcare Improvement
ILR	Implantable loop recorder
IMSN	International Medication Safety Network
IMV	Invasive mechanical ventilation
INACSL	International Nursing Association of Clinical Simulation and Learning
INR	International normalized ratio [test]
IOM	Institute of Medicine
IPC	Intermittent pneumatic compression
IPSS	International Pediatric Simulation Society
ISCR	Improving Surgical Care and Recovery [program]
ISMP	Institute for Safe Medication Practice
IU	International unit
IV	Intravenous
IV-PCA	Intravenous patient-controlled analgesia
JCAHO	Joint Commission on Accreditation of Healthcare Organizations
JCI	Joint Commission International
LDUH	Low-dose unfractionated heparin
LFT(s)	Liver function test(s)
LMA	Laryngeal mask airway
LMICs	Low- and middle-income countries
LMWH	Low molecular weight heparin
LOS	Length of stay
LOSA	Line Operations Safety Audit
LT	Laryngeal tube
LVEF	Low ventricular ejection fraction
M & M	Morbidity and mortality
MAP	Mean arterial pressure

MATTERs	Military Application of Tranexamic Acid in Trauma Emergency Resuscitation study
MBSAQIP	Metabolic and Bariatric Surgery Accreditation and Quality Improvement Program
ME(s)	Medication error(s)
MELD	Model for end-stage liver disease
MGH	Massachusetts General Hospital
MI	Myocardial infarction
mL	Milliliter
MOCA®	Maintenance of Certification in Anesthesiology
MPs	Microparticles
MRSA	Methicillin-resistant *S. aureus*
MSF	Médecins Sans Frontières
MT	Massive transfusion
MTP(s)	Massive transfusion protocol(s)
MTS	Massive transfusion score
MTT	Medical team training
MV	Mask ventilation
NAPBC	National Accreditation Program for Breast Centers
NASA	National Aeronautics and Space Administration
NCC MERP	National Coordinating Council for Medication Error Reporting and Prevention
NDA	New drug approval
NDMR	Non-depolarizing muscle relaxation
NHSN	National Healthcare Safety Network
NIBP	Non-invasive blood pressure
NICE	National Institute for Health and Care Excellence
NIOSH	National Institute for Occupational Safety and Health
NMBA(s)	Neuromuscular blocking agent(s)
NRC	Nuclear Regulatory Commission
NSP	National Simulator Program
NSQIP	National Surgical Quality Improvement Program
NTDB	National Trauma Data Bank
NQF	National Quality Forum
O/E	Observed to expected [events]
OR	Operating room
OR	Odds ratio
OSCE	Objective Structured Clinical Exam
OSHA	Occupational Safety and Health Agency
PAC	Pre-anesthesia clinic
PACU	Post-anesthesia care unit
PALS	Pediatric advanced life support
PA-PSRS	Pennsylvania Patient Safety Reporting System
PBM	Patient blood management

PCA	Patient-controlled analgesia
PCI	Percutaneous coronary intervention
PDSA	Plan, do, study, act
PE	Pulmonary emboli
PEP	Post-exposure prophylaxis
PFO	Patent foramen ovale
PM	Pacemaker
POMR	Perioperative mortality rate
PPE	Personal protective equipment
PPM	Preventative periodic maintenance
PPV	Pulse pressure variation
PROMMTT	PRospective, Observational, Multicenter, Major Trauma Transfusion [study]
PROPPR	Pragmatic, randomized Optimal Platelet and Plasma Ratios [trial]
PSIs	Patient Safety Indicators
PT	Prothrombin time
PTSD	Post-traumatic stress disorder
PVC	Polyvinyl chloride
PWH	Prince of Wales Hospital/Rainer [score]
QA	Quality assurance
QI	Quality improvement
QIP(s)	Quality improvement program(s)
QL	Quadratus lumborum
RA	Regional anesthesia
RACE	Rescue, alarm, confine, extinguish
RAS-ACS	Resident and Associate Society of the American College of Surgeons
RBC(s)	Red blood cell(s)
RCA	Root cause analysis
RCRI	Revised cardiac risk index
RCT(s)	Randomized controlled trial(s)
RF	Radio frequency
RFDS	Radio-frequency detection systems
RFID	Radio-frequency identification
RI	Resuscitation intensity
RIOT	Return to intended oncologic therapy
ROTEM	Rotational thromboelastometry
RPI	Robust process improvement
RR	Recovery room
RSI(s)	Retained surgical item(s)
SAD	Supraglottic airway device
SAGES	Society of American Gastrointestinal and Endoscopic Surgeons
SAQ	Safety Attitudes Questionnaire
SBAR	Situation, Background, Assessment, and Recommendation

SCD	sequential compression device
SCIP	Surgical Care Improvement Project
SCORE	Surgical Council on Resident Education
SDB	Sleep disordered breathing
SDGs	Sustainable Development Goals
SEN	Simulation Education Network
SGA	Supraglottic airway
SMART	Specific, Measurable, Achievable, Relevant, and Timely
SOR	Safe operating rooms
SP	Source patient
SPSC	Saudi Patient Safety Center
SSH	Society for Simulation in Healthcare
SSI(s)	Surgical site infection(s)
S-TEAMS	Surgical Teamworking in Emergency and Acute Medical Situations
STPC	Standardization, Technology, Pharmacy / Prefilled / Premixed, and Culture
SURPASS	SURgical PAtient Safety System
SV	Stroke volume
SVV	Stroke volume variation
TACO	Transfusion-associated circulatory overload
TAP	Transversus abdominus plane
TASH	Trauma-associated severe hemorrhage [score]
TBSS	Traumatic bleeding severity score
TEA	Thoracic epidural anesthesia
TeamSTEPPS™	Team Strategies and Tools to Enhance Performance and Patient Safety
TEG	Thromboelastography
THA	Total hip arthroplasty
TID	Three times a day [dose]
TKA	Total knee arthroplasty
TQIP	Trauma Quality Improvement Program
TRALI	Transfusion-related acute lung injury
TRIM	Transfusion-related immunomodulation
TTI(s)	Transfusion-transmitted infection(s)
TXA	Tranexamic acid
UFH	Unfractionated heparin
UHC	United Health Care
UHC	University HealthSystem Consortium
UHC	Universal health overage
US	Ultrasound
USMLE	United States Medical Licensing Examination
UTI(s)	Urinary tract infection(s)
VA	Veterans Affairs
VEST©	Virtual Electrosurgery Skill Trainer

VET	Viscoelastic testing
ViSIOT	Video-Supported Simulation of Interactions in the Operating Theater
VL	Video laryngoscope
VRE	Vancomycin-resistant *Enterococci*
VTE	Venous thromboembolism
WFSA	World Federation of Societies of Anaesthesiologists
WHO	World Health Organization

Part I

Perioperative Optimization

1 Human Factors and Principles of Patient Safety: The James Reason Model

Ryan Howard and Justin B. Dimick

Introduction

The case scenario below, which will be revisited throughout this chapter, is an example of a situation in which people working within a complex system precipitate an adverse event despite nobody intending to do so. The traditional approach to this situation tends to focus on the individuals involved. The emergency department is to blame for not notifying the surgery service at the time of the patient's initial presentation. The radiology resident is to blame for not remarking on the presence of mesenteric swirling on her initial interpretation. The medicine team is to blame for not seeing that the imaging interpretation had been updated with critical information.

There is widespread cultural underpinning to this "person approach." It fulfills a desire for compensation and allows individuals to match the degree of blame with the harm of an error. This approach, however, fails to recognize that error is part of the human condition [1, 2]. Moreover, this approach fails to address the critical issues that can lead to prevention of a similar situation in the future [3]. Quite often, investigation of what appears to be an error on the part of an individual leads to the conclusion that the individual is not to blame. In aviation maintenance, it has been reported that up to 90% of lapses in quality are "blameless" [3, 4]. To focus exclusively on the individuals involved in an error fails to recognize the context of the larger system within which the error occurred. This is evidenced by the fact that the person approach rarely leads to action that can improve the system in which an error occurs, and rarely leads to systematic improvement [5].

R. Howard (✉)
Department of Surgery, University of Michigan, Ann Arbor, MI, USA
e-mail: rhow@med.umich.edu

J. B. Dimick
Frederick A. Coller Distinguished Professor and Chair Department of Surgery, Michigan Medicine, University of Michigan, Ann Arbor, MI, USA

J. J. Hoballah et al. (eds.), *Principles of Perioperative Safety and Efficiency*,
https://doi.org/10.1007/978-3-031-41089-5_1

In contrast to the person approach is the "system approach," which recognizes that humans are fallible and human error is inevitable. Rather than view human errors as the cause of an adverse event, human errors are viewed as the consequences of failures of systemic safeguards and barriers. In this light, the fatigued resident who orders the wrong dose of medication for a patient is a reflection of failures in reasonable work-hour limitations, appropriate supervision, and even lack of pharmacist support. Within the system approach, error analysis seeks to discover the systematic failures that lead to an adverse outcome in order to design better safeguards. Importantly, because the system approach analyzes the entire framework within which humans perform their duties, potential weaknesses can be identified and fixed before they result in an adverse event, as opposed to retrospectively trying to identify which individual is at fault once an adverse event has occurred. This is the cornerstone of human factors analysis and the Swiss cheese model of human error.

Case Scenario

A 45-year-old woman presents to the emergency department of a large academic medical center with nausea, vomiting, and severe abdominal pain. She has a history of a Roux-en-Y gastric bypass. She is evaluated by an emergency medicine resident, and her initial laboratory workup is largely unremarkable. A CT scan is performed, but the radiology resident does not specifically remark on any evidence of an internal hernia. Therefore, the patient is admitted to a general medicine service for further evaluation and management. The following day, the attending radiologist reads the CT scan, and notes a swirled appearance to the central mesentery and vasculature. While the interpretation is subsequently updated in the medical record, the patient's team is not notified of this change, and does not revisit the CT scan results. The following night, the patient's condition deteriorates—she develops worsening abdominal pain, tachycardia, and hypotension. At this point, the surgical service is consulted, after the patient had been in the hospital for 3 days. Their review of her clinical presentation and imaging are immediately concerning for an internal hernia with vascular compromise, and she is taken emergently to the operating room. An exploratory laparotomy is performed, revealing extensive ischemic and necrotic bowel, which requires resection, leaving the patient with less than 100 cm of viable small bowel, and TPN-dependent indefinitely.

James Reason and the Swiss Cheese Model of Human Error

The "Swiss cheese model" was a metaphor proposed by James Reason to explain and analyze the occurrence of adverse events within a complex system (Fig. 1.1) [3, 6–10]. In this model, there are hazards and losses. Hazards are the potential harms to patients that can occur because of human error—a wrong medication dose, wrong-site surgery, iatrogenic harm. Losses are the end result that occurs when a

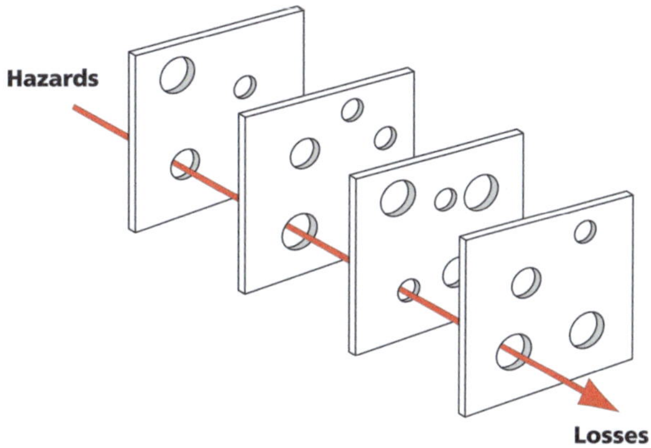

Fig. 1.1 Swiss cheese model

harm reaches a patient—pain, disability, and even death. Because human error is inevitable, complex systems such as hospitals have innumerable "defenses, barriers, and safeguards" to help prevent errors from occurring [6, 7, 9]. In 1990, Reason proposed that these barriers to mistakes are not infallible, but rather have weaknesses or "holes" that make them vulnerable to failure. Because these holes are inconsistent or sometimes temporary, they usually do not align, and errors still do not occur. An example would be a medication verification system being offline, but a pharmacist still reviewing that the correct dosage is dispensed. Another hole in a defense against harm may be a fatigued resident at the end of a shift, but the additional layer of appropriate oversight on the part of a teammate or nurse provides a barrier to prevent harm. In the Swiss cheese model, however, there are occasionally situations in which the transient holes in each level of defense align and allow a hazard to reach the patient. A situation may arise where the resident is fatigued, the medication verification system is offline, and the pharmacist is attending to another matter. As Reason points out, "When an adverse event occurs, the important issue is not who blundered, but how and why the defenses failed" [3].

Within the Swiss cheese model, human errors can be divided into *active failures* and *latent conditions*. The active failures are the unintentional, actual mistakes committed by the healthcare provider that result in patient harm. This could be failing to recognize a critical change in patient condition or performing the wrong procedure. Active failures have an immediate effect but are typically limited to a single instance (i.e., one active failure does not go on to harm other patients). These active failures are also referred to as being at the "sharp end" on Reason's model. The individual at the sharp end of an error may be the actual surgeon who is holding the scalpel and performs a wrong-site surgery, even while she may entirely think that she is performing the correct procedure. Active human failures can occur in a variety of forms, and within human factor analysis are typically divided into skill-based errors and mistakes (Fig. 1.2) [11, 12].

A skill-based error can occur due to a *slip* or a *lapse*. A slip is essentially performing the wrong action, or an error in the execution stage of an action. This could also be known as an error of *commission*. For example, this may involve performing

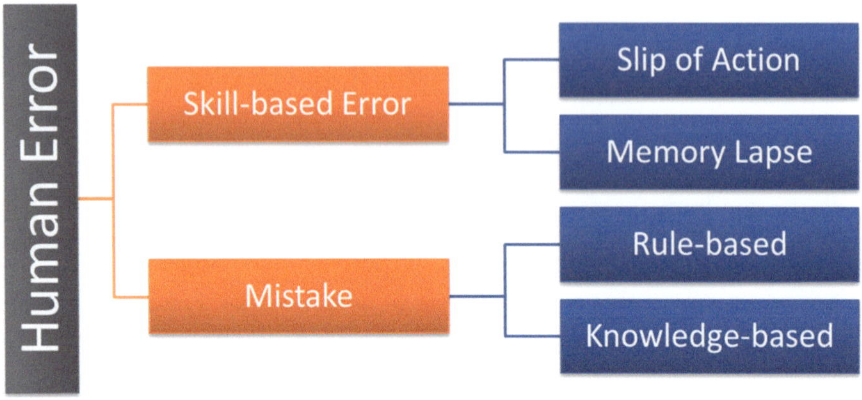

Fig. 1.2 Human factor analysis

wrong-site surgery while having no actual intent to do so, or giving the right medication to the wrong patient. On the other hand, a lapse is essentially a failure of memory, such as forgetting to restart an intravenous infusion after pausing it to transport a patient. This could also be known as an error of *omission*. These skill-based errors typically occur with tasks that require little active thought and are carried out mostly automatically. In both of these errors, the provider intends to perform the right action but fails to do so.

A mistake is a failure of the decision-making or planning stage of an action. The provider succeeds in carrying out the intended action, but the intended action is based on an incorrect assumption. In our case study, the emergency department resident not immediately consulting the surgery service may be an example of a mistake. Reason divides mistakes into rule-based and knowledge-based [7]. A rule-based mistake results when a rule or set of conditions is applied to a situation but results in a poor outcome. A classic example of a rule-based mistake is ignoring a fire alarm during a real fire because you've come to realize that the last 20 fire alarms were false alarms or drills. In our original scenario, the medicine team may have made a rule-based mistake in assuming that a patient who was determined not to have a surgical problem by the emergency department truly does not have a surgical problem. On the other hand, a knowledge-based mistake is probably what is most universally understood when we talk about someone "making a mistake." In this case, a lack of knowledge results in an error: a radiology resident misses a diagnosis of mesenteric ischemia because they are unfamiliar with its appearance on a CT scan. Knowledge-based mistakes can also be procedural, such as a trainee who causes a pneumothorax when placing a central line, or causes bleeding due to an insecure surgical knot. Skill-based errors and mistakes are examples of active failures.

Arguably, the more important element of a medical error within the context of the Swiss cheese model are the latent conditions that allow human error to occur and to result in patient harm. Metaphorically, latent conditions are the holes in the slices of cheese which, when aligned, allow a potential harm to reach a patient. Reason called latent conditions the "resident pathogens" within a system that exist due to how the system is designed or managed. In contrast to active failures, the impact of latent conditions is not limited to a single patient or event. The unsafe design of a piece of medical equipment could result in harm to a great number of patients. These conditions may exist and lie dormant for years before conditions align to result in an actual error or may result in a number of adverse events before being recognized. Critical to the idea of latent conditions is that because they exist in the design of a complex system such as a hospital, they can be identified and remedied before causing any adverse event through safety analysis strategies.

Many industries—from healthcare to aviation to nuclear power—share similar latent conditions that can result in error. If the slices of cheese in Reason's model represent the barriers and defenses to human error, one slice may represent the barrier of clear communication. The next may represent adequate training. Subsequent slices, or defenses, may be adequate supervision, appropriate staffing, safe procedures, safe design, fatigue prevention, and so on. Therefore, the latent conditions, or holes, are gaps in these defenses. A nursing unit may be understaffed due to a hiring freeze. A supervisor may be unavailable for part of a critical procedure due to an emergency involving another patient. In our case of the surgical patient with an internal hernia, the design of the radiology software does not create any kind of alert once results are updated (even when the update represents an important diagnostic change).

Reason likened active failures—slips, lapses, and mistakes—to mosquitos, which could be swatted again and again, but would invariably keep coming back. A more durable solution is to address and remove the conditions that allow the mosquitos to breed in the first place, namely, by fixing the "ever-present latent conditions."

Mitigating Human Error

If human error is an inevitable part of healthcare, what measures can be taken to improve outcomes and minimize the losses caused by human error? The following section reviews the principles of a reporting or just culture, human factors engineering strategies, failure mode and effect analysis (FMEA), and root cause analysis (RCA).

Reporting Culture/Just Culture

A key element to detecting and fixing the latent conditions in a system that can lead to patient harm is what Reason described as the creation of a "just culture." A just culture is "an atmosphere of trust in which people are encouraged, even rewarded, for providing essential safety-related information, but in which they are also clear about where the line must be drawn between acceptable and unacceptable behavior." [8, 10] This is in juxtaposition to "blame" and "no blame" cultures. Whereas a "blame culture" punishes the individual for mistakes and leads to potential hazards going unreported for fear of retribution, a "no blame" culture leads to a lack of accountability and a feeling that if no line has been crossed, nothing needs to change. A just culture, on the other hand, is an environment in which there is a clear distinction between inevitable human error and reckless behavior, but in which a provider is not punished simply for reporting a safety incident. Unfortunately, the U.S. Agency for Healthcare Research and Quality's 2018 Patient Safety Survey database revealed that 47% of respondents felt like reporting an unsafe event would be held against them, and that it was the individual, not the event, that was being "written up" once an event was reported [13].

Leadership engagement and support is central to creating a just culture. When health system leaders serve as models for a reporting culture and are willing to report mistakes themselves, other managers and staff are more likely to model this accountability [14]. Once leadership is engaged in promotion of a culture of incident reporting without retribution, tools can be implemented to make it easy for employees to report safety concerns. An example of the effectiveness of these tools is found in this case report published by the Joint Commission:

> Montefiore Medical Center created a user-friendly version of the just culture decision tree to encourage its use in everyday situations. The use of this tool and the rollout of an electronic event reporting system were a part of a transformational change to a just and learning culture that improved reporting of adverse events from 6097 in 2014 to nearly 9000 in 2017, including increased reporting by groups that traditionally would not be involved in reporting, such as attending physicians, who made 542 reports in 2017. Through training and empowering staff across the health system, including members of 50 peer review committees, Montefiore increased root cause analyses from 60 a year to several every day. Near-miss and unsafe conditions reporting went up from 681 in 2014 to 2493 in 2017. This improved reporting has saved lives and has pointed to additional systemic safety issues that the organization can address and improve [15].

Revisiting the case scenario presented at the beginning of this chapter, we can see that a just culture may have provided several opportunities for residents and faculty to report a safety concern. A just culture may have encouraged the emergency medicine resident to speak up and ask whether it would have been appropriate to consult a surgical service; the medicine team may have felt empowered to voice their lack of familiarity with caring for a patient who may have a surgical complication; and the radiology team certainly could have pointed to the lack of any kind of further notification to other providers once their subsequent interpretation had been changed.

Central to creating the just culture that Reason describes is the use of error- or incident-reporting systems within healthcare systems. In 1999, when the Institute of Medicine estimated that up to 98,000 patients died each year due to medical errors, they called for these reporting systems as a crucial strategy to learn from adverse events and prevent their recurrence [16, 17]. These systems allow healthcare employees to anonymously voice safety concerns without fear of retribution. In a just culture, such reporting is even viewed as a positive contribution to the safety culture of an organization rather than an admission of guilt. Implementation of one such system, The University of Texas Close Call Reporting System, which is funded by the Agency for Healthcare Research and Quality (AHRQ), collected nearly 26,000 safety reports in just under 2 years, which resulted in a number of targeted quality improvement initiatives that redesigned processes in order to maximize safety [18]. Additionally, while it may appear that hospitals or units with a higher number of safety reports are performing poorly, it has been shown that higher reporting rates are associated with a more positive safety culture and identification of unsafe events [19].

Human Factors Engineering Strategies

There are a number of systemic strategies that can be employed to mitigate human errors. Case studies of institutional implementation have demonstrated that the outcomes of measures can range from least reliable to most reliable [20].

Some of the least reliable strategies include additional education and training, or creating new rules, policies, or procedures. While these approaches attempt to help providers perform the correct action, they nevertheless result in providers relying on memory to perform a task. For example, having a new surgical resident complete a computer-based module about how to place a central line may in fact familiarize the resident with the steps of completing this task. However, when it time to carry this out, the resident may not remember, or may incorrectly remember, certain portions of how to safely insert the catheter, and her previous training does not offer any hard stops or useful checklists during the task to ensure that a mistake is not made. The same is true for new rules and policies, which may try to raise awareness about how to correctly carry out a task, but fail to ensure any kind of enforcement.

More reliable strategies to mitigate human errors involve standardizing processes so that variability is minimized as much as possible. Standardization means that the same process is completed the same way, regardless of the different providers or teams who are completing the process [21]. It has been demonstrated that when processes and equipment are standardized across institutions and the same steps are followed to complete the same task, errors are reduced and efficiency is increased [22]. Therefore, in the example of a surgical resident inserting a central line, human error can be mitigated by ensuring that this process is standardized and performed the same way every time. In this specific example, the dramatic impact of standardization can be highlighted by the widespread practice of requiring ultrasound use for all central line placements, regardless of an individual provider's previous training or preference. This practice has been shown to reduce iatrogenic complications associated with this practice [23].

A critical tool in improving standardization is the use of checklists. While rules and education sessions are ultimately limited by human memory, checklists ensure that the steps of a given procedure are carried out in the same way regardless of the provider or team performing them. In the central line example, this would involve a checklist of the exact steps and order that should be observed to complete the action. Within surgery specifically, checklists have been shown to significantly reduce mortality and complications by nearly half [24]. A particular example of a surgical checklist is the "timeout" that is performed prior to any invasive procedure. These "timeout" procedures are now ubiquitous at virtually all health systems and are endorsed as a best practice by the World Health Organization. Standardization of the timeout procedure is ensured by providers using a pre-made card or poster with a list of items that should be verified and discussed during the timeout. Common items discussed prior to beginning an operation include verifying the correct patient, procedure, surgical site, positioning, and medications.

One of the most important realms in which human error takes place is in communication. The Joint Commission estimates that communication errors are one of the three most common root causes of sentinel events in hospitals and play a role in 65% of these adverse events [21]. These errors typically occur during transitions of care ("handoffs") between providers or patient care groups [25]. Therefore, checklists or other means of standardization are now routinely employed during handoff situations. A popular example of this standardization is the use of the SBAR format, or "situation, background, assessment, and recommendation," which is widely used among nurses [26]. This often templated format strives to ensure that all key pieces of information are discussed during a transition of care.

One of the most effective strategies for mitigating human error—which human factors analysis acknowledges is inevitable—is referred to as "forcing functions," or designing a system in such a way that it is virtually impossible to perform an incorrect action. A classic example of this, which demonstrates the effect of these various safety strategies, is the management of medical gasses that are used in many areas of patient care. On March 5, 2002, the Veterans Health Administration issued a Patient Safety Advisory addressing the critical issue of incorrect administration of a medical gas. This was issued due to a variety of sentinel events in which patients who required oxygen, for example, were administered a different gas, such as compressed air or carbon dioxide. It is not hard to imagine how an error like this could occur—the wrong canister is brought into a patient's room from storage, or tubing is connected to the wrong gas outlet on the wall. Ineffective measures at preventing this error would be educating providers how to recognize which medical gas is being administered (perhaps by use of a color code). A provider who is in haste or who does not remember the training may still inadvertently make a mistake. A more effective countermeasure would be using an aforementioned checklist that may involve verifying which medical gas is about to be administered to a patient. Lastly, however, the practice of "forcing functions" would involve making the physical regulator on a carbon dioxide cannister—which would never be administered directly to a patient—functionally incompatible with any device or tubing that would deliver a medical gas to a patient. In this case, even if the provider obtains the wrong equipment, fails to recognize the mistake, and tries to connect face mask tubing to the canister, they would be physically prevented from carrying out the task and causing patient harm. Another example of a forcing function is administration of epinephrine for an anaphylactic reaction. In order to prevent administration of the wrong dose, a premeasured dose is provided in an EpiPen injector, leaving any decision about the dose out of the hands of the provider [27].

Prospective and Retrospective Error Analysis

While the above strategies are designed to prevent errors from happening in the moment, knowing what strategies and measures to implement requires identification of weaknesses in a system that are vulnerable to human error. A strategy to evaluate the safety of new or existing processes in healthcare is healthcare failure mode and effect analysis (HFMEA), which is an extension of a safety analysis process commonly used within the engineering community [28]. A description of this entire process is beyond the scope of this chapter, but what follows is a brief outline of this process and an example of a specific case, drawn from work conducted at the VA. There are five steps to HFMEA:

1. **Define the topic under investigation.** This should be a high-risk and high-vulnerability area within the health system.
2. **Assemble a team.** Convening a multidisciplinary team comprised of individuals both familiar and unfamiliar with the process under investigation will ensure critical review.
3. **Describe the process.** This is typically done graphically with the use of a process flow diagram.
4. **Conduct hazard analysis.** This is the heart of HFMEA and involves listing all of the potential failure modes of a given process, determining the probability of failure, the severity of failure, and the downstream effects of a potential failure. An example found in an HFMEA tutorial published by the Joint Commission would be hazard analysis of confirming drug allergies. Failure modes would include (1) not recording drug allergies and (2) incompletely recording drug allergies. The cause, in this case, may be poor integration of allergy confirmation into automated medical record systems. There are a number of freely available worksheets that outline the steps to completely capture the modes and effects of healthcare process failure.
5. **Develop actions and outcomes measures**. The final step of HFMEA involves developing countermeasures to mitigate potential failures. In the allergy confirmation example, the countermeasure may be developing an automated hard stop in the medical record system that requires confirmation of drug allergies prior to ordering a medication.

Root Cause Analysis

Root cause analysis (RCA), on the other hand, is a way to retrospectively analyze an adverse event. RCA is a systematic approach to investigating a sentinel event in order to prevent similar events from occurring in the future. Although RCA focuses on identifying both the errors that were committed by the individuals involved in a sentinel event, as well as the latent errors inherent in the system, the overriding goal is to recognize and correct the systematic weaknesses that allowed a major error to occur [29, 30].

Much like HFMEA, RCA can be conducted in a stepwise manner as follows: categorizing the level of harm due to an incident, gathering information, identifying the problems in care delivery that led to the problem, analyzing these problems to identify root causes, generating recommendations and solutions, and ultimately implementing these solutions [29]. A team should be convened to conduct the RCA, typically composed of at least one administrator, one patient representative, and an individual skilled in RCA [31].

Categorization of an incident includes no harm (a "near miss"), severe harm or death, or severe harm or death with public interest (such as a "never event" that becomes newsworthy). In the case of our initial scenario, we would categorize the incident as one that resulted in severe harm to the patient.

Gathering information is a multifaceted process that involves obtaining as much data about the incident as possible. Facts are obtained by verifying actions and orders that occurred within the medical record system. A hospital's paging system can be queried to look at the timing of communication between teams. Interviews are conducted to collect each provider's perspective on the event. Interviews are particularly important in ascertaining institutional biases or opinions as to why certain procedures were carried out a certain way. Again, in our case scenario, some critical information gathering would involve the timing of when the emergency department contacted the medicine team, when the medicine team contacted the surgery team, the language of the pages used to notify other teams of the patient, the patient's vital signs and clinical condition during these events, and the orders that were placed for the patient.

Next, the care delivery problems are identified, which in our case, are numerous: the failure of the emergency department physician to recognize and diagnose a patient with mesenteric ischemia due to an internal hernia; the failure of the radiologist to comment on radiographic findings concerning for an acute surgical pathology; the inappropriate admission of a patient with a surgical pathology to a medical service without notifying a surgical team; the failure to notify the medicine team once the radiographic interpretation of mesenteric ischemia had been updated; and even the delay in notifying the surgical team until the patient's condition had significantly deteriorated.

Identifying the root causes of each of these problems involves recognizing the factors that contribute to each of these problems. Strategies for conducting this analysis are commonly described as part of the Lean Thinking methodology, the two most popular of which are "the five whys" and creating a fishbone diagram. The five whys is an exercise in going beyond the most superficial explanations for an adverse event. A simple answer to the question "Why did this adverse event happen?" may be "Because the team caring for this patient missed the correct diagnosis." But stopping there results in a situation in which there is no real room for improvement, other than to perhaps have a teaching session about mesenteric ischemia, which is an ineffective solution. Conducting the five whys forces the group conducting the RCA to reach explanations that may have more actionable remedies. For example:

Problem: A patient underwent highly morbid, emergency surgery because her mesenteric ischemia was not diagnosed until she was clinically unstable.

Why?

Because the medicine team did not realize that she had a surgical problem.

Why?

Because they were only aware of the initial radiology interpretation, which did not comment on any findings suggestive of internal hernia or mesenteric ischemia.

Why?

Because once the interpretation was updated, the team was not made aware of this.

Why?

Because when radiologic interpretations are updated in the electronic medical record system, no notification is sent to any provider that the interpretation has been changed. It is up to the provider to go back and review the radiology findings.

Why?

Because this kind of notification system has never been implemented.

The ultimate conclusion to that exercise identifies the lack of a notification system for changed radiology results as one of the root causes of this event. The countermeasure or remedy to prevent future events like this, therefore, becomes obvious: implementing a notification system that updates providers when a radiographic interpretation is changed. In this case, had the medicine team been notified the following day that there was radiographic evidence of a surgical emergency, the patient would have likely been taken to the operating room 48 h before she ultimately was, and in a much more stable condition.

Lastly, the solutions identified following RCA should be implemented in a systematic manner. One strategy to achieve this is by using "SMART" goals, or goals that are specific, measurable, achievable, relevant, and timely. Simply having the solution of "don't miss a critical diagnosis again" has no way to guarantee its enforcement. However, the goal of "implementing a radiology notification system in the next 6 months" gives a very measurable outcome and timeframe by which to assess whether the root cause of this incident has been corrected. Another strategy is the use of a "plan, do, study, act" (PDSA) cycle, which is also described commonly in quality improvement in Lean Thinking.

References

1. Runciman WB, Merry AF, Tito F. Error, blame, and the law in health care—an antipodean perspective. Ann Intern Med. 2003;138(12):974–9.
2. Caplan RA, Posner KL, Cheney FW. Effect of outcome on physician judgments of appropriateness of care. JAMA. 1991;265(15):1957–60.
3. Reason J. Human error: models and management. BMJ. 2000;320(7237):768–70.
4. Marx D. Discipline: the role of rule violations. Ground Effects. 1997;2:1–4.
5. Holden RJ. People or systems? To blame is human. The fix is to engineer. Prof Saf. 2009;54(12):34–41.

6. Reason J. Understanding adverse events: human factors. Qual Health Care. 1995;4(2):80–9.
7. Reason JT. Human error. Cambridge: Cambridge University Press; 1990. p. xv, 302.
8. Reason JT. Managing the risks of organizational accidents. Aldershot: Ashgate; 1997. p. xvii, 252.
9. Reason JT. The human contribution : unsafe acts, accidents and heroic recoveries. Farnham: Ashgate; 2008. p. x, 295.
10. Reason JT. Organizational accidents revisited. 2nd ed. Burlington: Ashgate; 2015.
11. Armitage G. Human error theory: relevance to nurse management. J Nurs Manag. 2009;17(2):193–202.
12. Rasmussen J, Jensen A. Mental procedures in real-life tasks: a case study of electronic trouble shooting. Ergonomics. 1974;17(3):293–307.
13. Famolaro T, Dyer Yount N, Hare R, Thornton S, Meadows K, Fan L, et al. Hospital survey on patient safety culture 2018 user database report. AHRQ Publication No. 18-0025-EF. Rockville: Agency for Healthcare Research and Quality; 2018. https://psnet.ahrq.gov/issue/hospital-survey-patient-safety-culture-2018-user-database-report
14. O'Connor S, Carlson E. Safety culture and senior leadership behavior: using negative safety ratings to align clinical staff and senior leadership. J Nurs Adm. 2016;46(4):215–20.
15. Developing a reporting culture: learning from close calls and hazardous conditions. Sentinel Event Alert. 2018;(60):1–8.
16. Kohn LT, Corrigan J, Donaldson MS. To err is human: building a safer health system. Washington: National Academy Press; 2000. p. xxi, 287.
17. Brunsveld-Reinders AH, Arbous MS, De Vos R, De Jonge E. Incident and error reporting systems in intensive care: a systematic review of the literature. Int J Qual Health Care. 2016;28(1):2–13.
18. Simmons D, Mick JA, Graves K, Martin SK. 26,000 close call reports: lessons from the University of Texas close call reporting system. In: Henriksen K, Battles JB, Keyes MA, Grady ML, editors. Advances in patient safety: new directions and alternative approaches (vol 1: assessment). Rockville: Agency for Healthcare Research and Quality; 2008.
19. Hutchinson A, Young TA, Cooper KL, McIntosh A, Karnon JD, Scobie S, et al. Trends in healthcare incident reporting and relationship to safety and quality data in acute hospitals: results from the National Reporting and learning system. Qual Saf Health Care. 2009;18(1):5–10.
20. Wetterneck TB, Karsh B-T. Human factors applications to understanding and using close calls to improve health care. In: Wu A, editor. The value of close calls in improving patient safety: learning how to avoid and mitigate patient harm. Oak Brook: Joint Commission Resources; 2011. p. 39–53.
21. Siewert B, Hochman MG. Improving safety through human factors engineering. Radiographics. 2015;35(6):1694–705.
22. Wood DL, Brennan MD, Chaudhry R, Chihak AA, Feyereisn WL, Woychick NL, et al. Standardized care processes to improve quality and safety of patient care in a large academic practice: the Plummer project of the department of medicine, Mayo Clinic. Health Serv Manage Res. 2008;21(4):276–80.
23. Saugel B, Scheeren TWL, Teboul JL. Ultrasound-guided central venous catheter placement: a structured review and recommendations for clinical practice. Crit Care. 2017;21(1):225.
24. Haynes AB, Weiser TG, Berry WR, Lipsitz SR, Breizat AH, Dellinger EP, et al. A surgical safety checklist to reduce morbidity and mortality in a global population. N Engl J Med. 2009;360(5):491–9.
25. Rabol LI, Andersen ML, Ostergaard D, Bjorn B, Lilja B, Mogensen T. Descriptions of verbal communication errors between staff. An analysis of 84 root cause analysis-reports from Danish hospitals. BMJ Qual Saf. 2011;20(3):268–74.
26. Haig KM, Sutton S, Whittington J. SBAR: a shared mental model for improving communication between clinicians. Jt Comm J Qual Patient Saf. 2006;32(3):167–75.

27. Pennsylvania Patient Safety Advisory. Let's stop this "epi"demic! Preventing errors with epinephrine. PA PSRS Patient Saf Advis. 2006;3(3):16–7.
28. DeRosier J, Stalhandske E, Bagian JP, Nudell T. Using health care failure mode and effect analysis™: the VA national center for patient safety's prospective risk analysis system. Jt Comm J Qual Improv. 2002;28(5):248–67.
29. Jhugursing M, Dimmock V, Mulchandani H. Error and root cause analysis. BJA Educ. 2017;17(10):323–33.
30. Wachter RM, Gupta K. Understanding patient safety. 3rd ed. New York: McGraw-Hill Education; 2018. p. xviii, 510.
31. Joint Commission International. Root cause analysis in health care: tools and techniques. Joint Commission Resources; 2017.

Further Reading

Classic case report of sentinel event: Chassin MR, Becher EC. The wrong patient. Ann Intern Med. 2002;136(11):826–33.

The Joint Commission's recommendations for patient safety for accredited hospitals: "Patient Safety Systems" chapter. Joint Commission Accreditation. Comprehensive accreditation manual 2019: CAMH for Hospitals Effective January 1, 2019: Standards elements of performance scoring accreditation policies. Jt Comm Accred Health; 2018.

Outline and examples of healthcare failure mode and effect analysis: DeRosier J, Stalhandske E, Bagian JP, Nudell T. Using health care failure mode and effect analysis™: the VA national center for patient safety's prospective risk analysis system. Jt Comm J Qual Improv. 2002;28(5):248–67.

An overview of Reason's "just culture" in healthcare: Developing a reporting culture: learning from close calls and hazardous conditions. Sentinel Event Alert. 2018;(60):1–8.

Primer on conducting root cause analysis in healthcare: Joint Commission International. Root cause analysis in health care: tools and techniques: Joint Commission Resources; 2017.

2 Preoperative Testing in the Era of Cost Containment: Is There a Limit?

Georgios Tsoulfas

Introduction

This chapter aims to help the reader understand the rationale for approaching preoperative testing in an evidence-based manner. Essentially, the goal is to decide when preoperative testing is not indicated, which is really most of the time! Preoperative testing is commonly ordered for most patients scheduled to undergo general, regional or (even) local anesthesia, and it usually includes a panel of tests used for all patients, or tests used for specific patient groups (i.e., elderly) or for patients undergoing specific procedures. This is one side of the equation, which is also the most commonly practiced one, whereas the other is doing no preoperative testing or doing tests based on the clinician's evaluation of the patient's condition. In order to make the decision about which strategy to follow regarding preoperative testing, it is important to consider a series of factors.

On the one hand, those advocating in favor of routine preoperative testing argue that this strategy may help identify latent health issues that can ultimately affect the course and outcome of the surgical procedure or impact the anesthesia risk. In addition, this strategy allows for the accumulation of data, which can be used postoperatively for comparison, as well as possibly predict the possibility of postoperative complications. On the other hand, we have all come across false-positive testing, which can then lead to further tests, thus not only delaying a necessary surgical procedure, but also subjecting the patient to unnecessary care and psychological stress. Other times, even if a preoperative test is "positive," it may have absolutely nothing to do with the upcoming operation, and thus lead to an unnecessary delay. Additionally, there is the human factor, which is something that we have all been witnesses to, and which is exemplified by the positive preoperative test that goes unnoticed and for which nothing is done—by itself a patient safety issue at the

G. Tsoulfas (✉)
Department of Transplantation Surgery, Center for Research and Innovation in Solid Organ Transplantation, Aristotle University School of Medicine, Thessaloniki, Greece

J. J. Hoballah et al. (eds.), *Principles of Perioperative Safety and Efficiency*,
https://doi.org/10.1007/978-3-031-41089-5_2

system level. Obviously, on top of all this, one has to consider the financial aspect of the testing, as the higher number of preoperative testing means increased and likely unnecessary utilization of valuable resources. All of the above essentially means that clinicians have to balance the urgency and complexity of the surgical procedure, the cost involved, the patient's overall health, their personal experience, and last but not least, medico-legal concerns. An evidence-based approach has the potential to provide the necessary roadmap in this challenging situation, thus balancing both the patient's and society's well-being.

Risk Classification

In order to decide what preoperative testing should be done, one of the first things to consider is the risk(s) involved. Specifically, this has to do with the risk and complexity of the procedure and the health of the patient.

Type of Procedure

Different procedures have different degrees of complexities having to do with the part of the anatomy or the organ involved and the nature of the procedure. This has been documented in several studies, including a large analysis of 68,831 patients from Veterans Affairs hospitals and another one involving more than 400,000 major surgeries, again from the Veterans Affairs system [1, 2]. As a result, it is possible to classify procedures into high-, intermediate-, and low-risk ones during the perioperative period, based on the type of the procedure, as can be seen in Table 2.1.

Table 2.1 Perioperative risk classifications for surgical procedures [1, 2]

Low (<1%)	Intermediate (1–5%)	High (≥5%)
Superficial surgery	Intrathoracic (nonmajor)	Aortic, major vascular surgery, peripheral vascular surgery
Breast	Intraperitoneal	Major abdominal surgery, prolonged procedures with large fluid shifts or blood loss
Dental	Carotid endarterectomy	Esophagectomy
Cataract	Endovascular aneurysm repair	Pneumonectomy
Endoscopic	Head and neck surgery	Lung, liver, or pancreas transplantation
Thyroid	Neurologic or orthopedic, major	Adrenal resection
Gynecologic, minor	Urologic or gynecologic major	
Orthopedics, minor	Renal transplantation	
Urologic, minor		
Reconstructive or cosmetic		

Existing Chronic Comorbidities

It should come as no surprise that chronic conditions and comorbidities can increase the perioperative risk of complications. This is especially true today with an increasing elderly patient population. One of the most practical ways to evaluate this increased perioperative risk is to use the American Society of Anesthesiologists (ASA) physical status classification system, which is presented in Table 2.2 [3]. This uses the preoperative functional status of the patient, with examples provided in order to classify the perioperative risk involved. Such comorbidities include, but are not limited to, ischemic heart disease, cerebrovascular disease, heart failure, diabetes mellitus, chronic kidney disease, liver disease, bleeding disorders, and pulmonary disease. The degree of these comorbidities and whether they are under adequate treatment can play a significant role in the perioperative outcome.

Table 2.2 American Society of Anesthesiologists classification system [3]

ASA PS classification	Definition	Examples, including, but not limited to:
ASA I	A normal healthy patient	Healthy, non-smoking, no or minimal alcohol use
ASA II	A patient with mild systemic disease	Mild diseases only without substantive functional limitations. Examples include (but not limited to): current smoker, social alcohol drinker, pregnancy, obesity (30 < BMI < 40), well-controlled DM/HTN, mild lung disease
ASA III	A patient with severe systemic disease	Substantive functional limitations; One or more moderate to severe diseases. Examples include (but not limited to): poorly controlled DM or HTN, COPD, morbid obesity (BMI ≥40), active hepatitis, alcohol dependence or abuse, implanted pacemaker, moderate reduction of ejection fraction, ESRD undergoing regularly scheduled dialysis, premature infant PCA < 60 weeks, history (>3 months) of MI, CVA, TIA, or CAD/stents
ASA IV	A patient with severe systemic disease that is a constant threat to life	Examples include (but not limited to): recent (<3 months) MI, CVA, TIA, or CAD/stents, ongoing cardiac ischemia or severe valve dysfunction, severe reduction of ejection fraction, sepsis, DIC, ARD, or ESRD not undergoing regularly scheduled dialysis
ASA V	A moribund patient who is not expected to survive without the operation	Examples include (but not limited to): ruptured abdominal/thoracic aneurysm, massive trauma, intracranial bleed with mass effect, ischemic bowel in the face of significant cardiac pathology or multiple organ/system dysfunction
ASA VI	A declared brain-dead patient whose organs are being removed for donor purposes	

Social, Obesity, and Functional Status Factors

Social factors may include habits such as tobacco, alcohol, or illicit substance use; or factors such as nutritional status, obesity, ability to exercise, and even level of stress. These factors need to be quantified for each patient in order to determine the threat posed. Examples include measuring tobacco use in packets per year (how many packets of cigarettes multiplied by the number of years), whether it is cigarettes or other types of tobacco, the type, frequency, and amount of alcohol that the patient uses or, in the case of obesity, measurement of the patient's body mass index (BMI). These can increase the risk for cardiopulmonary complications.

Preoperative Testing

Before the decision is made to conduct preoperative tests, there are several questions that need to be asked and considered.

1. ***Why do we need to test preoperatively?*** In 2010, the Committee on Standards and Practice Parameters of the American Society of Anesthesiologists, in an effort to evaluate the need for changes in the then existing recommendations in the Practice Advisory from 2001, formed a task force on preanesthesia evaluation. The result was an updated Practice Advisory for Anesthesia Evaluation, which was eventually published in 2012 [4]. We have to remember that practice advisories are not the same as guidelines or standards, because they are not supported by scientific literature to the same extent as guidelines, given the lack of an adequate number and quality of randomized controlled trials. They are meant to be treated as useful suggestions, which are the result of consensus and synthesis between experts on the topic.

   Having identified the limitations of the practice advisory, we also need to understand its importance. The reasoning behind preoperative testing is that it can help identify acute or chronic conditions that may interfere with the anesthesia or the surgical plan, as well as confirm the existence and degree of severity of known health problems. The information from the preoperative testing can be useful in formulating the best anesthesia plan for the specific procedure and for the specific patient. At the same time, it is supposed to help delineate the overall health status of the patient, so that the surgical team can also decide whether the patient can be operated upon, and what the best procedure for the specific patient is. All of this is important in order to provide the patient with the best possible information regarding the upcoming procedure and the various alternatives (especially regarding the anesthesia plan) in an effort to obtain a truly informed consent.

   The main reason for the need to reevaluate existing protocols is the importance of periodically examining new data and information in anesthesia and adjusting the relevant policies accordingly. Specifically, although the rationale behind preoperative testing appears to be solid, there have been studies going back to the 1990s questioning the existing practices. One of the more interesting papers is by Kaplan et al. from 1985, where the authors reviewed the data on routine preoperative testing done on 2000 patients scheduled to undergo elective surgery [5]. The authors found that 60% of the routinely performed tests would not have been done if indications were part of the decision-making process. More astonishing is the fact that only 0.22% of these tests actually revealed an abnormality that could influence the anesthesia and/or surgical plan; and to make things worse, a review of the charts confirmed that none of these small number of abnormalities were actually acted upon and none of them had any effect on the outcome. In another study from 1997, the authors reviewed the records of 1044 patients who underwent surgical or diagnostic procedures at the Mayo Clinic in 1994 without any preoperative laboratory tests within a timeframe of 90 days prior to the procedure [6]. The authors found that there were no deaths, and only 17 intraoperative laboratory tests were required, with three of them being eventually abnormal. None of the perioperative laboratory tests changed the patient management in any manner.

As with most things in life, the truth lies somewhere in the middle. That is to say, neither the policy of multiple, routine preoperative laboratory testing, nor the one of no testing at all, may be the best for patients. Essentially, using the best available evidence, we have to decide which tests are needed for a specific patient, based on the overall anesthesia evaluation. This brings us to our next question.

2. ***Who do we need to test preoperatively? How do you decide?*** There are several different ways of deciding which patients need to be tested, some better than others. Physicians, and perhaps surgeons more so, are creatures of habit and of the "$n = 1$" phenomenon. Specifically, given the fact that "habit" essentially provides a feeling of safety, it is not unusual to get the following responses to the question of why does this patient need to do preoperative testing: "Because that's our routine" or "Because that's what we always do" or "Because the chief resident told us to do that." The "$n = 1$" phenomenon has to do that frequently, and despite any literature to the contrary, our decisions are influenced by the last case that had a complication. Obviously, this is not optimal and begs the question of how do we choose between existing guidelines originating from different specialties (e.g., surgery, anesthesia, subspecialties), and who is the one developing hospital policies (physicians, administration) and with what criteria (purely medical, medico-legal, medico-economico-legal). Just as this discussion becomes increasingly more confusing by creating more questions than answers, we have to remember to get back to the basics in order to make an evidence-based decision.

The answer to the question of who should get preoperative evaluation is rather simple: ALL patients scheduled for surgery should undergo preoperative evaluation. However, here is where we need to be very clear that preoperative evaluation is NOT the same as preoperative testing. Specifically, all patients scheduled to undergo a surgical procedure, no matter how "small," should be *evaluated* preoperative either by their surgeon (e.g., if the plan is to use only local anesthesia) or by an anesthesiologist. However, the exact type and extent of the evaluation varies depending on the extent of the procedure. For very low-risk procedures, it may be enough to obtain a history and physical exam to confirm the absence of any major medical issues or risk factors. In cases of minor procedures or surgery in a patient with no known medical history, it may be enough to obtain the same information, even during a telephone interview or with the use of telemedicine. In the case of a more complex procedure or surgery, or in the case of a patient with comorbidities, then it is necessary to have the patient evaluated by an experienced physician to assess the risk and determine which tests are necessary as part of the evaluation for this specific patient. The key point here is that preoperative ***testing*** is indicated only if, as part of the preoperative ***evaluation***, the type of surgery or the patient's overall condition and comorbidities or abnormal findings during the history and physical exam warrant a more detailed assessment. Additionally, we should also be cognizant of the fact that apart from having a clear indication for obtaining preoperative testing, we should also consider whether the result of such testing can affect the perioperative management of the patient or mitigate the risks involved. Later in this chapter, the specific indications will be analyzed according to the different organ systems.

3. ***Is preoperative testing a problem?*** As physicians we consider ourselves the biggest advocates of our patients, and as a result there is always the temptation to think that there is no such thing as "overdoing" it when it comes to preoperative testing for our patients. However, reality is very different, as we could be *not* helping our patients or society. Preoperative testing overuse can lead to wasting valuable resources, exposing our patients to needless blood work and procedures, creating anxiety for the patients and their families, and (always the bottom line) costing over $30 billion per year in 1987 calculations [7–9].
4. ***How do we decide which patients to test preoperatively?*** Several efforts have approached this question in an evidence-based manner to achieve consensus. One example is the guidelines by the National Institute for Health and Care Excellence (NICE). NICE was originally set up in 1999 as the National Institute for Clinical Excellence, a special health authority, to reduce variation in the availability and quality of treatments and care in the U.K. National Health System. In 2005, there was a merger with the Health Development Agency, which led to increased involvement in the development of public health guidelines.

   Let's examine under what circumstances should the "main" preoperative tests be ordered, if at all. Specifically:

   Electrocardiogram (ECG): There are no prospective, randomized clinical controlled trials regarding the utility of preoperative ECG and, as such, we are lacking prospective, good-quality data on whether it is useful or not. There are several studies of lower quality, such as retrospective reviews or case series, as well as consensus statements, which are often conflicting and complicated. It is not surprising that the prevalence of an abnormal ECG increases with age, as almost 75% of people older than 75 years old have an abnormal ECG, given the accumulated changes over time having to do with cardiac anatomy, function, and conductivity [10]. Although the patients mentioned above may be asymptomatic, there is evidence suggesting poorer outcomes in patients with abnormal ECGs. In a retrospective study of 23,036 patients who underwent 28,457 surgical procedures in the Netherlands, patients with abnormal ECG findings had a greater incidence of cardiovascular death compared to those with normal ECGs, with a 4.5 relative risk (3.3–6.0) of death [11]. This finding was much less evident in patients undergoing low- or low-to-intermediate-risk surgery, as in these patients the difference in the incidence of cardiovascular death between those with and without ECG abnormalities was only 0.5%. Although recommendations from several organizations such as the American College of Cardiology/American Heart Association (ACC/AHA), the American Society of Anesthesiologists (ASA), the European Society of Cardiology/European Atherosclerosis Society (ESC/EAS) and others may vary and are often conflicting, there seems to be agreement that an ECG is warranted when: (a) there are signs and symptoms of cardiovascular disease, (b) there is stable known cardiac disease, (c) there are risk factors; and the surgery will be intermediate- or high-risk with revised cardiac risk index (RCRI) ≥ 1 [12–14]. On the other hand, ECG can be safely avoided when the surgery and the patient are both low risk or in cases such as cataract surgery. As always, there remain gray areas regarding the utility of ECG. These include the combination of a low-risk patient who is scheduled to undergo an intermediate-risk procedure or that of a patient with risk factors who is scheduled to undergo a low-risk procedure.

Coagulation studies: There is indeed significant pressure on this issue, given the multitude of anticoagulation medications available (and continuously increasing), the complex nature of the hemostasis process with its numerous mediators and different phases, the hereditary nature of several of these problems, and the large number of available coagulation tests. Early literature on the topic supported the use of prothrombin time (PT) and the activated partial thromboplastin time (aPTT) as part of the preoperative assessment of the patient's coagulation [15, 16]. However, what became apparent is that clinical history and physical exam are more than adequate in terms of predicting bleeding or coagulation problems, an opinion that is shared by the ASA and the British Committee for Standards in Hematology [17–21]. Given all this, it is obvious that the history and the clinical exam need to be very thorough and should include information such as family history of coagulation problems, history of abnormal bleeding with other procedures or during various activities, and use of any anticoagulation medication.

Complete blood count (CBC): There should be a reason behind ordering a preoperative CBC, which has to do either with the patient or with the type of surgery. Specifically, if there are clinical history or physical exam findings suggestive of an abnormality, such as known cytopenia, a history of bleeding, immunosuppressed state as in the case of medications or recent chemotherapy, pallor or excessive or unexplained fatigue among others, then obtaining a CBC could affect the management of the patient. Additionally, if significant blood loss is anticipated given the complexity of the surgery, or if there are existing comorbidities (such as ischemic heart disease) that could affect the transfusion threshold, then a CBC is justified.

Electrolytes, creatinine, glucose: If a patient has renal failure or is on medications (i.e., diuretics, digoxin) that can lead to loss or retention of electrolytes, or there is concern over the fluid status of the patient, then testing for electrolytes and creatinine can provide valuable information. The decision of whether or not to include these tests is a matter of estimating the overall risk based on the combination of the complexity of the surgery (minor, intermediate, high-risk) and the overall condition of the patient (ASA status; see Table 2.2). So, ASA 1 or ASA 2 patients scheduled for a minor procedure do not need them, whereas ASA 3 or ASA 4 patients scheduled for an intermediate procedure should be offered them. Still, the gray areas remain, such as in the case of ASA 2 and intermediate procedure, where the overall risk for acute kidney failure needs to be taken into consideration [21, 22]. Regarding blood glucose, there really is no good evidence for routine inclusion in the preoperative workup, other than what the history and physical might dictate.

Chest X-ray (CXR): Although the predictive value of the history and physical remains strong, a CXR is part of most preoperative evaluations. Interestingly enough, although abnormalities are relatively frequent (10–20%), they influence the management of the patient in less than 3% of cases [23].

Liver function tests (LFTs): LFTs should be included as part of the preoperative evaluation only if there is suspicion of liver disease on the basis of the patient's history, physical exam, or any prior laboratory abnormalities [24]. In such a case that LFTs are warranted, then it may be wise to obtain INR and creatinine as well, so that the patient's model for end-stage liver disease (MELD) score can be calculated. The latter is a useful indicator of the severity of the acute or chronic liver disease, as well as predictive of mortality in the near future.

Pregnancy Testing: Unrecognized pregnancy when someone presents for an elective, or even an emergency, procedure, can cause significant clinical and medico-legal problems. As such, the overall tendency is to err on the side of caution, unless the history and physical can fully exclude this possibility. However, the literature to support such a strategy is rather limited and the argument is based on the fear of missing a pregnancy. In a very interesting study from the Mayo Clinic in Arizona, the authors reviewed the records of 8245 women with preoperative pregnancy tests and identified 11 positive tests, of which six were false positives [25]. Of the five true positives, three decided to cancel elective surgery, one had surgery under local anesthesia, and the other proceeded with the procedure, as it involved a malignancy, and subsequently had the pregnancy terminated. The positive pregnancy test rate was 0.13%, which essentially meant that the estimated cost for each of the true positive tests was around $49,000 [25]. The very low incidence of unrecognized pregnancies together with the sensitive nature of the topic led the ASA in a practice advisory for preanesthesia evaluation in 2012 to declare "…the literature is inadequate to inform patients or physicians on whether anesthesia causes harmful effects on early pregnancy. Pregnancy testing *may* be offered to female patients of childbearing age *and* for whom the result would alter the patient's management." [4].

Geriatric population: The part of the population over the age of 65 years deserves special mention, as it represents a continuously increasing percentage of the whole population with increased needs. There are several reasons for this demographic change, including the baby boom generation crossing the 65-year-old threshold, decreased birth rates, and people living longer [26]. The American College of Surgeons (ACS) National Surgical Quality Improvement Program (NSQIP)/American Geriatrics Society (AGS) Best Practices Guidelines in 2012 in an evidence-based manner presented guidelines regarding the preoperative assessment of the geriatric population, with special emphasis on the several issues that are unique to the geriatric patient [26]. Specifically, this includes assessment of the cognitive ability and capacity of the patient, screening for depression, identifying risk factors for postoperative delirium, documenting functional status and risk of falls, determining baseline frailty score and nutritional status, obtaining a detailed medication history, and evaluating the family and social support system, in addition to the standard history and physical.

Key Points

An overview of the topic helps identify certain critical points. Specifically, with the help of a thorough history and physical, we can avoid routine preoperative testing for low-risk surgeries without a clinical indication. The reason is that if we tested everybody, any findings (and IF they were followed up appropriately) would influence the management in under 3% of the patients tested. Additionally, in almost all cases, there are no adverse outcomes when patients who are clinically stable undergo elective surgery, irrespective of the testing. Examples of low-risk surgeries include eye surgery, endoscopic surgery, superficial surgery, breast surgery, and most types of ambulatory surgery. Also, patients who have no cardiac history and a good functional status do not require preoperative stress testing when scheduled to undergo non-cardiac thoracic surgery.

Determining when to do preoperative anesthetic evaluation and testing has to do with the clinical condition of the patient and the invasiveness of the procedure. For a disease of high severity and a highly invasive procedure, it is best to always perform the evaluation before the day of surgery, whereas in a disease of low severity and a less invasive procedure, the evaluation could be performed on the day of the surgery.

It is extremely important to remember the following three key points:

1. ALL preoperative testing should be dictated and guided by the preoperative history and physical exam.
2. There are NO guidelines suggesting preoperative routine laboratory testing for everybody.
3. Preoperative *evaluation* is NOT the same as preoperative *testing*; the latter should take place only when indicated.

Conclusion

In this chapter, we had the opportunity to review the decision-making process involved (or at least that should be involved) in the preoperative evaluation, with special emphasis on when and why to order preoperative testing.

References

1. Khuri SF, Daley J, Henderson W, Hur K, Demakis J, Aust JB, et al. The Department of Veterans Affairs NSQIP: the first national, validated, outcome-based, risk-adjusted, and peer-controlled program for the measurement and enhancement of the quality of surgical care. National VA surgical quality improvement program. Ann Surg. 1998;228(4):491–507.
2. Smetana GW. Preoperative pulmonary evaluation. N Engl J Med. 1999;340(12):937–44.
3. Mayhew D, Mendonca V, Murthy BVS. A review of ASA physical status—historical perspectives and modern developments. Anaesthesia. 2019;74(3):373–9.
4. Committee on Standards and Practice Parameters, Apfelbaum JL, Connis RT, Nickinovich DG, American Society of Anesthesiologists Task Force on Preanesthesia Evaluation, Pasternak LR, et al. Practice advisory for preanesthesia evaluation: an updated report by the American Society of Anesthesiologists task force on preanesthesia evaluation. Anesthesiology. 2012;116(3):522–38.
5. Kaplan EB, Sheiner LB, Boeckmann AJ, Roizen MF, Beal SL, Cohen SN, et al. The usefulness of preoperative laboratory screening. JAMA. 1985;253(24):3576–81.
6. Narr BJ, Warner ME, Schroeder DR, Warner MA. Outcomes of patients with no laboratory assessment before anesthesia and a surgical procedure. Mayo Clin Proc. 1997;72(6):505–9.
7. Katz RI, Dexter F, Rosenfeld K, Wolfe L, Redmond V, Agarwal D, et al. Survey study of anesthesiologists' and surgeons' ordering of unnecessary preoperative laboratory tests. Anesth Analg. 2011;112(1):207–12.
8. Lichtor JL, Johanson CE, Mhoon D, Faure EA, Hassan SZ, Roizen MF. Preoperative anxiety: does anxiety level the afternoon before surgery predict anxiety level just before surgery? Anesthesiology. 1987;67(4):595–9.
9. Guttikonda N, Nileshwar A, Rao M, Sushma TK. Preoperative laboratory testing—comparison of National Institute of Clinical Excellence guidelines with current practice—an observational study. J Anaesthesiol Clin Pharmacol. 2019;35(2):227–30.
10. Strait JB, Lakatta EG. Aging-associated cardiovascular changes and their relationship to heart failure. Heart Fail Clin. 2012;8(1):143–64.
11. Noordzij PG, Boersma E, Bax JJ, Feringa HH, Schreiner F, Schouten O, et al. Prognostic value of routine preoperative electrocardiography in patients undergoing noncardiac surgery. Am J Cardiol. 2006;97(7):1103–6.
12. NICE guideline [NG45]. Routine preoperative tests for surgery. 2016. https://www.nice.org.uk/guidance/NG45. Accessed 2019 Nov 2010.
13. Fleisher LA, Fleischmann KE, Auerbach AD, Barnason SA, Beckman JA, Bozkurt B, et al. 2014 ACC/AHA guideline on perioperative cardiovascular evaluation and management of patients undergoing noncardiac surgery: executive summary: a report of the American College of Cardiology/American Heart Association task force on practice guidelines. J Nucl Cardiol. 2015;22(1):162–215.
14. Kristensen SD, Knuuti J, Saraste A, Anker S, Bøtker HE, De Hert S, et al. 2014 ESC/ESA guidelines on non-cardiac surgery: cardiovascular assessment and management: the joint task force on non-cardiac surgery: cardiovascular assessment and management of the European Society of Cardiology (ESC) and the European Society of Anaesthesiology (ESA). Eur J Anaesthesiol. 2014;31(10):517–73.

15. Wahlberg T, Blombäck M, Hall P, Axelsson G. Application of indicators, predictors and diagnostic indices in coagulation disorders. I. Evaluation of a self-administered questionnaire with binary questions. Methods Inf Med. 1980;19(4):194–200.
16. Eika C, Havig O, Godal HC. The value of preoperative haemostatic screening. Scand J Haematol. 1978;21(4):349–54.
17. Velanovich V. The value of routine preoperative laboratory testing in predicting postoperative complications: a multivariate analysis. Surgery. 1991;109:236–43.
18. Narr BJ, Warner ME, Schroeder DR, Warner MA, editors. Outcomes of patients with no laboratory assessment before anesthesia and a surgical procedure. In: Mayo Clinic Proceedings. Philadelphia: Elsevier, vol 124; 1997. p. 428.
19. Thiruvenkatarajan V, Pruett A, Adhikary SD. Coagulation testing in the perioperative period. Indian J Anaesth. 2014;58(5):565–72.
20. Chee YL, Crawford JC, Watson HG, Greaves M. Guidelines on the assessment of bleeding risk prior to surgery or invasive procedures. British Committee for Standards in Haematology. Br J Haematol. 2008;140(5):496–504.
21. Kozek-Langenecker SA, Afshari A, Albaladejo P, Santullano CA, De Robertis E, Filipescu DC, et al. Management of severe perioperative bleeding: guidelines from the European Society of Anaesthesiology. Eur J Anaesthesiol. 2013;30(6):270–382.
22. Czoski-Murray C, Lloyd Jones M, McCabe C, Claxton K, Oluboyede Y, Roberts J, et al. What is the value of routinely testing full blood count, electrolytes and urea, and pulmonary function tests before elective surgery in patients with no apparent clinical indication and in subgroups of patients with common comorbidities: a systematic review of the clinical and cost-effective literature. Health Technol Assess. 2012;16(50):i–xvi, 1–159.
23. Qaseem A, Snow V, Fitterman N, Hornbake ER, Lawrence VA, Smetana GW, et al. Risk assessment for and strategies to reduce perioperative pulmonary complications for patients undergoing noncardiothoracic surgery: a guideline from the American College of Physicians. Ann Intern Med. 2006;144(8):575–80.
24. Teh SH, Nagorney DM, Stevens SR, Offord KP, Therneau TM, Plevak DJ, et al. Risk factors for mortality after surgery in patients with cirrhosis. Gastroenterology. 2007;132(4):1261–9.
25. Gong X, Poterack KA. Retrospective review of universal preoperative pregnancy testing: results and perspectives. Anesth Analg. 2018;127(2):e4–5.
26. Chow WB, Rosenthal RA, Merkow RP, Ko CY, Esnaola NF, American College of Surgeons National Surgical Quality Improvement Program; American Geriatrics Society. Optimal preoperative assessment of the geriatric surgical patient: a best practices guideline from the American College of Surgeons National Surgical Quality Improvement Program and the American Geriatrics Society. J Am Coll Surg. 2012;215(4):453–66.

3 Preventing Never Events: Checklists, Timeouts, Debriefings, and Skin Marking

George Molina and Alex Haynes

Introduction

There were two seminal events in the late 1990s that laid the groundwork for subsequent quality and safety efforts in healthcare in the United States. In 1999, the Institute of Medicine published a pioneering report titled, "To Err is Human: Building a Safer Health System" [1]. The report estimated that about 98,000 deaths were attributable to medical errors. This estimate was jarring and served as the necessary shock to the system that sparked numerous initiatives to make the delivery of healthcare in the United States safer. These have been multi-pronged in their aims, including improving the delivery of healthcare and promoting the reporting of medical errors. Since its publication, multiple concepts and tools in the healthcare quality and safety space have been developed including, but not limited to, never events, timeouts, debriefings, skin marking, and checklists.

The second seminal event was the creation of the National Quality Forum (NQF). In 1997, President Bill Clinton created the President's Advisory Commission on Consumer Protection and Quality in the Healthcare Industry. The purpose of the panel was to "draft a bill of rights for healthcare consumers and to assess the need for the federal government to regulate private health insurance plans" [2]. In 1999, the commission made more than 50 recommendations, including the creation of a nonpartisan organization that would be representative of all stakeholders in the delivery, management, and utilization of healthcare and whose mission would be "to promote and ensure patient protections and healthcare quality through measurement and public reporting" [3]. This led to the creation of the NQF, "the only consensus-based healthcare organization in the nation as defined by the Office of

G. Molina
Brigham and Women's Hospital, Boston, MA, USA

A. Haynes (✉)
Department of Surgery and Perioperative Care, University of Texas Austin, Austin, TX, USA
e-mail: alex.haynes@austin.utexas.edu

J. J. Hoballah et al. (eds.), *Principles of Perioperative Safety and Efficiency*,
https://doi.org/10.1007/978-3-031-41089-5_3

Management and Budget" [4]. The NQF endorses reporting measures and evidence-based healthcare practices that are then adopted by the public and private healthcare sectors.

Never Events

The Institute of Medicine's report and the founding of the NQF brought into focus the need to improve the quality and safety of healthcare in the United States. "To Err is Human" contextualized what we have always known in our daily lives—humans make mistakes. This pioneering report made this commonly accepted human reality a core tenet of quality and safety efforts in healthcare. This notion does not imply that all mistakes lead to significant patient harm. However, there are medical errors that do lead to significant patient morbidity and, at times, death. This led to the concept of "never events," which the NQF defined as medical errors or complications in healthcare that should never occur. With regard to surgery, never events can be understood as complications that are not "acceptable risks of surgery" [5]. The NQF has further developed the concept of never events and now refers to these events as "serious reportable events." There are currently 29 NQF-defined serious reportable events, categorized into seven groups: (1) surgical or procedural events, (2) product or device events, (3) patient protection events, (4) care management events, (5) environmental events, (6) radiologic events, and (7) criminal events (Table 3.1).

Another important entity that has further expounded on the concept of never events is the Joint Commission, which is an independent, not-for-profit organization that evaluates and accredits healthcare organizations and programs throughout the United States. The Joint Commission, which is the "nation's oldest and largest standards-setting and accrediting body in healthcare" [6], defines never events as sentinel events in patient care that result in death, permanent harm, or severe temporary harm that requires life-sustaining interventions. In 1996, the Joint Commission adopted a policy that encouraged accredited facilities to report sentinel events. According to the Joint Commission, these events should be investigated with a root cause analysis, and a response should be formulated by the accredited facility [7]. It is important to note that the Joint Commission also considers the 29 events listed by the NQF as sentinel events.

Many states have since adopted statewide reporting requirements for never events or serious reportable events. The National Academy for State Health Policy reported that as of 2015 there were 27 states and the District of Columbia that had adverse-event reporting systems that were authorized and that had a documented focus on adverse events with an intent to improve patient safety. Unfortunately, this number of adverse-event reporting systems in the United States has remained static since 2007 [8]. Although the number of adverse-event reporting systems has not increased, these systems have embraced technological advancements and are facilitating the exchange and sharing of important information that is leading to improved care by addressing areas in need of improvement (Fig. 3.1).

Table 3.1 National quality forum list of serious reportable events, 2016

Surgical events	Product or device events	Care management events	Environmental events	Radiologic events	Criminal events
• Surgery or other invasive procedure performed on the wrong body part • Surgery or other invasive procedure performed on the wrong patient • Wrong surgical or other invasive procedure performed on a patient • Unintended retention of a foreign object in a patient after surgery or other procedure • Intraoperative or immediately postoperative/post-procedure death in an American Society of Anesthesiologists Class I patient	• Patient death or serious injury associated with the use of contaminated drugs, devices, or biologics provided by the healthcare setting • Patient death or serious injury associated with the use or function of a device in patient care, in which the device is used for functions other than as intended • Patient death or serious injury associated with intravascular air embolism that occurs while being cared for in a healthcare setting	• Patient death or serious injury associated with a medication error (e.g., errors involving the wrong drug, wrong dose, wrong patient, wrong time, wrong rate, wrong preparation, or wrong route of administration) • Patient death or serious injury associated with unsafe administration of blood products • Maternal death or serious injury associated with labor or delivery in a low-risk pregnancy while being cared for in a healthcare setting • Death or serious injury of a neonate associated with labor or delivery in a low-risk pregnancy • Artificial insemination with the wrong donor sperm or wrong egg • Patient death or serious injury associated with a fall while being cared for in a healthcare setting • Any stage 3, stage 4, or unstageable pressure ulcers acquired after admission/presentation to a healthcare facility • Patient death or serious disability resulting from the irretrievable loss of an irreplaceable biological specimen • Patient death or serious injury resulting from failure to follow up or communicate laboratory, pathology, or radiology test results	• Patient or staff death or serious disability associated with an electric shock in the course of a patient care process in a healthcare setting • Any incident in which a line designated for oxygen or other gas to be delivered to a patient contains no gas, the wrong gas, or is contaminated by toxic substances • Patient or staff death or serious injury associated with a burn incurred from any source in the course of a patient care process in a healthcare setting • Patient death or serious injury associated with the use of restraints or bedrails while being cared for in a healthcare setting	• Death or serious injury of a patient or staff associated with introduction of a metallic object into the MRI area	• Any instance of care ordered by or provided by someone impersonating a physician, nurse, pharmacist, or other licensed healthcare provider • Abduction of a patient/resident of any age • Sexual abuse/assault on a patient within or on the grounds of a healthcare setting • Death or significant injury of a patient or staff member resulting from a physical assault (i.e., battery) that occurs within or on the grounds of a healthcare setting

Source: National Quality Forum. List of Serious Reportable Events. https://www.qualityforum.org/Topics/SREs/List_of_SREs.aspx

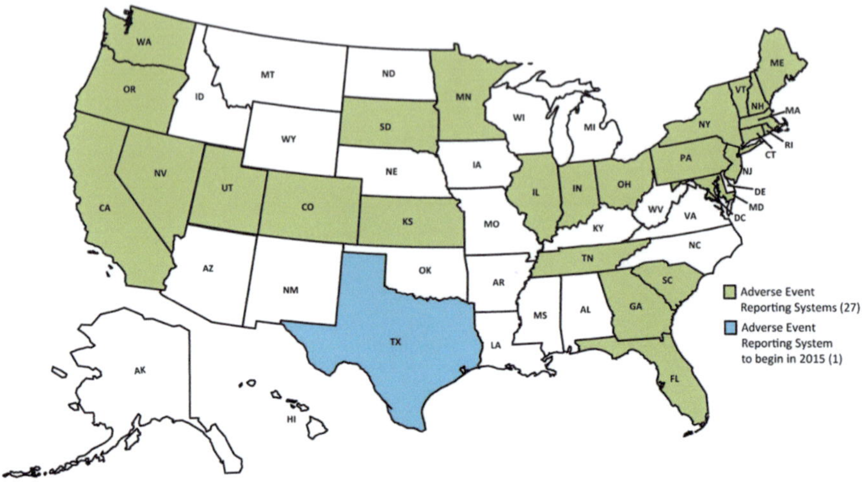

Fig. 3.1 Adverse event reporting systems. (From Hanlon C, Sheedy K, Kniffin T, Rosenthal J. Guide to State Adverse Event Reporting Systems. November 2014. Used with permission from the National Academy for State Health Policy. https://nashp.org/wp-content/uploads/2015/02/2014_Guide_to_State_Adverse_Event_Reporting_Systems.pdf)

Although the classification of events as never events, serious reportable events, and/or sentinel events is instructive when creating solutions to ameliorate or prevent these events, the degree to which they are preventable should be taken into account. The concept of preventable medical errors establishes an additional layer of granularity to how we report, investigate, and create solutions to medical errors. In 2013, more than 400,000 deaths per year were attributed to preventable medical errors occurring in hospitals [9]. Additionally, the NQF estimated that 90,000 deaths can be attributed to healthcare-associated infections, and that these infections cost the healthcare system more than $4.5 billion [10]. In response to these staggering statistics and associated costs, in 2008 the Centers for Medicare and Medicaid Services (CMS) implemented a nonpayment policy for costs associated with preventable errors and medical mistakes [11]. Studies evaluating the effect of the CMS nonpayment policy have shown mixed results. After implementation of the CMS nonpayment policy, there were no significant changes in the incidence of catheter-associated urinary tract infections or catheter-associated bloodstream infections [12]. However, there was a significant reduction in the incidence of hospital-acquired pressure ulcers after implementation of the CMS nonpayment policy [13].

The concept of never events provided a powerful incentive to develop quality-improvement initiatives and programs that targeted the reduction of medical errors and consequently improved the safety of healthcare. These initiatives have taken the form of timeouts, debriefings, skin marking, and checklists. Throughout this chapter we will review these concepts and provide guidance from lessons learned on how to more effectively implement these programs to make healthcare safer for all.

Timeouts and Debriefings

Creating a work-environment culture that promotes safety requires intentional steps that invite members of the team to share their insights and expertise. Many organizations have adopted the concepts of timeouts, briefings, and debriefings. These can be used in the context of an organization or an operating room at the start and conclusion of the workday. Conversely, timeouts, briefings, and debriefings can be used in reference to a surgical procedure. We will predominantly focus our discussion of these concepts to the latter context, that of a patient undergoing a surgical procedure.

A timeout usually takes the form of reviewing pertinent information before the start of a surgical procedure. A timeout is similar to a briefing, which can take the form of a coming together to discuss potential issues that may occur before that start of a shift or a surgical procedure. The Institute for Healthcare Improvement developed the concept of "safety briefings," which were designed to "increase safety awareness among front-line staff and to help develop a culture of safety" [14]. Thinking of a timeout as a "safety briefing" can be instructive, and appropriately highlights to participants its value in keeping the patient safe. A debriefing can take the form of discussing what procedure was performed, whether there were any unexpected events, and whether there are any specific post-procedure aspects of care that should be discussed with all team members. Timeouts and debriefings are essential components of safe surgical care that promote exchange of critical information at important points in time during the care of surgical patients, sometimes referred to as pause points. A timeout must occur before the surgical procedure begins, and a debriefing typically occurs before the patient is transported to the next location of care, such as the post-anesthesia care unit (PACU) or Intensive Care Unit (ICU). Timeouts and debriefings allow for a routine pause point to discuss and review important information that all team members should be aware of, either before the start of or at the end of a surgical procedure, before moving onto the next stage of care.

Furthermore, timeouts and debriefings can be components of a program to improve the safety of surgical care at a facility. A comprehensive program to improve the safety of surgical care at a hospital or facility is multifactorial and can include multiple interventions. Timeouts and debriefings can serve as "entry" interventions since their contribution to the safety of patient care and to the improvement of workflow systems can be clearly outlined to prospective participants. The lessons learned in implementing timeouts and debriefings can inform future efforts to improve other aspects of patient care, including implementing more transparent reporting systems for medical errors, team crisis simulation, and/or implementation of surgical safety checklists.

Fundamental Elements

Fundamental elements of effective timeouts and debriefings include the following characteristics: (1) they should be a psychologically safe environment for all participants; (2) they should be routine and expected at the beginning (e.g., timeouts) and conclusion (e.g., debriefing) of every procedure and, in the case of debriefing, before the patient is transported to the next level of care; (3) they should be led by at least one of the participants; (4) all profession-specific teams should contribute; (5) they need to take priority over all other activities; and (6) they should be adapted and modified as needed according to the hospital, facility, specialty, etc. We will further elaborate on each of these six fundamental elements of an effective timeout and debriefing.

Safe Environment

Team psychological safety, a construct first introduced by Edmondson, is defined as "a shared belief held by members of a team that the team is safe for interpersonal risk taking" [15]. Timeouts and debriefings, therefore, should be characterized as being a safe space for all participants to take part in. These team activities should not feel rushed or rehearsed. They should never take on the tone of being judgmental or of identifying who to blame for what may have gone wrong or for lack of knowledge. When participating in a timeout or a debriefing, members of each profession in the operating room should contribute essential information that is pertinent to their respective roles. For example, in a debriefing, the surgeon should state what procedure was performed, whether there were any unexpected aspects of the procedure, and whether there are any aspects of the post-procedure care that are non-routine or out of the ordinary. Additionally, the surgeon can use his/her judgment on whether to share other aspects of the post-procedure care that may not be intuitive or that may not be known by all the team members present. The surgeon should feel comfortable in voicing any additional information that he/she feels would be important to share. The same principles apply to an effective timeout. Additionally, these moments are opportunities to share ideas for possible process improvements through discussions of what went well and what would make things better next time.

Routine and Expected

Timeouts and debriefings should be routine and an expected aspect of what happens before the start of the procedure and at the conclusion of every procedure or team activity. Specific to debriefings, they should happen when all critical aspects of care have been provided and before the patient is transported to the next level of care. When all participants expect a debriefing at the end of a procedure, it serves as a pause point for the exchange of information that team members can save until this point of the case. By making this routine, participants can save questions about the name of the procedure, where the patient is going, and other questions related to the care of the patient that is perceived to be essential. This also allows for these activities to be incorporated into the workflow and for the development of a culture of communication that prioritizes explicit information sharing and focus on patient safety.

Led by a Member of the Operating Room Staff

One member of the operating room staff should be the designated person to initiate and lead the timeout and debriefing although it is not necessary that it be the same person who leads both activities. At many hospitals, the circulating nurse is the designated person who customarily initiates and leads the timeout and debriefing. The circulating nurse will ask if this is an appropriate time to perform the timeout before the patient is brought into the operating room, and then the debriefing at the conclusion of the procedure. These questions are targeted to all staff in the operating room, ensuring that each member has an opportunity to speak. Many times, it is clear that it is an appropriate time to perform the timeout or debriefing, and other times it is not. Having the person who has been designated to initiate these activities ask whether it is an appropriate time to perform them allows all members the opportunity to confirm that they are able to solely focus on the task at hand.

Invitation to Speak and Contribute

By designating the person who will initiate and lead the timeout and debriefing, this person can be instructed to ask each of the respective teams to contribute to the discussion. At many institutions, the circulating nurse asks the surgeon to state the name of the procedure as the initiation for the debriefing. The circulating nurse then confirms the specimens that were sent (or are being sent, depending on institutional policies) to pathology. He or she then confirms whether the instrument, needle, and gauze/sponge count were correct. Finally, he or she will ask the surgeon and anesthesiologist if there were any unforeseen aspects of the surgery and anesthesia and whether there are any foreseen issues with recovery. Although it is essential that one participant be the designee for initiating and leading the debriefing, this should not prevent any member of the operating room staff from speaking up or contributing information that he/she identifies as being important to share with the group. Of note, a qualitative analysis of implementation of debriefing programs at four hospitals identified that oftentimes the surgeon was looked upon as having the responsibility to create an environment that promoted open communication [16]. Therefore, it is essential for the surgeon to ensure that his or her behavior is contributing to an environment conducive to effective communication. Brindle and colleagues found that the surgeon could accomplish this by actively asking all members to contribute to the debriefing, giving voice to all team members.

Priority over all Other Activities

A timeout should occur before any aspect of the surgical procedure is performed and is part of the Joint Commission Universal Protocol. Operating room team members should not be distracted with other tasks while performing the timeout. Therefore, the timeout should be performed immediately before the surgical incision is made, at a point where plans can still be changed if information revealed so dictates. Conversely, the debriefing should occur at the conclusion of the procedure or team activity. There should be no remaining critical tasks. This is essential because all participants should be solely focused on the debriefing. If there are other critical tasks to be performed, then participants are not able to exclusively focus on debriefing. This may lead to failure to properly share or receive information that all team members should know, and it might also lead to misinformation if the patient's condition changes. It would be helpful if institutions clarify when debriefings should occur in relation to extubation of the patient and closure of the skin incision. Performing the debriefing before these two tasks may be appropriate, but all members should be prepared to debrief again if the patient cannot be extubated as was originally expected, or if there are issues with wound closure that change the management of the patient postoperatively.

Adapted and Modified

Like most quality and safety tools, the timeout and debriefing processes should be modified and adapted to the level of the institution, facility, or specialty. At the level of the institution or facility, there are critical components of the timeout and debriefing processes that pertain to all procedures and ought not to be significantly modified. These critical components include (1) name of procedure, (2) non-routine aspects of the procedure, and (3) non-routine aspects of the anesthetic care. Furthermore, debriefings may include the following other critical components: (a) confirmation that the instrument, needle, and sponge/gauze count were correct; (b) identification of the specimens that were sent or are being sent to pathology; (c) location to which the patient will be transported after he/she leaves the operating room, and (d) aspects of the postoperative care plan that may be out of the ordinary or specific for the procedure at hand. Furthermore, the debriefing can also include aspects of care that are pertinent to the procedure that was just performed. This could include activity restrictions for vascular or orthopedic procedures, pain control, or any aspect of care that is important at the facility level or for the specific procedure.

Successful Implementation of a Timeout or Debriefing Program

A timeout or debriefing program can be part of a larger quality-improvement initiative or program that is being implemented across a facility or hospital or a standalone program to test the success of implementing larger programs in the future. Implementation of a debriefing program is enhanced by having many of the following [16]:

1. Early and strong leadership support
2. Active involvement and participation by senior clinical leadership through participation in, or observation of, debriefings
3. Relevant strategies to sustain the practice of performing effective debriefing after the initial implementation phase (e.g., aligning participation in debriefing training with credentialing and/or granting/maintenance of operating room privileges)
4. Engagement of on-the-ground clinician leaders

Many, if not all, of these factors are also important for successful implementation of any type of quality and safety intervention, including implementation of a timeout program.

Skin Marking

Skin marking has become a universally accepted aspect of the pre-procedure process to ensure that the right procedure is being performed on the right patient, on the right side, and on the right site. The Joint Commission has incorporated skin marking into the Universal Protocol, which they have called their "Speak Up" initiative [17]. The Universal Protocol, or "Speak Up" includes the following three components: (1) conducting a pre-procedure verification process, (2) marking the procedure site, and (3) performing a timeout. The Joint Commission states that the Universal Protocol has the aim of "preventing wrong site, wrong procedure, wrong person surgery."

The Joint Commission through its Universal Protocol outlines several aspects of skin marking which, in our opinion should always be observed. For starters, there are few surgical procedures for which a skin marking should be omitted. For surgical procedures on sites and/or patients that cannot be easily or safely preoperatively marked, an alternative form of confirming the right location preoperatively should be employed. The Joint Commission lists potentially extraneous sites or situations that may not be conducive to preoperative site marking and these include: (1) mucosal surfaces or perineum, (2) minimal access procedures treating a lateralized internal organ (percutaneous or through a natural orifice), (3) teeth, and (4) premature infants (since skin marking may lead to permanent marks/tattoos). For these procedures/patients, an alternative process should be created, adopted, and effectively implemented at the facility level. The alternative should come as close to as possible to marking the site of interest. In these circumstances, all members of the operating room team should be present, especially all members of the surgical team who will be performing the procedure. The goal is to correctly identify the site that will undergo a surgical procedure. The other important aspects of the Universal Protocol that are identified by the Joint Commission should also be kept in mind when formulating this alternative process for patients/procedures/surgical sites that cannot be readily or safely marked preoperatively.

Patient Involvement

An important recommendation that the Universal Protocol includes is encouraging the involvement of the patient when the planned site for the surgical procedure is marked. Involving the patient serves multiple purposes, including making sure the patient understands the surgical procedure that is being prepared for, and making everyone aware of the patient's expectations. Furthermore, this action empowers the patient to take an active role in their surgical care, something he/she cannot do when they are under general anesthesia. However, it also should be recognized that patient identification alone is insufficient for site identification, as patients may have variable understanding of the location of lesion or targets for procedures. Ultimately, all these measures, including surgical marking and the Joint Commission Universal Protocol, center on keeping the patient safe during surgery. Involving the patient ensures that the patient is invested and actively participating in ensuring their own safety. This can serve as a powerful message to not only the patient, but also to all healthcare providers involved in the surgical care of the patient.

Other Important Aspects of Skin Marking

Other important aspects of skin marking that should be addressed include the following: (1) making sure that the skin marking happens preoperatively, and (2) making sure that how the site is marked follows a hospital/facility standard. Ideally, we recommend that the site be marked in the pre-induction/preoperative area. This allows for the patient to confirm that indeed the correct site is marked, and for collateral information to be checked (e.g., photos, radiographs, other documentation) to confirm location for the procedure. Furthermore, this also allows for all members of the operating room, including the circulating nurse and anesthesiologist, to understand the site that will be operated on and/or voice any concerns they may have. In particular, the circulating nurse and/or the anesthesiologist may have had a different understanding of what the surgery was going to entail, based on the patient chart compared to the site that was marked by the surgeon and/or surgeon-assistant (e.g., resident, fellow, or physician assistant). Secondly, there should be a hospital/facility-level standard on how the site marking is performed. For example, the site marking may take the form of the initials of the person doing the marking or take the form of an okay sign or something similar. We argue that circling the site or drawing an arrow to the site plus placing your initials is the best way to mark the site. We suggest such steps because they ensure that the site itself is marked or easily pointed to and they also ensure that anyone who visualizes the site marking can then identify who did the marking. This therefore requires that the initials be clear and easily readable. Although skin marking may be implemented as a stand-alone intervention, it works best when it is part of a larger quality and safety initiative. In particular, incorporating skin marking with timeouts and debriefing can be synergistic. The surgical safety checklist, which we will learn more about in the following section, incorporates many of the concepts we have already addressed, including never events, timeouts, debriefings, and skin marking.

Checklists

Checklists are a relatively recent addition to the toolkit for quality and safety in healthcare. Pronovost and colleagues produced an early example of a team-based procedural checklist in healthcare with their work toward reducing catheter-associated bloodstream infections in intensive care units through the use of an evidence-based intervention [18]. Building on the success of checklists for central line placement, the World Health Organization (WHO) brought together an international group of experts who developed the WHO Surgical Safety Checklist. The pilot study of this innovation was the first international, multi-center study of a surgical checklist that demonstrated significant reductions in postoperative mortality and postoperative complications. Since that time, checklists have proliferated as tools for team communication and perioperative safety and are used in a large proportion of operations all over the world [19]. Checklists have evolved to include all aspects of a surgical patient's experience; for example, the SURgical PAtient Safety System (SURPASS) checklist is a comprehensive set of checklists that aims to improve the entire surgical pathway before, during, and after the operation itself [20].

Origins of the WHO Surgical Safety Checklist

Checklists in healthcare have been inspired by the pilot preflight checklist created in response to the fatal crash on October 30, 1935, of the Boeing 299, referred to as the "Flying Fortress" and later as the B-17 bomber [21, 22]. The United States Army Air Corps, the precursor to the United States Air Force, held a competition for a technologically advanced bomber aircraft. The major aircraft manufacturers of the day—Boeing, Douglas, and Martin—entered the competition for the contract. On October 30, 1935, a test flight competition was held in Dayton, Ohio; the Boeing 299, a four-engine airplane, was the favored aircraft. Unfortunately, at 300 feet above the ground the "Flying Fortress" stalled and crashed during its second flight and two of Boeing's senior test pilots died. Analysis of the crash found that the five-member crew had neglected to switch off the elevator locking mechanism, which controls the movement of the airplane nose. Previous airplanes had historically had this switch on the outside of the airplane. However, this technologically advanced aircraft, the first of its kind, had the elevator locking mechanism inside the airplane. The pilots were not able to level off the airplane because they had failed to switch off the elevator locking mechanism, and the airplane's nose kept climbing. This led to the plane stalling during takeoff and fatally crashing. The pilot preflight checklist was then created to avert mistakes when flying complex airplanes. The checklist did not instruct the pilot on how to fly a plane, instead it prompted the pilot to perform essential tasks every time when flying a plane. This became important as the complexity of flying airplanes increased with more technologically advanced aircraft. Crew resource management training, which focuses on improving teamwork and communication among the aviation crew, was developed in tandem with the creation and implementation of the pilot preflight checklist. The pilot preflight checklist has been expanded to more extensive checklists that cover all aspects of safety and quality when operating an airplane. Furthermore, crew resource management training has become the standard when training aviation crews on how to work together effectively (Fig. 3.2).

Although there was no single event in surgical care that paralleled the fatal Boeing 299 crash, the WHO Surgical Safety Checklist was the product of an effort

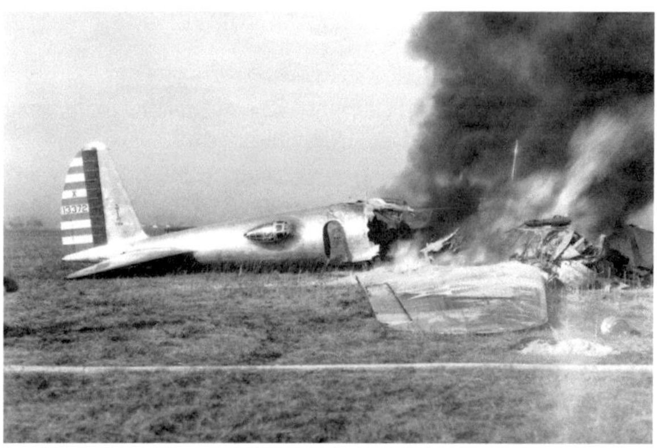

Fig. 3.2 The XB-17 (Model 299) crashed during its test flight at Wright Field on October 30, 1935. U.S. Air Force photo. (Used with permission from: https://www.nationalmuseum.af.mil/Visit/Museum-Exhibits/Fact-Sheets/Display/Article/610002/model-299-crash/)

to improve the safety and quality of surgical care throughout the world. A convening was organized of experts from around the world in surgery, anesthesia, nursing, and other aspects of perioperative care. This convening led to the creation of ten essential objectives that were considered fundamental to the delivery of safe and high-quality surgical care (Table 3.2).

The ten essential objectives are common to all surgical procedures, and they are essential steps in the care of a surgical patient. They have the common underlying quality that if they are not performed, the patient could be placed in serious risk of harm. Importantly, none of them instruct healthcare providers on how to perform their duties. Instead, they highlight important pieces of information that need to be communicated among the operating room team members.

The first objective is to ensure that the operation is being performed on the correct patient, side and site. The second and third objectives center on safe anesthesia delivery. The fourth and fifth objectives ensure readiness to respond to potential emergencies during an operation, such as discussion of anticipated blood loss, and acknowledgment of allergic reactions. The sixth objective addresses preventing or controlling existing infections, and complications that may ensue. The seventh objective covers the importance of correctly counting all surgical sponges and instruments to ensure that surgical sponges and instruments are not left behind inside the patient. The eighth objective highlights the importance of labeling all specimens so that they reach their correct destination and so that they can be attributed to the correct patient. The final two objectives address the importance of communication and exchanging critical patient information in a timely and effective

Table 3.2 Ten essential objectives for safe surgery

Objective 1	The team will operate on the correct patient at the correct site
Objective 2	The team will use methods known to prevent harm from anesthetic administration, while protecting the patient from pain
Objective 3	The team will recognize and effectively prepare for life-threatening loss of airway or respiratory function
Objective 4	The team will recognize and effectively prepare for risk of high blood loss
Objective 5	The team will avoid inducing an allergic or adverse drug reaction known to be a significant risk to the patient
Objective 6	The team will consistently use methods known to minimize risk of surgical site infection
Objective 7	The team will prevent inadvertent retention of sponges or instruments in surgical wounds
Objective 8	The team will secure and accurately identify all surgical specimens
Objective 9	The team will effectively communicate and exchange critical patient information for the safe conduct of the operation
Objective 10	Hospitals and public health systems will establish routine surveillance or surgical capacity, volume, and results

Used with permission from World Alliance for Patient Safety: The Second Global Patient Safety Challenge, Safe Surgery Saves Lives. © 2008. Used with permission from World Health Organization (WHO). https://www.who.int/patientsafety/safesurgery/knowledge_base/SSSL_Brochure_finalJun08.pdf manner, along with measurement of surgical outcomes. These ten essential objectives were then transformed into a checklist with three pause points. These three pause points are: (1) before induction of anesthesia, (2) before the skin incision is made, and (3) before the patient leaves the operating room (Fig. 3.3).

These three pause points were selected because they represented critical points in the care of a patient in the operating room. These three pause points represent moments of "no turning back." For example, once anesthesia is induced, the patient has undergone a critical aspect of care in the operating room that carries potential risks and complications. The same concept applies to the other two pause points—making the skin incision and the patient leaving the operating room for the next phase of care (e.g., ICU or PACU). The checklist was structured around these three pause points because certain actions should be performed every single time before these points of "no turning back," when intervention(s) to ameliorate lapses or problems is still possible. Similarly, certain critical pieces of information should be communicated to all healthcare members in the operating room before each of these three pause points. For example, in the first pause point, it is paramount to confirm that the patient has provided consent for the planned procedure. Additionally, it is important to identify and confirm the patient's medication allergies, whether the patient has a difficult airway, and what the expected risk of blood loss is. Similarly, there are other essential tasks that should be performed at the other two pause points before proceeding.

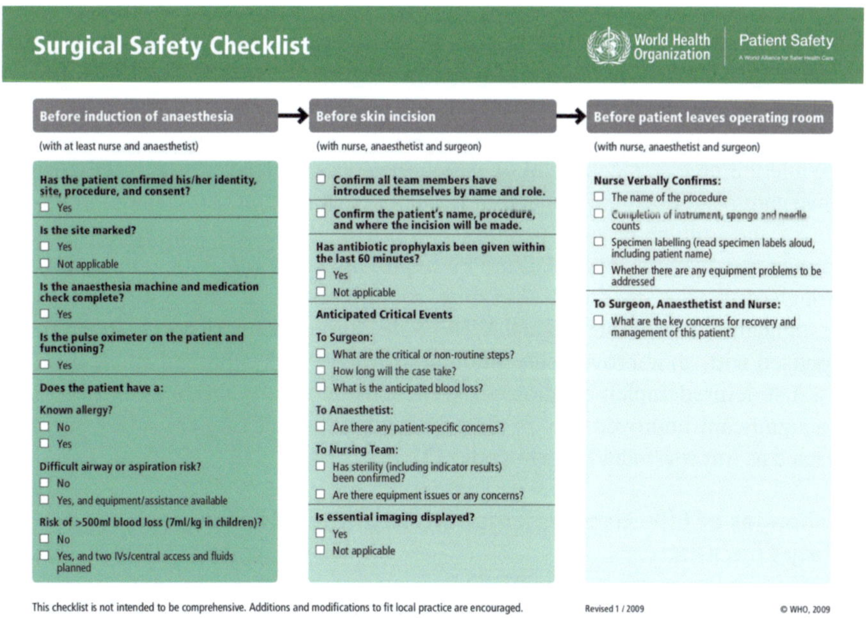
Surgical Safety Checklist

World Health Organization | Patient Safety

Before induction of anaesthesia

(with at least nurse and anaesthetist)

Has the patient confirmed his/her identity, site, procedure, and consent?
- ☐ Yes

Is the site marked?
- ☐ Yes
- ☐ Not applicable

Is the anaesthesia machine and medication check complete?
- ☐ Yes

Is the pulse oximeter on the patient and functioning?
- ☐ Yes

Does the patient have a:

Known allergy?
- ☐ No
- ☐ Yes

Difficult airway or aspiration risk?
- ☐ No
- ☐ Yes, and equipment/assistance available

Risk of >500ml blood loss (7ml/kg in children)?
- ☐ No
- ☐ Yes, and two IVs/central access and fluids planned

Before skin incision

(with nurse, anaesthetist and surgeon)

- ☐ **Confirm all team members have introduced themselves by name and role.**
- ☐ **Confirm the patient's name, procedure, and where the incision will be made.**

Has antibiotic prophylaxis been given within the last 60 minutes?
- ☐ Yes
- ☐ Not applicable

Anticipated Critical Events

To Surgeon:
- ☐ What are the critical or non-routine steps?
- ☐ How long will the case take?
- ☐ What is the anticipated blood loss?

To Anaesthetist:
- ☐ Are there any patient-specific concerns?

To Nursing Team:
- ☐ Has sterility (including indicator results) been confirmed?
- ☐ Are there equipment issues or any concerns?

Is essential imaging displayed?
- ☐ Yes
- ☐ Not applicable

Before patient leaves operating room

(with nurse, anaesthetist and surgeon)

Nurse Verbally Confirms:
- ☐ The name of the procedure
- ☐ Completion of instrument, sponge and needle counts
- ☐ Specimen labelling (read specimen labels aloud, including patient name)
- ☐ Whether there are any equipment problems to be addressed

To Surgeon, Anaesthetist and Nurse:
- ☐ What are the key concerns for recovery and management of this patient?

This checklist is not intended to be comprehensive. Additions and modifications to fit local practice are encouraged. Revised 1 / 2009 © WHO, 2009

Fig. 3.3 World Health Organization, Surgical Safety Checklist in English. https://apps.who.int/iris/bitstream/handle/10665/44186/9789241598590_eng_Checklist.pdf

History of Implementation of the WHO Safe Surgery Checklist

The WHO Surgical Safety Checklist was trialed in a limited set of operating rooms in eight hospitals located throughout the world, representing all WHO regions and a diversity of environments: Toronto, Canada; London, England; Amman, Jordan; Manila, Philippines; Auckland, New Zealand; New Delhi, India; Ifakara, Tanzania; and Seattle, USA (Table 3.2).

This pre-post study evaluated the change in 30-day, in-hospital postoperative mortality rate and 30-day complication rate before and after implementation of the WHO Safe Surgery Checklist. The study found that implementation of the checklist was associated with a 47% reduction in postoperative mortality and a 36% reduction in postoperative complications [23]. The WHO Safe Surgery Checklist was also found to be effective when used in urgent surgical procedures [24]. Since the initial pilot study of the WHO Surgical Safety Checklist, several other studies have shown similar reductions in postoperative complications and/or mortality [25–29]. However, not all large- and limited-scale implementation of the WHO Surgical Safety Checklist have demonstrated the reductions in postoperative morbidity and mortality that were seen in the initial international, multi-center study. Limited-scale implementation of the checklist in Moldova, for example, did demonstrate significant and sustained reductions in postoperative morbidity [25, 26]. A limited-scale implementation study that demonstrated mixed results included a stepped wedge cluster randomized trial performed in Norway that found a statistically significant reduction in postoperative complications, but not in postoperative mortality, after implementation of the surgical safety checklist [27]. In Ontario, Canada, a mandatory adoption across the entire province of the surgical safety checklist was not associated with reductions in postoperative complications or mortality [30]. Conversely, a large-scale implementation initiative in the state of South Carolina in the U.S. was associated with a 22% reduction in postoperative mortality in hospitals that effectively implemented the checklist [28].

While the precise mechanism by which the checklist leads to improved postoperative care is still being evaluated, it is mediated at least in part through improvement of the culture in the operating room. The WHO Safe Surgery Checklist improves the operating room culture by improving communication and teamwork. Through use of a modified operating room version of the Safety Attitudes Questionnaire (SAQ), the original WHO Safe Surgery Checklist was found to be associated with an improved perception of teamwork and culture of surgical safety [31]. A structured implementation of the checklist in South Carolina was associated with significant improvements in the perceived culture of surgical safety that was reflected as improvement in teamwork [32].

Challenges of Effective Implementation of the WHO Surgical Safety Checklist

Effective implementation of the WHO Surgical Safety Checklist requires intentionality and active participation by all stakeholders. An important and necessary step in effective implementation of the WHO Surgical Safety Checklist is modification of the checklist to meet local needs and practices. The Ontario, Canada, mandatory adoption experience demonstrated that such a top-down strategy to implement innovative tools like the surgical safety checklist may not be effective in leading to the necessary change in practice that is needed to achieve favorable reductions in postoperative morbidity and mortality. Of 92 hospitals (out of 101 hospitals in the Ontario, Canada, study) that provided copies of the checklist they used after mandatory adoption, only 10% modified the Canadian Patient Safety Institute checklist [33]. The majority of hospitals used an unmodified version of these checklists. There was no measurement of how well or poorly these checklists were used. It is unclear if the checklists were used as they are intended, which are to create an atmosphere in the operating room that requires effective and clear communication. Although the concept of a surgical safety checklist is simple, the practice of effectively implementing the checklist can be difficult if there isn't support and promotion by hospital leadership.

Lessons Learned on How to Effectively Implement the Checklist

Effective implementation of the checklist requires an intentional and structured approach. In the *Safe Surgery Checklist Implementation Guide*, published by Ariadne Labs (https://www.ariadnelabs.org/resources/downloads/), a joint health systems innovation center of Brigham and Women's Hospital and Harvard T.H. Chan School of Public Health, the work of effective implementation of the surgical safety checklist is divided into four phases that include preparing, owning, expanding, and improving [34]. These four phases encompass 11 essential steps that include (1) recruiting a team, (2) understanding the work, (3) assessing your environment, (4) deciding if you are ready to implement the checklist, (5) customizing and testing the checklist, (6) planning the expansion of the checklist, (7) having 1-on-1 conversations about implementing the checklist with on-the-ground users, (8) promoting the checklist, (9) training and spreading of checklist use, (10) watching and coaching checklist use, and (11) continually improving (Fig. 3.4) [34].

Additionally, some facilities have already implemented the surgical safety checklist, but may not have done so effectively, or it is not currently in use. Resistance to implementation of the checklist may lie in the fact that the checklist was implemented previously, but unsuccessfully. The distinction of whether the checklist was implemented before is important because it will guide the approach of how the checklist is implemented, but not necessarily the framework that has been proposed by Ariadne Labs. In these settings, the purpose should be to improve the existing checklist (Fig. 3.5).

The essential components to effective implementation of a surgical safety checklist program are similar to those needed for effective implementation of any quality-improvement initiative. These include strong and early leadership support, the creation of a team of "champions" who are respected and are regarded as being collegial, a progressive and iterative implementation approach, and continual evaluation and monitoring of how effective the checklist is being used. Nevertheless, a major challenge in effective checklist implementation is accurate monitoring and evaluation of checklist use. Effective checklist use is more than just checking off boxes on a paper or electronic checklist; it should entail active participation by all

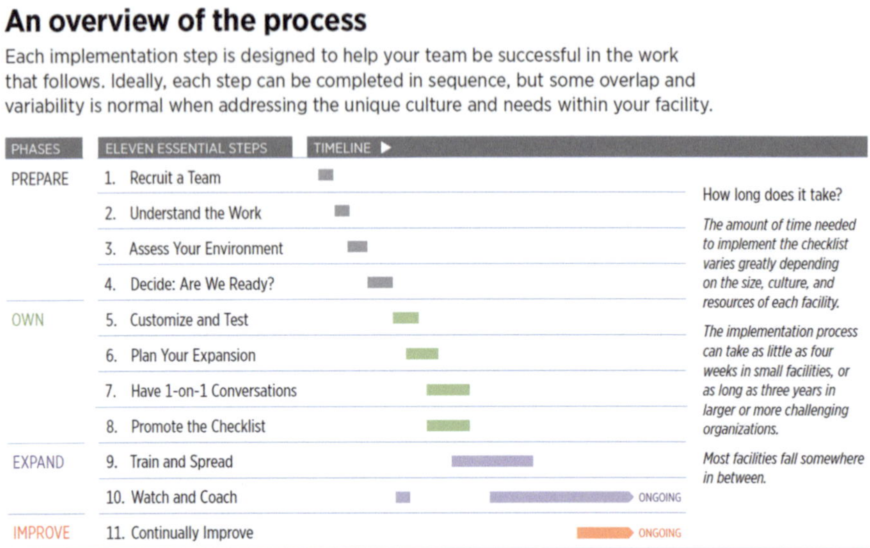
An overview of the process
Each implementation step is designed to help your team be successful in the work that follows. Ideally, each step can be completed in sequence, but some overlap and variability is normal when addressing the unique culture and needs within your facility.
PHASES
ELEVEN ESSENTIAL STEPS
TIMELINE
PREPARE
1. Recruit a Team
2. Understand the Work
3. Assess Your Environment
4. Decide: Are We Ready?
OWN
5. Customize and Test
6. Plan Your Expansion
7. Have 1-on-1 Conversations
8. Promote the Checklist
EXPAND
9. Train and Spread
10. Watch and Coach
ONGOING
IMPROVE
11. Continually Improve
ONGOING
How long does it take?
The amount of time needed to implement the checklist varies greatly depending on the size, culture, and resources of each facility.
The implementation process can take as little as four weeks in small facilities, or as long as three years in larger or more challenging organizations.
Most facilities fall somewhere in between.

Fig. 3.4 "An overview of the process" from Chap. 2 of the Ariadne Labs *Safe Surgery Checklist Implementation Guide*. (Reproduced with kind permission of Ariadne Labs 2019. All Rights Reserved)

members of the operating room team in discussing the case and voicing their concerns. The checklist should serve as a tool to foster closed-loop communication and to ensure that all professionals in the operating room feel empowered to be active participants. Although electronic integration of checklists into the electronic medical record has a role in facilitating the use of checklists, it does not replace or more accurately capture the difficult-to-measure qualities of effective checklist use, including teamwork and effective communication. Nevertheless, electronic integration of checklists can improve checklist use compliance by facilitating the availability of the checklist and also allowing for accurate measurement of whether the checklist was used. Electronic integration of checklists to reduce central line-associated bloodstream infections demonstrated improved compliance and reductions in the incidence of infections [35, 36].

The surgical safety checklist has been a success story for surgical safety efforts in general. The checklist is a tool in the ever-growing toolbox of surgical safety measures and initiatives. Efforts to improve the safety of surgical patients now include work on coaching of surgeons [37], team simulation trainings [38], and artificial intelligence to improve recognition of surgical errors and facilitate training of surgeons [39]. These initiatives and research all have the central goal of improving the safety of surgical patients. The landscape of quality and safety in healthcare has expanded since the publication of the Institute of Medicine report, "To Err is Human: Building a Safer Health System," and it is our responsibility to make sure we remain vigilant on the ongoing need to make healthcare safer for all.

DIAGRAM 2.2 **Using the framework to improve your existing checklist**

The implementation framework is also useful for facilities that already use a surgical safety checklist. The sequence of steps remains the same, but the focus may be slightly different, as shown below.

STEP	FOCUS FOR FACILITIES ALREADY USING A SURGICAL CHECKLIST
1. Recruit a Team	Always start by checking that you have the right mix of enthusiastic people on your implementation team. Adding or changing members can help give your effort a boost.
2. Understand the Work	As a team, compare the recommended implementation process with the process you have followed so far, and look for gaps.
3. Assess Your Environment	Look at how your existing checklist is actually being used, to highlight opportunities for improvement. Conduct the Safe Surgery Culture Survey.
4. Decide: Are We Ready?	As a team, and with the input of facility leadership, decide whether you have the resources and support you need to recommit to your checklist effort.
5. Customize and Test	Compare your organization's checklist to the Safe Surgery Checklist template. Evaluate your checklist design. Make changes if needed, and always test new versions before putting them into use.
6. Plan Your Expansion	Based on a review of your situation and these best practices, plan specific actions you will take to close any gaps or to make changes.
7. Have 1-on-1 Conversations	Have 1-on-1 conversations with each surgical team member before launching the updated version of your checklist. Even if you had these previously, talk to everyone again and let them know about the project and which aspects of checklist use your facility is aiming to improve. There is no substitute for this step, and it is never too late to connect with people personally.
8. Promote the Checklist	Promote your new checklist effort widely. Advertise what this project is about, and how it is different from what your teams were previously doing. Focus on positive stories or the improvements you will be making.
9. Train and Spread	The key to training is practice. Create opportunities for surgical team members to practice using your new checklist.
10. Watch and Coach 11. Continually Improve	Coaching is absolutely critical for helping people learn how to properly use the checklist and for maintaining high-quality use over time. If you do not have an ongoing program for coaching your checklist, create a plan and process now.

Fig. 3.5 "Using the framework to improve your existing checklist" from Chap. 2 of the Ariadne Labs *Safe Surgery Checklist Implementation Guide*. (Reproduced with kind permission of Ariadne Labs 2019. All Rights Reserved)

References

1. Kohn LT, Corrigan JM, Donaldson MS, Institute of Medicine. To err is human: building a safer health system. Washington: National Academy Press; 2000.
2. Pear R. Clinton names panel to draft health consumer bill of rights. The New York Times. 1997;Sect. B:11.

3. President's advisory commission on consumer protection and quality in the health care industry. Executive summary—quality first: better health care for all Americans. govinfo.library.unt.edu/hcquality/final/execsum.html. Accessed 26 Aug 2019.
4. National Quality Forum. NQF's history. www.qualityforum.org/about_nqf/history/. Accessed 26 Aug 2019.
5. Hempel S, Maggard-Gibbons M, Nguyen DK, Dawes AJ, Miake-Lye I, Beroes JM, et al. Wrong-site surgery, retained surgical items, and surgical fires: a systematic review of surgical never events. JAMA Surg. 2015;150(8):796–805.
6. The Joint Commission. History of the Joint Commission. https://www.jointcommission.org/about_us/history.aspx. Accessed 26 Aug 2019.
7. The Joint Commission. Patient safety systems chapter, sentinel event policy and RCA2. https://www.jointcommission.org/sentinel_event.aspx. Accessed 19 Aug 2019.
8. Hanlon C, Sheedy K, Kniffin T, Rosenthal J, National Academy for State Health Policy. 2014 guide to state adverse event reporting systems. 2015. https://nashp.org/wp-content/uploads/2015/02/2014_Guide_to_State_Adverse_Event_Reporting_Systems.pdf. Accessed 19 Aug 2019.
9. James JT. A new, evidence-based estimate of patient harms associated with hospital care. J Patient Saf. 2013;9(3):122–8.
10. National Quality Forum. Patient safety. www.qualityforum.org/Topics/Patient_Safety.aspx. Accessed 19 Aug 2019.
11. Centers for Medicare and Medicaid Services. Hospital-acquired conditions (present on admission indicator). https://www.cms.gov/Medicare/Medicare-Fee-for-Service-Payment/HospitalAcqCond/index.html?redirect=/HospitalAcqCond/01_Overview.asp. Accessed 19 Aug 2019.
12. Lee GM, Kleinman K, Soumerai SB, Tse A, Cole D, Fridkin SK, et al. Effect of nonpayment for preventable infections in U.S. hospitals. N Engl J Med. 2012;367(15):1428–37.
13. Padula WV, Makic MB, Wald HL, Campbell JD, Nair KV, Mishra MK, et al. Hospital-acquired pressure ulcers at academic medical centers in the United States, 2008-2012: tracking changes since the CMS nonpayment policy. Jt Comm J Qual Patient Saf. 2015;41(6):257–63.
14. Institute for Healthcare Improvement. Safety briefings. http://www.ihi.org/Engage/Memberships/Passport/Documents/SafetyBriefings.pdf. Accessed 23 Aug 2019.
15. Edmondson A. Psychological safety and learning behavior in work teams. Adm Sci Q. 1999;44(2):350–83.
16. Brindle ME, Henrich N, Foster A, Marks S, Rose M, Welsh R, et al. Implementation of surgical debriefing programs in large health systems: an exploratory qualitative analysis. BMC Health Serv Res. 2018;18(1):210.
17. The Joint Commission. The universal protocol: speak up. https://www.jointcommission.org/assets/1/18/UP_Poster1.PDF. Accessed 20 Aug 2019.
18. Pronovost P, Needham D, Berenholtz S, Sinopoli D, Chu H, Cosgrove S, et al. An intervention to decrease catheter-related bloodstream infections in the ICU. N Engl J Med. 2006;355(26):2725–32.
19. Delisle M, Pradarelli JC, Panda N, Koritsanszky L, Sonnay Y, Lipsitz S, et al. Variation in the global uptake of the surgical safety checklist. Br J Surg. 2020;107(2):e151–60.
20. de Vries EN, Hollmann MW, Smorenburg SM, Gouma DJ, Boermeester MA. Development and validation of the SURgical PAtient Safety System (SURPASS) checklist. Qual Saf Health Care. 2009;18(2):121–6.
21. A piece of history: the 1935 plane crash that almost destroyed Boeing. 2019. https://theweek.com/speedreads/828848/1935-plane-crash-that-almost-destroyed-boeing. Accessed 11 Aug 2019.
22. Vedantam S, Boyle T, Klahr R, National Public Radio. The trick to surviving a high-stakes, high-pressure job? Try a checklist. https://www.npr.org/2017/10/30/559996276/the-trick-to-surviving-a-high-stakes-high-pressure-job-try-a-checklist. Accessed 11 Aug 2019.

23. Haynes AB, Weiser TG, Berry WR, Lipsitz SR, Breizat AH, Dellinger EP, et al. A surgical safety checklist to reduce morbidity and mortality in a global population. N Engl J Med. 2009;360(5):491–9.
24. Weiser TG, Haynes AB, Dziekan G, Berry WR, Lipsitz SR, Gawande AA, et al. Effect of a 19-item surgical safety checklist during urgent operations in a global patient population. Ann Surg. 2010;251(5):976–80.
25. Kwok AC, Funk LM, Baltaga R, Lipsitz SR, Merry AF, Dziekan G, et al. Implementation of the World Health Organization surgical safety checklist, including introduction of pulse oximetry, in a resource-limited setting. Ann Surg. 2013;257(4):633–9.
26. Kim RY, Kwakye G, Kwok AC, Baltaga R, Ciobanu G, Merry AF, et al. Sustainability and long-term effectiveness of the WHO surgical safety checklist combined with pulse oximetry in a resource-limited setting: two-year update from Moldova. JAMA Surg. 2015;150(5):473–9.
27. Haugen AS, Softeland E, Almeland SK, Sevdalis N, Vonen B, Eide GE, et al. Effect of the World Health Organization checklist on patient outcomes: a stepped wedge cluster randomized controlled trial. Ann Surg. 2015;261(5):821–8.
28. Haynes AB, Edmondson L, Lipsitz SR, Molina G, Neville BA, Singer SJ, et al. Mortality trends after a voluntary checklist-based surgical safety collaborative. Ann Surg. 2017;266(6):923–9.
29. Ramsay G, Haynes AB, Lipsitz SR, Solsky I, Leitch J, Gawande AA, et al. Reducing surgical mortality in Scotland by use of the WHO surgical safety checklist. Br J Surg. 2019;106(8):1005–11.
30. Urbach DR, Govindarajan A, Saskin R, Wilton AS, Baxter NN. Introduction of surgical safety checklists in Ontario, Canada. N Engl J Med. 2014;370(11):1029–38.
31. Haynes AB, Weiser TG, Berry WR, Lipsitz SR, Breizat AH, Dellinger EP, et al. Changes in safety attitude and relationship to decreased postoperative morbidity and mortality following implementation of a checklist-based surgical safety intervention. BMJ Qual Saf. 2011;20(1):102–7.
32. Molina G, Jiang W, Edmondson L, Gibbons L, Huang LC, Kiang MV, et al. Implementation of the surgical safety checklist in South Carolina hospitals is associated with improvement in perceived perioperative safety. J Am Coll Surg. 2016;222(5):725–36.e5.
33. Leape LL. The checklist conundrum. N Engl J Med. 2014;370(11):1063–4.
34. Safe surgery checklist implementation guide. Boston: Ariadne Labs; 2015. www.SafeSurgery2015.org. Accessed 27 2019.
35. Quan KA, Cousins SM, Porter DD, O'Brien M, Rudkin S, Lambertson B, et al. Electronic health record solutions to reduce central line-associated bloodstream infections by enhancing documentation of central line insertion practices, line days, and daily line necessity. Am J Infect Control. 2016;44(4):438–43.
36. Pageler NM, Longhurst CA, Wood M, Cornfield DN, Suermondt J, Sharek PJ, et al. Use of electronic medical record-enhanced checklist and electronic dashboard to decrease CLABSIs. Pediatrics. 2014;133(3):e738–46.
37. Hu YY, Peyre SE, Arriaga AF, Osteen RT, Corso KA, Weiser TG, et al. Postgame analysis: using video-based coaching for continuous professional development. J Am Coll Surg. 2012;214(1):115–24.
38. Arriaga AF, Bader AM, Wong JM, Lipsitz SR, Berry WR, Ziewacz JE, et al. Simulation-based trial of surgical-crisis checklists. N Engl J Med. 2013;368(3):246–53.
39. Hashimoto DA, Rosman G, Witkowski ER, Stafford C, Navarette-Welton AJ, Rattner DW, et al. Computer vision analysis of intraoperative video: automated recognition of operative steps in laparoscopic sleeve gastrectomy. Ann Surg. 2019;270(3):414–21.

Reducing Perioperative Medication Errors: How to Build Safer Systems

4

Petra Khoury and Ulfat Usta

Introduction: What Is Medication Error?

The National Coordinating Center for Medication Error Reporting and Prevention (NCC MERP) in the United State defines medication errors as "Any preventable event that may cause or lead to inappropriate medication use or patient harm while the medication is in the control of the healthcare professional, patient, or consumer. Such events may be related to professional practice, healthcare products, procedures, and systems, including prescribing, order communication, product labeling, packaging, and nomenclature, compounding, dispensing, distribution, administration, education, monitoring, and use" [1].

Adverse drug events (ADEs)—unintended or excessive responses to a drug that occur at doses normally used—are considered nonpreventable, but, like medication errors, they can cause untoward harmful effects [2]. Errors and adverse events may overlap. "Near misses" are errors or precursor acts corrected in a timely manner and not considered as adverse events.

Medication Management in the Perioperative Setting

Compared to other patient care areas, medication prescribing, preparation, administration, and recording in the perioperative setting bypasses the standard safety checks, such as electronic physician order entry, with decision support, prospective pharmacy verification, and multiple nursing checks at the time of medication

P. Khoury
Health and Care Department, International Federation of Red Cross Red Crescent, Geneva, Switzerland

U. Usta (✉)
Pharmacy Department, Aman Hospital, Doha, Qatar
e-mail: U.usta@amanhospital.org

J. J. Hoballah et al. (eds.), *Principles of Perioperative Safety and Efficiency*,
https://doi.org/10.1007/978-3-031-41089-5_4

administration [3]. Moreover, multiple providers are involved in the perioperative care as patients move across a continuum of healthcare settings such as operating room (OR), anesthesia, and post-anesthesia care unit, leading to a high probability of communication failure and medication errors.

Prevalence of Medication Errors in Anesthesia

The Institute of Medicine (IOM) reported that more than 1.5 million Americans are injured every year in US hospitals [4]. The prevalence of medication errors in the perioperative setting is markedly high. In anonymous surveys, 80–85% of anesthesiologists admit having made at least one medication administration error or having a "near miss," with 12% of these causing patient injury [5]. The most common reasons were "syringe swap" that involved a muscle relaxant instead of a reversal agent (70.4%) and the misidentification of the label (46.8%). In a large prospective observational study, a total of 277 operations were observed with 3671 medication administrations, of which 193 (5.3%) involved a medication error (ME) and/or adverse drug event (ADE); 40 (20.7%) were nonpreventable, and 153 (79.3%) were deemed preventable; 70 (45.8%) had the potential for patient harm, and 3 (2.0%) were life-threatening. The authors concluded that more than one-third of MEs led to observed ADEs, and the remaining two-thirds had the potential for harm [6]. The analysis of 1137 reports from the Pennsylvania Patient Safety Reporting System (PA-PSRS) database showed that almost three-quarters (73.0%, $n = 830$) of reported events were from the intraoperative setting, concerning potential or actual medication errors in the perioperative setting [7].

Errors in that study were stratified according to the NCC MERP harm index (Fig. 4.1) [8]. Of the errors reported, 54.6% (n = 621) reached the patient (harm score = C through I) and 1.6% (n = 18) resulted in patient harm (harm score = E through I). In both studies, the most common types of errors were incorrect dosing, omission error (e.g., failure to administer perioperative prophylactic antimicrobial agent or re-dose when indicated) followed by wrong time, wrong drug administration (e.g., syringe or ampoule swap), and poor medication labeling practice. The most common classes of medications involved in the errors were analgesics, including opioids and antibiotics, followed by anticoagulants, steroids, vasoactives, and sedatives.

Multiple factors that increase the risk for medication errors in the perioperative setting were identified [9] such as:

- Newly trained or inexperienced staff
- Production pressures
- Emergency/trauma cases
- Multiple medications administered throughout perioperative period
- High-risk medications (opioids, neuromuscular blocking agents, volatile anesthetics, cardiovascular drugs)
- Fast-paced, distracting, complex, dynamic perioperative environment

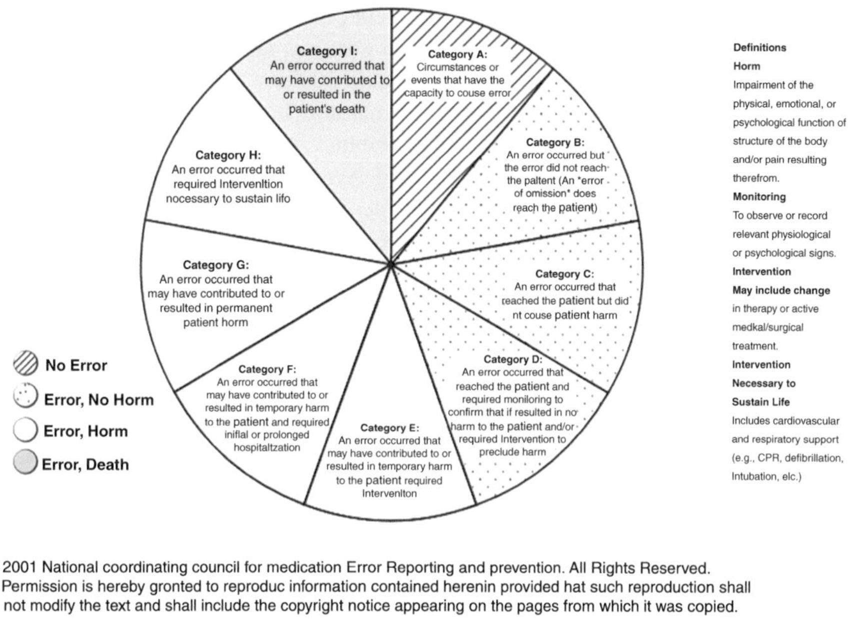

Fig. 4.1 NCC MERP Index for Categorizing Medication Errors. (Reproduced with permission of the National Coordinating Council for Medication Error Reporting and Prevention. © 2001)

- High-risk patients (geriatric, pediatric, trauma, oncology, renal- and liver-impaired patients, etc.)
- Inability of patients to respond due to sedation and anesthesia
- Anesthesia providers solely prescribing, dispensing, administering, and monitoring
- Verbal orders

Initiatives of Quality and Safety in Anesthesia and Perioperative Care

Quality and safety in the operating room (OR) continues to gain attention at almost all professional and safety organizations and impacts hospital accreditation. Agencies such as the Anesthesia Patient Safety Foundation (APSF) aim to ensure that no patient is harmed by the effects of anesthesia by encouraging and conducting safety research and education, patient safety programs, and exchange of information at the national and international level.

Consensus statements regarding medication safety strategies have been published by the Institute for Safe Medication Practice (ISMP) and Association of peri-Operative Registered Nurses (AORN). Due to the scarcity of randomized controlled trials that demonstrate the ability of a specific technique to reduce the rate of medication errors, healthcare institutions struggled to determine which strategy will produce the optimal patient safety environment [10]. The Joint Commission added the improvement of medication safety in the OR (i.e., labeling medications on the sterile field) as a National Patient Safety Goal in 2007.

A mandate for improving effectiveness of communication, including implementing a standardized approach to handoff communications, was added in 2006 and remained in the 2017 update [7]. The 2013 Accreditation Council for Graduate Medical Education (ACGME) endorsed the recommendation and specified that programs must ensure residents are proficient in the handoff process.

Prevention of Medication Errors

Medication Reconciliation

Medication reconciliation is a formal process in which healthcare providers obtain the most complete and accurate list possible of the patient's current and regularly taken medications, known as the Best Possible Medication History (BPMH) ensuring accurate and complete medication information transfer at interfaces of care (e.g., outpatients to inpatients or OR setting). This step is crucial in the perioperative setting since the management of some medications may change (e.g., anticoagulants). Kantelhardt et al. found that failure to discontinue anticoagulants resulted in case cancellation in 19% of patients receiving those drugs, highlighting the importance of medication reconciliation in the perioperative setting. [11]

Limit Verbal Orders

In the perioperative setting, reliance on verbal communication is frequent since the patient requires rapid intervention, and it helps avoid the need to break sterility when involving the surgeon. AORN recommend limiting verbal orders as much as possible and, when really needed, secure accuracy before execution using digit-by-digit read back, or writing the order on a whiteboard to be validated by the prescribing physician [12].

Checklists

The World Health Organization (WHO) "Safe Surgery Save Lives" program launched in 2007 introduced checklists to the operating room (OR) using safety concepts borrowed from aviation to improve patient safety [13]. The checklist identified a list of tasks to be completed by the surgery, anesthesia, and nursing teams before each of the three phases of an operation (the induction, incision, and exit from the OR) known as "sign in," "time out," and "sign out." WHO highlighted that the checklist may be modified and more elements might be added to fit local practices.

Another group of anesthesia professionals in Germany devised a complementary briefing template that includes a section about medications to communicate action plans and expectations [14] (e.g., type and estimated dosage of drugs and requirement for additional drugs to be available based on the existing medical conditions, such as availability of vasopressors for patients with cardiac conditions).

Clear Process in Case of Medication Shortage

Medication shortage can have a substantial impact on patient care and is responsible for creating an environment conducive to an increase in MEs. Anesthesiologists, in particular, were acutely affected by the drug shortage in the past two decades. In a recent survey on drug shortages in the United States from August through October 2017, most respondents confirmed that drug shortages during the 6 months prior to the survey were a daily struggle. Shortages were reported across all treatment categories, but more than two-thirds of respondents reported shortages that impacted anesthesia care (85%) and pain management (81%). The shortage of medications (e.g., ephedrine) may be due to the shortages of raw material [15]. The current shortage in the United States of some formulations of fentanyl, vecuronium, midazolam, etomidate, dexmedetomidine, and rocuronium has been reported to be the result of manufacturing-related issues [16]. The decrease in medication supply due to voluntary recalls is another important factor that can initiate an abrupt decrease in medication supply. Medication shortages have led to unsafe practices that have increased the risk of an error, thus impairing patient safety. Medication substitutes with higher concentration or potency than the ones routinely used can lead to overdosing. For example, fentanyl overdosing can and has resulted in respiratory arrest because the shortage of 2-mL (50 μg/mL) formulation of the drug and the purchase of the larger 5-mL ampoule size (total dose 250 μg) created confusion for the healthcare providers. Similarly, respiratory arrests requiring subsequent intensive care unit admission have occurred because sufentanil was used in substitution for fentanyl during a fentanyl shortage. Other similar errors can occur when healthcare providers use the higher concentration single-use vials for multiple patients. For example, an incident was reported recently where 50-mL vials of propofol were used for multiple endoscopy patients, resulting in the transmission of hepatitis C to some patients, and thousands of patients were exposed to human immunodeficiency virus, hepatitis B, and hepatitis C [17]. Because of the pivotal role pharmacists play in dealing with medication shortages, the American Society of Health-System Pharmacists (ASHP) has developed a guideline to help institutions deal more effectively with medication shortages (Fig. 4.2). This guideline involves three phases: identification and assessment, preparation, and contingency. During shortages, pharmacists should play a key role in a multidisciplinary approach for the preparation, standardization, communication, and monitoring of medications to ensure patients' safety.

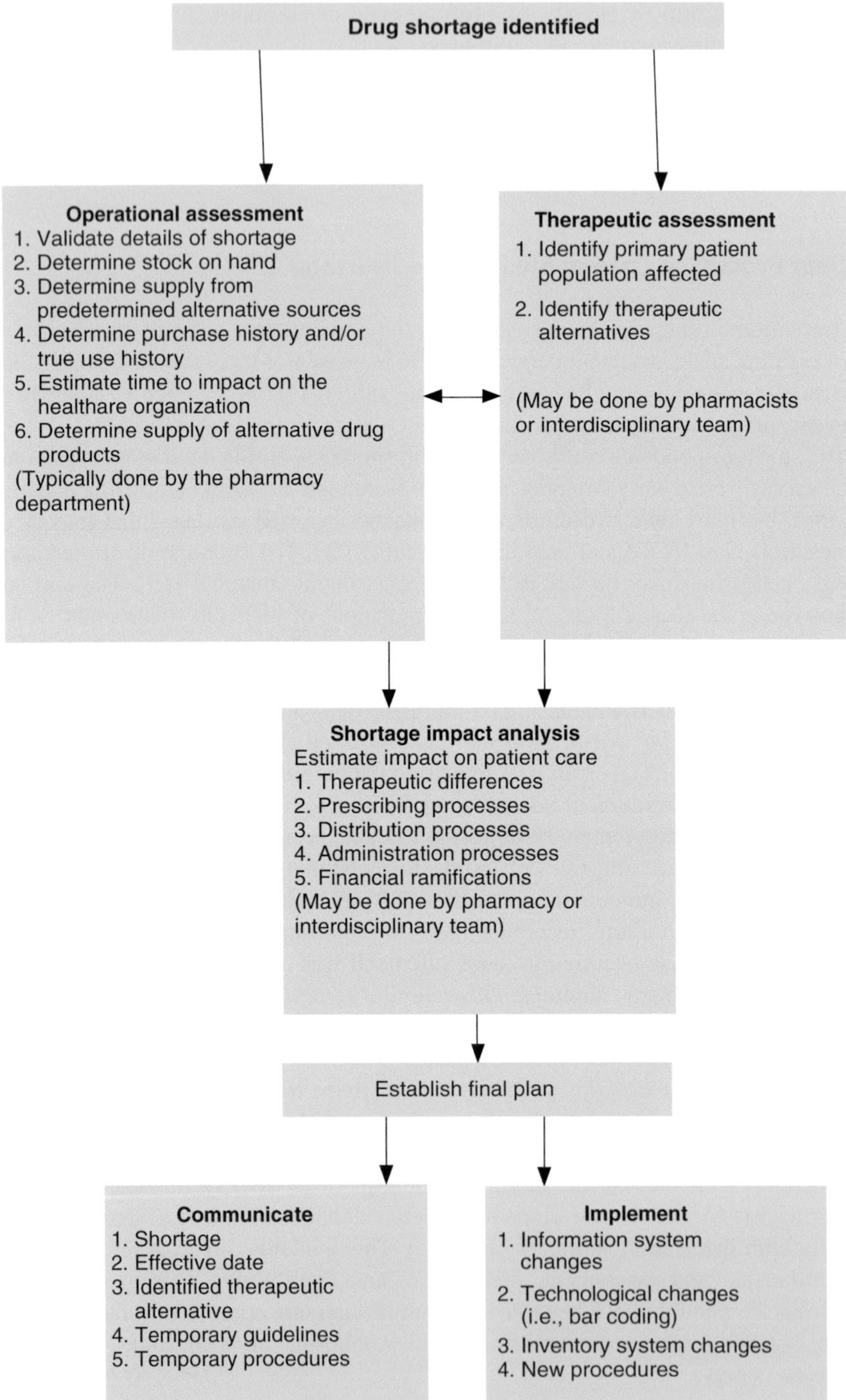

Fig. 4.2 American Society of Health-System Pharmacists (ASHP) guidelines to assist healthcare institutions in managing drug shortages. (Originally published in ASHP Expert Panel on Drug Product Shortages ©2009, American Society of Health-System Pharmacists, Inc. All rights reserved)

New Paradigm for Medication Safety: Standardization, Technology, Pharmacy/Prefilled/Premixed, and Culture (STPC)

The Anesthesia Patient Safety Foundation (APSF) convened a multidisciplinary consensus conference on January 26, 2010. The conference called for a "new paradigm" for future safety efforts to include four critical elements: standardization, technology, pharmacy/prefilled/premixed, and culture (STPC) [18]. Awards are considered for organizations that implement best practices in any element.

Standardization

Labeling

Drug names, dosage form, vials, and label color similarities have been reported as major reasons of medication errors in the hectic perioperative environment, where most of the drugs used are "high alert medications" as per the Institute for Safe Medication Practice (ISMP), such as muscle relaxants, vasopressors, and vasodilators [19].

Tall man lettering is the safety practice of partially writing a drug's name in uppercase letters to highlight the differences between similar sounding drugs and avoid MEs (e.g., predniSONE and predniSOLONE). Tall man lettering has been endorsed by The Joint Commission (recommended, not required), the US Food and Drug Administration (FDA) (as part of its Name Differentiation Project), as well as other national and international organizations, including the WHO and the International Medication Safety Network (IMSN). [20] Despite the fact that some have suggested that the strategy is ineffective [21, 22] other studies showed that the implementation of this technique may mitigate the risk of errors due to similar drug names [23].

The lack of or incomplete labeling of prepared medications can lead to administration errors. For example, Santell [24] described how an anesthesiologist was interrupted while preparing syringes of midazolam and rocuronium. He administered the rocuronium syringe to a patient in the holding area, believing it contained midazolam. He was again called away, and when he returned, the patient was unresponsive. The patient was intubated and given a reversal agent, and surgery was postponed.

The American Society of Anesthesiologists (ASA) has developed a medication color labeling standard; the colors are based upon an American Society for Testing and Materials (ASTM) standard for user-applied labels in the OR (Fig. 4.3). These are used to specify a particular drug class (e.g., labels are blue for all opiates).

The label contains the generic name of the drug, concentration, diluent name and volume, date and time of preparation, expiration date when not used within 24 h, or expiration time when expiration occurs in less than 24 h (not necessary for short procedures, as defined by the organization).

Similar tragic events of mix-ups between unlabeled solutions or medications on the sterile field such as the injection of undiluted **EPINEPH**rine injection instead of

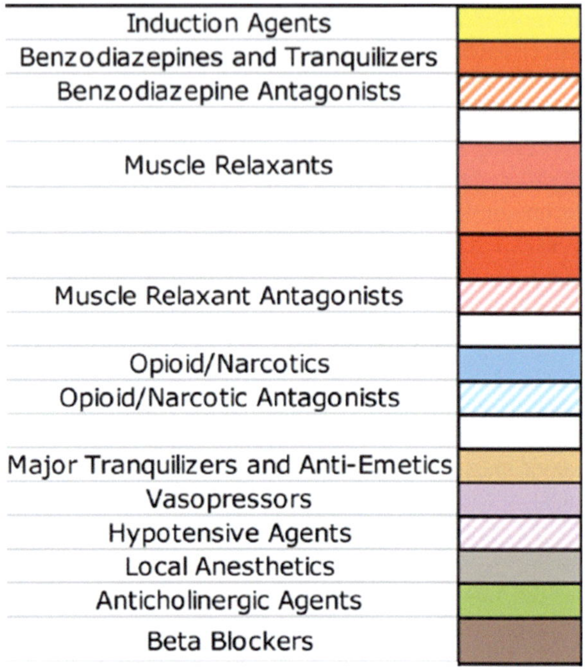

Fig. 4.3 Standard Background Colors for User-Applied Syringe Drug Labels. (American Society of Anesthesiologists Statement on creating labels of pharmaceuticals for use in anesthesiology' last amended October 2015)

lidocaine with **EPINEPH**rine 1:100,000 to a 7-year-old boy occurred [25]. The Joint Commission has since developed national patient safety goals to promote safe administration of medications with specific requirements for labeling medications as "Label all medications, medication containers (syringes, medicine cups, basins), or other solutions on and off the sterile field." [26, 27].

ISMP supports color labeling practice when anesthesia providers prepare drugs in the OR, after picking the correct drug and applying a color-coded adhesive label to the syringe. The ISMP recently raised concerns about commercially color-coded syringes packaged by pharmacies or outsourcing facilities, [17, 28] pointing out that drug mix-ups can happen and result in serious harm if commercial systems are used to the fullest extent outside anesthesia (e.g., morphine, fentaNYL, and HYDROmorphone, each with significant potency variations, all in blue syringes in the same physical area) [29].

The ISMP stressed the need to issue FDA guidance to assure safe labeling practices by 503A and 503B compounders to follow USP <7> labeling standards (the strength per total volume should be the primary and prominent expression on the principal display panel of the label, followed by the amount per mL enclosed by parentheses). This is based on reports sent to ISMP of errors or potential errors related to labeling inconsistencies and similarities (look-alikes) (Figs. 4.4 and 4.5).

To prevent wrong route errors, the "labeling standard" color codes for container, infusion lines, and each point of entry in the line (stopcock, infusion hub) shall be followed according to the route of administration (e.g., red for intra-arterial, blue for

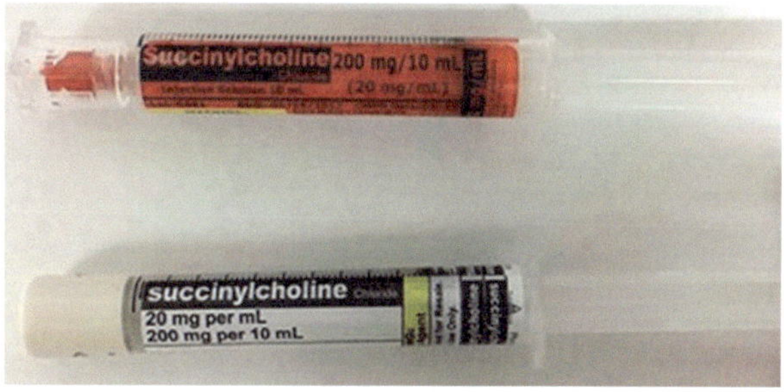

Fig. 4.4 Different display of strength (per total volume, versus per mL) for the same drug, strength, and volume manufactured by two different companies

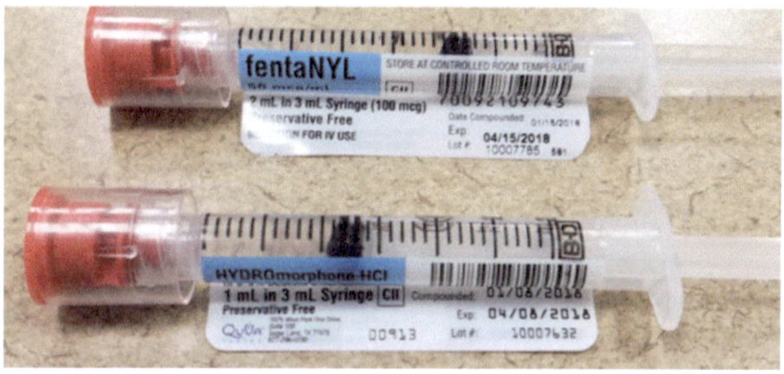

Fig. 4.5 Look-alike fentaNYL and HYDROmorphone syringes from QuVA Pharma, with ASTM international blue color on the label

intravenous, yellow for intrathecal, green for gastrointestinal) [30]. However, there are no data demonstrating error reduction with such labels [31]. To address the risk of wrong route administration, ISO 80369-6 medical device connectors NRFIT® are unique connectors with a yellow barrel devised for neuraxial and regional analgesia system, but these systems are not widely adopted. The Joint Commission published a sentinel event alert in 2014 highlighting the risks of incorrect connections and offered some strategies on how best to manage transitions to this system.

Standardizing the concentration of drugs, infusion concentrations, and dosing units for IV continuous medications throughout the institution, including perioperative areas, is crucial to avoid confusion and ensure maximum safety [32]. This will standardize the preparation of drugs between pharmacy, nursing, and the anesthesia providers and minimize calculation and preparation errors. In 2016, the FDA awarded ASHP a 3-year contract to develop and implement national standardized concentrations for intravenous (IV) and oral liquid medications. "Standardize 4 Safety" was the first inter-professional effort to standardize medication concentrations in the United States [31].

Standardized Drug Trays and Storage

Based on an extensive literature review and expert panel recommendations by Wahr et al. [32], standardization across the institution of the anesthesia cart inventory with tray divisions and clear labeling can minimize confusion and selection errors. Several factors must be taken into consideration when configuring the carts, including medication safety (e.g., look-alike drugs) mitigating controlled substance diversion.

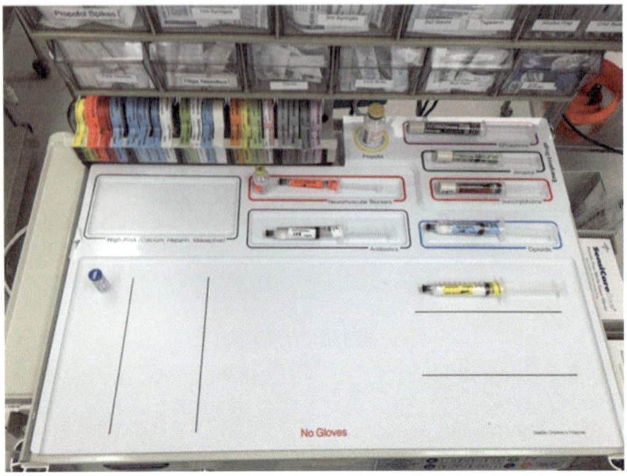

Fig. 4.6 Anesthesia Medication Template. (From Grigg E, et al. Assessing the impact of the anesthesia medication template on medication errors during anesthesia: a prospective study. Anesth Analg. 2017 May;124(5):1617–25)

Example of those strategies include storing uncommonly used drugs (e.g., insulin or protamine) in a separate color-coded bin rather than the standard workspace and removing at the end of the case [31]. A team of anesthesiologists and designers at the University of Washington created the anesthesia medication template (AMT) to organize the anesthesia workspace to reduce perioperative medication errors by anesthesia providers [33]. The layout primarily consists of a series of three-dimensional cells devoted to specific medications or medication classes (Fig. 4.6). In simulated emergencies, AMT significantly decreased the risk of MEs (odds ratio 0.21, 95% confidence interval [CI], 0.07, 0.66). The mean monthly error rate of reported swap, preparation, miscalculation, and timing errors decreased from 0.97 (95% CI, 0.64–1.48) to 0.35 (95% CI, 0.17–0.70) errors per 1000 anesthetics.

Technology Solutions

Computerized physician order entry (CPOE) systems with clinical decision support (CDS) have been shown to improve quality of care and reduce medical errors, but mistakes can still occur. For example, infusion pumps should be used to administer IV medications and fluids. These devices accept a wide range of programming parameters per rate (from 1 L per hour to one drop per hour) and volume (range from 0.1 to 9999 mL). Examples of fatal errors taken from published reports or professional meetings include a case in which morphine was entered as 90 mg/h instead of 9.0 mg/h, causing delivery of 10 times the intended dose. Incorrect entry of the drug concentration has also led to many of the tragic errors with patient-controlled analgesia (PCA) pumps. The common denominator in each of these cases was a single wrong entry or button press. The APSF now recommends the use of "smart infusion pumps" containing a drug library for drugs used within an institution with standardized concentrations, dosing units, dosage limits (maximum-minimum dose and bolus limits), and method of infusion (syringe or pumps) on a single platform. "Anesthesia mode" allows providers to access anesthesia-specific drugs with a common user interface with the anesthesia information management system, then the documentation of the infusion rate and drug dose can be automatically performed [34].

Technology-assisted drug identification and confirmation like bar coding can improve medication safety in healthcare facilities. Bar coding on purchased or compounded syringes, ampoules, or vials would prevent syringe or ampoule swap. Many US hospitals started the use of the "Safe Label System" which uses a bar code-assisted method of medication identification and labeling with audio and visual confirmation of the medication name, and printing of a label. This modality has been suggested to improve efficiency as well as compliance to 100% compared with standard methods [35].

Merry and colleagues demonstrated in a prospective randomized clinical evaluation that similar systems (bar coding, visual and auditory identification at administration, and electronic recording) reduce medication errors [36]. The rates of errors in drug administration were lower when anesthesiologists consistently applied two key principles of the new system (scanning the drug bar code before administering each drug, and keeping the voice prompt active) than when they did not.

Pharmacy

Pharmacy assistance helps reduce the medication errors in the perioperative setting, and pharmaceutical services in surgery and anesthesiology should be the standard of practice in healthcare organizations [37]. Pharmaceutical services should include drug preparation, distribution, and control in compliance with the accreditation standards, and clinical activities.

Drug Preparation

The Joint Commission suggests that the preparation of medications should be done by the pharmacy staff under aseptic technique, except in urgent care [38]. The APSF, during the Medication Safety Conference in 2010, recommended the use of labeled prefilled or premixed medications in the perioperative setting in order to discontinue the routine practice of anesthesia provider-preparing the medications [39].

The preparation/compounding of prefilled or premixed solutions with appropriate labeling eliminates miscalculation errors made by the healthcare providers in the perioperative setting. In addition, this process would decrease the waste of drugs by assigning an extended beyond-use date for drugs when prepared in an IV admixture unit meeting the USP<797> criteria [40]. There are inherent risks in sterile compounding, and quality assurance systems should be in place to avoid contamination of the final product (e.g., hand hygiene, aseptic technique, and microbial monitoring). Compounding of medications is costly, time consuming, and requires resources. In the United States, prefilled syringes are available by different manufacturers or by third-party medication distribution centers that repackage bulk drugs under the FDA section 503B of the Federal Food, Drug and Cosmetic Act exempted from the New Drug Approval (NDA) process. Pharmacists have a major role in validating the quality of the product and the labeling criteria to ensure safety.

Distribution

Services to perioperative areas as well as to procedural areas may be provided from an OR satellite pharmacy, but may also be provided from the central or other satellite pharmacy location.

The medication distribution system must be developed in a multidisciplinary approach with the end users to optimize efficiency and safety. One of two primary methods could be used for distribution of controlled substances in the OR: a per-case method or from a stock-replenishment method.

For the stock-replenishment method, drugs may be dispensed manually (i.e., direct delivery from pharmacy of compounded or unit-of-use medications) or through profiled or non-profiled automated dispensing device (ADD). Due to the critical nature of the perioperative setting, and the immediate need for the medications, profiled ADD orders are auto-verified bypassing the pharmacists' verification step.

The per-case method distribution is the use of a standardized pre-prepared medication kit by case type, dispensed either manually or through ADDs. The content of each kit is validated by another technician or pharmacist. Returning of kits and unused items and unusual drugs at the end of each operation/procedure is the best practice to ensure a "clean sweep" [41].

Recent use of the radiofrequency identification (RFID) technology has been shown to eliminate preparation errors of the kits and increases productivity by reducing time spent on restocking and verifying kits. RFID-tagged items can be scanned all at once by placing the items in an RFID-based scanning device to compare the contents of the kit with the contents specified by the database of the institution [41].

Clinical Pharmacy Services

Clinical pharmacists trained in basic perioperative skills (e.g., knowledge of drugs used, treatment of intraoperative emergencies, and bleeding) are especially suited to take leadership roles in medication-use management in the OR [42] andimprove patients' safety.

Previous research suggests that the introduction of standardized order sets, care protocols, or critical pathways has been found to reduce overall length of stay, postoperative length of stay, and total charges for multiple surgical procedures, including total knee arthroplasty [43], appendectomy [44], cholecystectomy [45], and gastrostomy [46].

Clinical pharmacists can lead the efforts to develop guidelines and incorporate them in the health information system, when available, for high-alert medications such as neuromuscular blocking agents, synthetic opioids, and propofol. They can be in charge of monitoring compliance and clinical outcomes.

Clinical pharmacists can play an important role in providing timely and accurate drug information to healthcare professionals as related to shortages, pharmacokinetics, incompatibilities, dosages and adverse effects of drugs, and to prevent purchase of look-alike medications. The clinical pharmacist can also play a key role in compliance with the Joint Commission standards, and ISMP-targeted medication safety best practices for perioperative drugs to avoid medication errors is mandatory. One example is the one related to neuromuscular blocking agents NMBAs [47]. In 2018–2019, the mandate was made to standardize storage practice throughout the organization, segregate NMBAs from other medications in the fridge, and place them in a lock-lidded pocket if the institution stored them in ADDs with auxiliary labels placed on storage containers.

Culture

Culture is the set of shared, implicit assumptions that a group holds and that determines how it perceives, thinks about, and reacts to its various environments, according to the Massachusetts Institute of Technology [48]. Healthcare literature defines a safety culture as an environment that encourages reporting, ends blame, involves senior leadership, and focuses on systems [49].

The culture of safety concept was first introduced by the aviation industry after a number of accidents attributable to human error and communication failure in the 1970s. After 30 years of true commitment to radical change of flight crews' culture, the aviation industry achieved an exemplary safety record. Healthcare, particularly hospital organizations, looked for examples from the aviation industry when deciding to formulate its own culture of safety.

Safety culture is generally measured by surveys of providers at all levels, and since 2009, the Joint Commission has required the leadership of all accredited healthcare organizations to "create and maintain a culture of safety" [50]. Available validated surveys include the Agency for Healthcare Research and Quality's (AHRQs) Patient Safety Culture survey (Table 4.1) [51]. It measures healthcare professionals' attitudes about six patient safety-related domains with yearly updated benchmarking data that allow the institution to compare themselves with other organizations, to prompt interventions to improve safety attitudes, and to measure the effectiveness of these interventions. The 2018 survey for 630 hospitals with 382,834 providers and staff respondents showed positive responses for three domains: teamwork within units (82% positive), supervisor/manager expectations and actions promoting patient safety (80% positive) and organizational learning—continuous improvement (72% positive). The areas with potential for improvement with the lowest average percent positive responses were: non-punitive response to error (47% positive), hand-offs and transitions (48% positive) and staffing (53% positive) [52].

Mature and highly reliable organizations create an environment that encourages reporting for unsafe conditions or practices, including medication administration, even for near misses, so they can be easily fixed before getting out of control. These organizations then accept responsibility for dealing with ethical or practice violations (zero tolerance for reckless behavior such as refusing to perform a "time-out" prior to surgery even if the patient was not harmed). This environment is called a "just culture."

Table 4.1 Patient safety culture survey composites and definitions

Patient safety culture composite	Definition: *The extent to which …*
1. Communication openness	Staff freely speak up if they see something that may negatively affect a patient and feel free to question those with more authority
2. Feedback and communication about error	Staff are informed about errors that happen, are given feedback about changes implemented, and discuss ways to prevent errors
3. Frequency of events reported	Mistakes of the following types are reported: (1) mistakes caught and corrected before affecting the patient, (2) mistakes with no potential to harm the patient, and (3) mistakes that could harm the patient but do not
4. Handoffs and transitions	Important patient care information is transferred across hospital units and during shift changes
5. Management support for patient safety	Hospital management provides a work climate that promotes patient safety and shows that patient safety is a top priority
6. Nonpunitive response to error	Staff feel that their mistakes and event reports are not held against them and that mistakes are not kept in their personnel file
7. Organizational learning—Continuous improvement	Mistakes have led to positive changes and changes are evaluated for effectiveness
8. Overall perceptions of patient safety	Procedures and systems are good at preventing errors and there is a lack of patient safety problems
9. Staffing	There are enough staff to handle the workload and work hours are appropriate to provide the best care for patients
10. Supervisor/manager expectations and actions promoting patient safety	Supervisors/managers consider staff suggestions for improving patient safety, praise staff for following patient safety procedures, and do not overlook patient safety problems
11. Teamwork across units	Hospital units cooperate and coordinate with one another to provide the best care for patients
12. Teamwork within units	Staff support each other, treat each other with respect, and work together as a team

The survey also includes two questions that ask respondents to provide an overall grade on patient safety for their work area/unit and to indicate the number of events they reported over the past 12 months. In addition, respondents are asked to provide limited background demographic information

High-Reliability Organization

Safety culture or "just culture" is one of the key domains critical to enhancing reliability. The other key domains are leadership engagement, and the use of effective process improvement tools.

High-reliability organizations (e.g., aviation) are organizations that operate in complex, high-hazard domains for extended periods without serious accidents or catastrophic failures. AHRQ and the Joint Commission advocated for achieving high reliability in healthcare [53]. The principles of high reliability go beyond standardization; it is a condition of persistent mindfulness by prioritizing safety over other performance pressures. Table 4.2 summarizes the characteristics that support this mindset. [54]

Table 4.2 Characteristics of high reliability organizations

Characteristic	Description
Preoccupation with failure	Everyone is aware of and thinking about the potential for failure. People understand that new threats emerge regularly from situations that no one imagined could occur, so all personnel actively think about what could go wrong and are alert to small signs of potential problems. The absence of errors or accidents leads not to complacency, but to a heightened sense of vigilance for the next possible failure. Near misses are viewed as opportunities to learn about systems issues and potential improvements, rather than as evidence of safety
Reluctance to simplify	People resist simplifying their understanding of work processes and how and why things succeed or fail in their environment. People in HROs understand that the work is complex and dynamic. They seek underlying rather than surface explanations. While HROs recognize the value of standardization of workflows to reduce variation, they also appreciate the complexity inherent in the number of teams, processes, and relationships involved in conducting daily operations
Sensitivity to operations	Based on their understanding of operational complexity, people in HROs strive to maintain a high awareness of operational conditions. This sensitivity is often referred to as "big picture understanding" or "situation awareness." It means that people cultivate an understanding of the context of the current state of their work in relation to the unit or organizational state—i.e., what is going on around them—and how the current state might support or threaten safety
Deference to expertise	People in HROs appreciate that the people closest to the work are the most knowledgeable about the work. Thus, people in HROs know that in a crisis or emergency the person with greatest knowledge of the situation might not be the person with the highest status and seniority. Deference to local and situation expertise results in a spirit of inquiry and de-emphasis on hierarchy in favor of learning as much as possible about potential safety threats. In an HRO, everyone is expected to share concerns with others, and the organizational climate is such that all staff members are comfortable speaking up about potential safety problems
Commitment to resilience	Commitment to resilience is rooted in the fundamental understanding of the frequently unpredictable nature of system failures. People in HROs assume the system is at risk for failure, and they practice performing rapid assessments of and responses to challenging situations. Teams cultivate situation assessment and cross-monitoring so they may identify potential safety threats quickly and respond either before safety problems cause harm, or by mitigating the seriousness of the safety event

HROs High reliability organizations
Sources: Weick et al. (2007) [54]; Chassin et al. (2013) [55]

Organizational Leadership and Commitment to Medication Safety

Patient safety should be clearly stated as an organizational goal, and resources must be devoted to maintain a viable safety program and create clear metrics and goals. The Crew Resource Management (CRM) program was developed by the aviation industry and extrapolated to healthcare practice to improve patient safety, including medication safety [56]. It includes: (a) building the team in charge, (b) improving teamwork skills, (c) stress and conflict management training, (d) enforced code of mutual respect and prohibit intimidating behaviors, (e) encouraging interdisciplinary awareness and education, (f) providing simulations, trainings, and recurrent trainings about clinical scenarios; and (g) using essential checklists in complementary role to teamwork.

Effective Process Improvement

The third key domain for reliability is the effective process improvement for medication safety plan. Failure modes and effects analysis, or a gap analysis, is the key step to identify causes of failures of safety processes and put in place an action plan using robust process improvement (RPI) tools. The Institute of Healthcare Improvement has a failure mode and effect analysis (FMEA) interactive tool, [57] and the AORN released an adult medication safety assessment [58]. RPI is defined as the blend of Lean Six Sigma plus formal change management and commitment to clear goals or outcomes supported by clear action.

Lean Six Sigma is a set of tools that identifies and removes wasted effort from a process and focuses on reducing the defects in a process (define, measure, analyze, improve, and control). The Joint Commission applied the RPI tools with teams from hospitals, and the rates of improvement demonstrated were consistent with other industries that applied the same tools [55, 59] (e.g., 81% of hand hygiene compliance after implementation versus 47.5%).

Summary

An interdisciplinary team—with significant representation from anesthesia, nursing, surgery, and pharmacy—should lead efforts to provide staff education and maintain and improve medication safety in the perioperative environment.

This chapter highlighted the recommendations of professional and safety organizations APSF, ASHP, AORN, and Joint Commission. These recommendations are based on standardization, technology, pharmacy services, and establishment of just culture around medication safety reporting and sharing the lessons learned.

Organizations can use the information in this chapter to assess safety gaps in their current perioperative workflows and processes. RPI tools are useful to define relevant improvement initiatives, to track the progress based on specific metrics to design systems, and to prevent errors from occurring.

References

1. National Coordinating Council for Medication Error Reporting Program. Council defines terms and sets goals for medication error reporting and preventing. Rockville: US Pharmacopoeia; 1995.

2. ASHP guidelines on adverse drug reaction monitoring and reporting. Am J Health Syst Pharm. 1995;52(4):417–419.
3. Merry AF, Anderson BJ. Medication errors—new approaches to prevention. Paediatr Anaesth. 2011;21(7):743–53.
4. Institute of Medicine. In: Kohn LT, Corrigan JM, Donaldson M, editors. To err is human: building a safer health system. Washington: National Academies Press; 1999.
5. Orser BA, Chen RJ, Yee DA. Medication errors in anesthetic practice: a survey of 687 practitioners. Can J Anaesth. 2001;48(2):139–46.
6. Nanji KC, Patel A, Shaikh S, Seger DL, Bates DW. Evaluation of perioperative medication errors and adverse drug events. Anesthesiology. 2016;124(1):25–34.
7. Cierniak KH, Gaunt MJ, Grissinger M. PA-PSRS. Perioperative medication errors: uncovering risk from behind the drapes. Patient Saf Advis. 2018;15(4)
8. National Coordinating Council for Medication Error Reporting and Prevention. NCC MERP index for categorizing medication errors. 2001.
9. Meyer TA, McAllister RK. Strategies for optimizing OR drug safety. Pharm Prac News. 2018;1–8.
10. Paparella S. Choosing the right strategy for medication error reduction—part II. J Emerg Nurs. 2008;34(3):238–40.
11. Kantelhardt P, Giese A, Kantelhardt SR. Medication reconciliation for patients undergoing spinal surgery. Eur Spine J. 2016;25:740.
12. Hicks RW, Wanzer LJ, Denholm B. Implementing AORN recommended practices for medication safety. AORN J. 2012;96(6):605–22.
13. Haynes AB, Weiser TG, Berry WR, Lipsitz SR, Breizat AH, Delinger EP, et al.; Safe Surgery Saves Lives Study Group. A surgical safety checklist to reduce morbidity and mortality in a global population. N Engl J Med. 2009;360:491–499.
14. Neuhaus C, Hofer S, Hofmann G, Wacher C, Weigand M, Lichtenstern C. Perioperative safety: learning, not taking from aviation. Anesth Analg. 2016;122:2059–63.
15. American Society of Health-System Pharmacists. Drug shortages list. 2010. http://www.ashp.org/shortages
16. American Society of Health-System Pharmacists. Drug shortages list. 2019. http://www.ashp.org/shortages
17. Hepatitis C virus infections from unsafe injection practices at an endoscopy clinic in Las Vegas, Nevada, 2007-2008. Clin Infect Dis. 2010;51(3):267–273.
18. Eichhorn JH. APSF hosts medication safety conference: consensus group defines challenges and opportunities for improved practice. APSF Newsletter. 2010;25:1.
19. Institute for Safe Medication Practices. Medication safety self assessment® for high-alert medications. https://www.ismp.org/assessments/high-alert-medications. Accessed June 2019.
20. International Medication Safety Network. Position statement on improving the safety of international non-proprietary names of medicines (INNs). 2011. https://www.intmedsafe.net/wp-content/uploads/2014/05/IMSN_position_on_INNs_2011_10_24.pdf
21. Schell KL. Using enhanced text to facilitate recognition of drug names: evidence from two experimental studies. Appl Ergon. 2009;40(1):82–90.
22. Irwin A, Mearns K, Watson M, Urquhart J. The effect of proximity, tall man lettering, and time pressure on accurate visual perception of drug names. Hum Factors. 2013;55(2):253–66.
23. Institute for Safe Medication Practices. Tall man lettering. https://www.ismp.org/recommendations/tall-man-letters-list
24. Santell JP. Medication errors involving neuromuscular blocking agents. Jt Comm J Qual Patient Saf. 2006;32(8):470–5, 417.
25. Grissinger M. Strengthen your resolve: no unlabeled containers anywhere, ever! P T. 2017;42(7):416–29.
26. Suyderhoud JP. Joint Commisssion on Accreditation of Healthcare Organizations requirements and syringe labeling systems. Anesth Analg. 2007;104:242.
27. The Joint Commission. National patient safety goals hospital accreditation. 2019. https://www.jointcommission.org/standards/national-patient-safety-goals/

28. Institute for Safe Medical Practices. FDA guidance needed to assure safe labeling practices by 503A and 503B compounders. 2018. https://www.ismp.org/resources/fda-guidance-needed-assure-safe-labeling-practices-503a-and-503b-compounders
29. Institute for Safe Medical Practices. Color-coded syringes for anesthesia drugs: use with care. 2008. https://www.ismp.org/resources/color-coded-syringes-anesthesia-drugs-use-care
30. Australian Commission on Safety and Quality in Health Care. National standard for user-applied labelling of injectable medicines, fluids and lines. https://www.safetyandquality.gov.au
31. American Society of Health-System Pharmacists. Standardize 4 safety. https://www.ashp.org/pharmacy-practice/standardize-4-safety-initiative?loginreturnUrl=SSOCheckOnly
32. Wahr JA, Abernathy JH 3rd, Lazarra EH, Keebler JR, Wall MH, Lynch I, et al. Medication safety in the operating room: literature and expert-based recommendations. Br J Aneaesth. 2017;118(1):32–43.
33. Grigg EB, Martin LD, Ross FJ, Roesler A, Rampersad SE, Haberkern C, et al. Assessing the impact of the anesthesia medication template on medication errors during anesthesia: a prospective study. Anaesth Analg. 2017;124:1617–25.
34. Merry AF, Anderson BJ. Medication errors—new approaches to prevention. Paediatr Anesth. 2011;21(7):743–53.
35. Caputo Nanji K, Vernest KA, Driscoll WD, et al. Smart labels: improving syringe labeling efficiency and accuracy in the operating room. Presented at the ASA conference, New Orleans (LA); October 17–21, 2009.
36. Merry AF, Webster CS, Hannam J, Mitchell SJ, Henderson R, Reid P, et al. Multimodal system designed to reduce errors in recording and administration of drugs in anaesthesia: prospective randomized clinical evaluation. BMJ. 2011;343:d5543.
37. ASHP guidelines on surgery and anesthesiology pharmaceutical services. Am J Health Syst Pharm. 1999;56(9):887–895.
38. Mansur J. The Joint Commission medication management update for 2018. http://www.njha.com/media/476876/EDU-1736-PPT-Mansur-Joint-Commission-Update-2018.pdf
39. Eichhorn JH. APSF hosts medication safety conference. Anesth Patient Saf Found Newsletter. 2010. https://www.apsf.org/newsletter/spring-2010/
40. USP. General chapter <797> pharmaceutical compounding—sterile preparations. https://www.usp.org/compounding/general-chapter-797
41. Summerfield MR, Xiao Y. Evaluation of medication kit processing time using radio frequency identification (RFID) technology. Innov Pharm. 2015;6(2):199.
42. Keicher PA, McAllister JC. Comprehensive pharmaceutical services in the surgical suite and recovery room. Am J Health Syst Pharm. 1985;42:2454–62.
43. Scranton PE Jr. The cost effectiveness of streamlined care pathways and product standardization in total knee arthroplasty. J Arthroplasty. 1999;14:182–6.
44. Takegami K, Kawaguchi Y, Nakayama H, Kubota Y, Nagawa H. Impact of a clinical pathway and standardization of treatment for acute appendicitis. Surg Today. 2003;33:336–41.
45. Greenwald JA, McMullen HF, Coppa GF, Newman RM. Standardization of surgeon-controlled variables: impact on outcome in patients with acute cholecystitis. Ann Surg. 2000;231:339–44.
46. Kiyama T, Tajiri T, Yoshiyuki T, Mitsuhashi K, Ise Y, Mizutani T, et al. [Clinical significance of a standardized clinical pathway in gastrectomy patients.] J Nippon Med Sch. 2003;70:263–9. [Japanese].
47. Institute for Safe Medication Practices. 2018–2019 targeted medication safety best practices for hospitals. https://www.ismp.org/sites/default/files/attachments/2019-01/TMSBP-for-Hospitalsv2.pdf
48. Schein EH. Organizational culture and leadership. 2nd ed. San Francisco: Jossey-Bass; 1992.
49. Larson L. Ending the culture of blame. A look at why medical errors happen—and what needs to change. Trustee. 2000;53(2):6–10, 1.
50. The Joint Commission. Sentinel event alert 57: the essential role of leadership in developing a safety culture. https://www.jointcommission.org/resources/patient-safety-topics/sentinel-

event/sentinel-event-alert-newsletters/sentinel-event-alert-57-the-essential-role-of-leadership-in-developing-a-safety-culture/. Accessed 20 July 2019.
51. Agency for Healthcare Research and Quality. Surveys on patient safety culture™ (SOPS)®. https://www.ahrq.gov/sops/index.html
52. Agency for Healthcare Research and Quality. Hospital survey on patient safety culture. 2018. https://www.ahrq.gov/sites/default/files/wysiwyg/sops/quality-patient-safety/patientsafetyculture/2018hospitalsopsreport.pdf
53. The toolkit for using the AHRQ quality indicators: how to improve hospital quality and safety. Rockville: Agency for Healthcare Research and Quality; 2016. https://www.ahrq.gov/patient-safety/settings/hospital/resource/qitool/index.html
54. Weick KE, Sutcliffe KM. Managing the unexpected. 2nd ed. San Francisco: Jossey-Bass; 2007.
55. Chassin MR, Loeb MJ. Joint Commission. High-reliability health care: getting there from here. 2013. https://psnet.ahrq.gov/issue/high-reliability-health-care-getting-there-here.
56. Gordon S, Mendenhall P, O'Toole BB. Beyond the checklist: what else health care can learn from aviation and safety. Ithaca: Cornell University Press; 2013.
57. Institute for Healthcare Improvement. Failure modes and effects analysis (FMEA) tool. http://www.ihi.org/resources/Pages/Tools/FailureModesandEffectsAnalysisTool.aspx. Accessed 16 July 2019.
58. Association of Perioperative Registered Nurses. AORN's safe medication administration tool kit, medication safety assessment, perioperative medications safety practices video. www.aorn.org. Accessed 16 July 2019.
59. Joint Commission Center for Transforming Healthcare. 2013. Robust Process Improvement. http://www.centerfortransforminghealthcare.org/about/rpi.aspx

Managing the Patient on Antiplatelet, Anticoagulation, Beta Blockers, Angiotensin-Converting Enzyme Inhibitors, Angiotensin-Receptors Blockers: The Anesthesia Perspective

5

Cynthia Karam, Wissam Maroun, and Marie T. Aouad

Introduction

Patients on anticoagulants and/or antiplatelet medications scheduled for elective or urgent surgical procedures may pose major clinical dilemmas throughout the perioperative period. Deep vein thrombosis prophylaxis, as well as primary or secondary prevention of cardiac or cerebral events with anticoagulants or antiplatelet therapy are very common scenarios in patients presenting for surgery. Withholding such medications is not without risk, which itself varies depending on the primary condition for which the medications are prescribed. On the other hand, maintaining such therapies may exacerbate the risk of perioperative bleeding. Patients receiving hemostasis-altering drugs are often considered high-risk patients. This may add an additional layer of complexity since neuraxial anesthesia may be favored over general anesthesia in this particular group of patients. However, hemostasis-altering drugs put the patients at a higher risk for spinal hematoma, a devastating complication that can cause irreversible neurological damage. The combination of surgical as well as patient-related perioperative risk factors may result in a wide spectrum of complicated clinical scenarios. A number of guidelines were issued to serve as a frame of practice during the perioperative period. However, level A evidence is lacking in this field with, at best, level B evidence in the form of observational and epidemiologic series. When data are sparse, level C evidence is derived from expert opinion and newer anticoagulant pharmacological models or kinetics. Most of the time, recommendations favor patients' safety and are rather conservative. As such, these guidelines do not define standard of care. Sound clinical judgment tailored to

C. Karam · W. Maroun
American University of Beirut Medical Center, Beirut, Lebanon

M. T. Aouad (✉)
Department of Anesthesiology, American University of Beirut Medical Center, Beirut, Lebanon
e-mail: mm01@aub.edu.lb

J. J. Hoballah et al. (eds.), *Principles of Perioperative Safety and Efficiency*,
https://doi.org/10.1007/978-3-031-41089-5_5

specific clinical scenarios should be exerted and may sometimes result in deviation from recommendations.

The management of medications in the perioperative period does not only concern drugs involved in coagulation hemostasis. Preexisting hypertension imposes the challenge of managing antihypertensive medications perioperatively. These patients are more likely to experience intraoperative blood pressure lability, which may lead to myocardial injury [1]. Adequate blood pressure control must be maintained in the perioperative setting, as its instability is associated with increased mortality, especially in the elderly population [2]. The goal is to maintain mean arterial pressure within acceptable ranges. To help achieve this measurable goal, management of antihypertensive medications, mainly angiotensin-converting enzyme (ACE) inhibitors and beta blockers, is a crucial part of the perioperative assessment.

In the first half of this review, we will present an overview of the following themes: patients on anticoagulants/antiplatelet medications scheduled for surgery under regional/neuraxial anesthesia, patients with recent cardiac stents undergoing non-cardiac surgery, and patients on chronic anticoagulation presenting for surgery. The second half will cover the management of antihypertensive medications in the perioperative period.

Regional Anesthesia in Patients Receiving Anticoagulants and Antiplatelet Medications

Incidence and Consequences of Spinal Hematomas

Hemorrhage within the spinal neuraxis is a devastating complication of spinal or epidural anesthesia or analgesia. Although it is difficult to have an accurate estimation of the magnitude of the problem, the calculated incidence derived from observational series [3] is approximated to be less than 1 in 150,000 epidural and less than 1 in 220,000 spinal anesthesia cases. The risk associated with epidural analgesia for labor (1 in 200,000) is significantly less than in elderly women receiving epidural anesthesia for knee arthroplasty (1 in 3600) [4]. Also, the risk of spinal hematoma in elderly women receiving spinal anesthesia for hip fracture is higher compared with the risk of hematoma associated with spinal anesthesia in the general population (1 in 480,000) [4]. In the presence of additional risk factors, such as anticoagulation, the incidence of this complication is expected to become higher. Spinal hematoma remains a rare occurrence. Nevertheless, its consequences are devastating unless prompt diagnosis and intervention are initiated. Risk factors for spinal hematomas include the presence of coagulation abnormalities or hemostasis-altering drugs, in addition to the presence of spinal pathologies and needle or catheter placement difficulties [4–6]. Furthermore, the risk seems to be higher with an epidural anesthetic, especially when a catheter is used as compared to a single-shot spinal anesthetic. In the presence of risk factors, bleeding in the epidural space may occur during catheter placement, but also during catheter removal. Therefore, clear time intervals between stopping hemostasis-altering drugs and epidural instrumentation are defined for both insertion and removal of the epidural catheter. A motor deficit is the most common initial manifestation of spinal hematomas, rather than back pain [5, 6]. In the setup of postoperative epidural analgesia, the confounding sensory and motor effect of local anesthetics can be confusing and may lead to a delay in the diagnosis of the neurologic deficit. Therefore, it is recommended to use dilute local anesthetic mixtures that would yield motor sparing, in addition to careful and frequent neurologic examinations. An early diagnosis and intervention are key for neurologic recovery. The shorter the interval between the onset of symptoms and surgical decompression, the better the neurologic outcome. For instance, a cutoff interval of 8 h resulted in the largest proportion of good neurologic outcome in the series of spinal hematomas reported by Vandemeulen et al. [5]

Vascular puncture during a peripheral nerve block is not a rare event; the incidence could be as high as 5.7% and 6.6% for femoral and sciatic catheters, respectively [7]. The use of ultrasound guidance has certainly led to a decrease in the rate of vascular puncture [8]. Yet, even with the risk of vascular puncture, significant bleeding and serious complications are rare. For instance, among 405 patients who received an axillary peripheral nerve block, only one patient developed hematoma, and that patient was on heparin [9]. Patients on anticoagulation may be at higher risk for hematoma development; however, there are no randomized controlled trials that specifically address this topic. Few case reports reported the occurrence of hematomas after catheter removal on patients treated with enoxaparin postoperatively [10, 11]. Nevertheless, major bleeding complications do not seem to be common during peripheral nerve blocks. Despite this reassuring fact, the relatively scarce data leads to the application of a conservative approach when a peripheral nerve block is contemplated in a patient receiving anticoagulation/antiplatelet therapy.

Effect of Regional Anesthesia on Postoperative Outcomes

With the ever growing proportion of elderly and high-risk patient populations, the number of patients receiving hemostasis-altering drugs presenting for surgery is on the rise. Respecting recommendations and guidelines regarding the acceptable time intervals between withholding these drugs and the performance of neuraxial anesthesia may result in delays of the surgical procedure, a time constraint that can by itself pose an additional risk factor for perioperative morbidity and mortality. For instance, confining an elderly patient with a hip fracture in bed waiting for the effect of anticoagulants or antiplatelet therapy to fade away in order to perform the hip surgery under spinal anesthesia may predispose the patient to a different set of morbidities and complications [12]. A clear understanding of the potential benefits of neuraxial or regional anesthesia (RA) over general anesthesia (GA) in terms of improved perioperative outcomes is required to be able to establish the most appropriate and evidence-based anesthesia plan. The choice of the anesthetic technique and its impact on postoperative outcomes remain a source of debate. RA results in improved analgesia as compared to GA with systemic opioids; however, its association with additional outcome benefits is less clear [13–15]. Beyond reducing acute postoperative pain, evidence suggests that epidural analgesia reduces post-thoracotomy chronic pain [16]. Surgeries conducted under peripheral nerve blocks result in less postoperative nausea and vomiting [17]. A clear reduction in pulmonary complications and, subsequently, intensive care unit admissions, are demonstrated with the use of epidural analgesia for abdominal, thoracic, and lower limb surgeries in patients with preexisting lung disease [15, 17]. The duration of postoperative ileus is also reduced with epidural analgesia [18]. Conversely, the impact of RA is less clear on the reduction of cardiac morbidity, postoperative cognitive dysfunction, reduction in cancer recurrence, and mortality [18]. When contemplating a neuraxial anesthesia technique in the presence of hemostasis-altering drugs, a clear benefit-to-risk ratio has to be determined.

Management of Hemostasis-Altering Drugs in Patients Receiving Neuraxial or Peripheral Nerve Blocks

As previously mentioned, no solid evidence that dictates the management of hemostasis-altering drugs in patients receiving neuraxial or peripheral blocks is available. Hence, pharmacological and physiological properties are used as guiding principles where evidence is lacking [19]. In the presence of therapeutic anticoagulation, it is assumed that five half-lives are needed to allow the resolution of 97% of anticoagulation effect (assuming normal kidney function and metabolism). Accordingly, subsequent neuraxial or peripheral block can be safely performed five half-life post-discontinuation of the drug [19]. The same concept applies for prophylactic anticoagulation, yet with a different time interval of two half-lives instead of five being required [19]. For patients on anticoagulation who need peripheral/neuraxial catheter removal, one has to take into account not only the pharmacokinetics of the given drug, but also the time needed to form a stable platelet plug that is somehow resistant to lysis by anticoagulation. It is estimated that approximately 8 h are needed for a platelet plug to become stable [20]; the safe time that would reduce the risk for bleeding post-catheter removal is calculated by subtracting the time to peak effect of the given drug from 8 h [21]. For example, given that the peak effect of low molecular weight heparin (LMWH) is 4 h, the time to subsequent dosing following catheter removal would be 4 h (8 h – 4 h). Of note, recommendations are usually given with time intervals rather than exact durations in order to account for normal variations in pharmacological activity. Patients with altered metabolism, such as a renal failure patient receiving a kidney-excreted medication may need longer time intervals than healthy individuals. Other factors, including patient characteristics (history of bleeding/bruising, medical comorbidities increasing the risk of bleeding) and the type of procedure (deep versus superficial block, continuous versus single injection technique) should also be considered. A summary of the major recommendations for specific medications based on the current evidence, and the major guiding principles, is presented in Table 5.1 [19]. Recommendations for neuraxial blocks and deep peripheral blocks are interchangeable [19]. Superficial peripheral blocks management is based on site compressibility, vascularity, and consequences of bleeding should it occur [19].

Table 5.1 Summary of the recommendations for the management of patients on anticoagulant/antiplatelet therapy, undergoing regional anesthesia [19]

Medication	Hold before neuraxial/deep peripheral block	Restart after neuraxial/deep peripheral block	Hold before neuraxial/peripheral catheter removal	Restart after neuraxial/peripheral catheter removal
Apixaban	72 h	At least 6 h	26–30 h	6 h
Aspirin	No restrictions	No restrictions	No restrictions	No restrictions
Bivalirudin	Avoid	Avoid	Avoid	Avoid
Cilostazol	2 days	6 h, avoid with indwelling catheter	Avoid	6 h
Clopidogrel	5–7 days	Immediately if no loading dose, 6 h if loading dose	Keep catheters for 1–2 days after restarting if no loading dose	Immediately if no loading dose, 6 h if loading dose
Dabigatran	5 days	6 h, avoid with indwelling catheters	34–36 h, or dTT/ECT testing	6 h
Enoxaparin BID, prophylaxis	12 h	12 h	Avoid	4 h
Enoxaparin QD, prophylaxis	12 h	12 h	12 h	4 h
Enoxaparin, therapeutic	24 h	24–72 h	Avoid	4 h
Fondaparinux	No recommendation	Avoid	Avoid	6 h
Heparin IV	4–6 h and normal coagulations status	1 h	4–6 h and normal coagulation status	1 h
Heparin SC, prophylaxis, high-dose BID and TID	12 h and assessment of coagulation status	Unknown risk; risk/benefit assessment required	Unknown risk; risk/benefit assessment required	Immediately
Heparin SC, prophylaxis, low-dose BID and TID	4–6 h or assessment of coagulation status	Immediately	4–6 h	Immediately
Heparin SC, therapeutic	24 h and assessment of coagulation status	Not recommended during indwelling catheter	Not recommended	Immediately
NSAIDs	No restrictions	No restrictions	No restrictions	No restrictions
Prasugrel	7–10 days	Immediately if no loading dose	Avoid	Immediately if no loading dose

(continued)

Table 5.1 (continued)

Medication	Hold before neuraxial/deep peripheral block	Restart after neuraxial/deep peripheral block	Hold before neuraxial/ peripheral catheter removal	Restart after neuraxial/ peripheral catheter removal
Ticagrelor	5–7 days	Immediately if no loading dose	Avoid	Immediately if no loading dose
Ticlopidine	10 days	Immediately if no loading dose	6 h, if loading dose is given	Immediately if no loading dose
tPA	Avoid	Avoid	No recommendation	No recommendation
Urokinase	Avoid	Avoid	No recommendation	No recommendation
Warfarin	5 days and normal INR	No delay	INR < 1.5, 12–24 h INR > 3, hold or reduce dose with indwelling catheters 1.5 < INR < 3, maintain catheter with caution	No delay

dTT/ECT dilute thrombin time/ecarin clotting time, *INR* international normalized ratio

Non-cardiac Surgery in Patients on Dual Antiplatelets or on Anticoagulation

Percutaneous coronary intervention (PCI) necessitates treatment with dual antiplatelet therapy (aspirin and $P2Y_{12}$ receptor inhibitors) for a variable duration after the procedure, depending on the type of PCI.

Certain conditions such as atrial fibrillation, history of deep vein thrombosis, and pulmonary embolism, or the presence of mechanical heart valves, require long-term anticoagulation to prevent the risk of thrombosis and embolism that may result in cerebrovascular accidents, heart failure, and death. Traditionally, warfarin is used for chronic anticoagulation, yet more recently, newer direct thrombin inhibitors or factor X inhibitors are becoming more popular.

In the case of either dual antiplatelet therapy or chronic anticoagulation, the risk of excessive surgical bleeding if the medications are continued versus the drastic consequences of withholding the medications has to be balanced.

Patients with Recent Cardiac Stents on Antiplatelet Therapy

Non-cardiac surgery following recent PCI with stenting is a risk factor for major cardiac events, including myocardial infarction and stent thrombosis [22]. Dual antiplatelet medications are usually prescribed after PCI to decrease the above risks. Hence, withholding dual antiplatelet therapy prematurely contributes to the risk of increased stent thrombosis, myocardial infarction, and death, especially during the prothrombin state associated with the perioperative period [23, 24]. Consequently, maintaining dual antiplatelet therapy may contribute to excessive surgical bleeding, which is more relevant in surgeries with high risk of bleeding like prostate and neurosurgical interventions. The risk for excessive surgical bleeding becomes less relevant if the surgery is minor, such as cataract extraction.

There are multiple types of stents used during PCI. The latter usually dictates the duration of dual antiplatelet therapy. While the detailed characteristics of the stent types goes beyond the scope of this discussion, it is important to note one major difference; as we progress from bare metal stents to newer drug-eluting stents, the risk of restenosis and late thrombosis decreases [25]. The decision to withhold or maintain dual antiplatelet therapy in the perioperative period depends not only on the type of cardiac stent, but also on the time elapsed between the PCI and the date of surgery, as well as the risk of bleeding associated with the specific surgery. In this regard, the American College of Cardiology /American Heart Association (ACC/AHA) task force provided guidelines in 2014. It is recommended that elective surgery be postponed 30 days and 360 days after PCI for bare metal stents and drug-eluting stents, respectively (Class 1 level B evidence) [23]. Of note, the period of 360 days or 30 days represents the optimal time associated with the lowest incidence of major cardiac events [26]. This also corresponds to the time after which dual antiplatelet therapy would have been stopped and the patient would be solely maintained on aspirin. Hence, both the risk of bleeding and major cardiac events is decreased. If stent implantation is less than 4–6 weeks before a necessary or a life-saving surgery, it is recommended to proceed with the surgery without stopping dual antiplatelet therapy, unless the risk of bleeding during the surgery outweighs the risk of stent thrombosis (Class 1 level C evidence) [23]. If stent placement is more than 30 days but less than 360 days for drug-eluting stents, it is recommended to proceed with the surgery after 180 days if and only if the risk of delaying the surgery is greater than the risk of stent thrombosis (Class 2B) [23]. If the risk of thrombosis is higher than the risk of delaying the surgery, it is recommended to postpone the surgery to the optimal time of 360 days (Class 1) [23]. If a patient with coronary stents needs to undergo a surgery that requires discontinuation of the $P2Y_{12}$ platelet receptor inhibitors, it is recommended that aspirin be continued if the type of surgery allows for that, and that the $P2Y_{12}$ platelet receptor inhibitors be resumed as soon as possible (Class 1 level of evidence C) [23]. In a patient without coronary stents, it may be reasonable to discontinue aspirin therapy before surgery (Class 3 level B evidence) [23]. However, if the risk of ischemic events outweighs the risk of bleeding, it may be reasonable to continue aspirin (Class 3 level of evidence C) [23].

With regard to clopidogrel/prasugrel, they need to be discontinued at least 5 days before surgery. Aspirin, on the other hand, needs to be discontinued for a minimum of 7 days if mandated by the risk of surgical bleeding. Antiplatelet therapy is typically resumed 24 h postoperatively [27].

With the development of the second-generation of drug-eluting stents, the risk of stent thrombosis was reduced. Accordingly, the ACC/AHA published in 2016 an update on their previous guidelines, stating that among patients who had a second-generation drug-eluting stent placement within 3–6 months of surgery, one may consider the discontinuation of the second antiplatelet drug, while maintaining aspirin, and accordingly proceed with the surgery if the risk of delayed surgery is greater than the risk of stent thrombosis [28] (as opposed to at least 180 days in the 2014 guidelines). As for elective non-cardiac surgery in patients treated with second-generation drug-eluting stents, proceeding with the surgery and discontinuation of one antiplatelet may be considered after 180 days [28] (as opposed to 360 days in 2014 guidelines). However, it is not only important to determine the time since the PCI was performed, but also one has to consider the reasons behind it, namely if it was electively placed or secondary to an acute coronary event. The 2014 European Society of Cardiology/European Society of Anesthesiology (ESC/ESA) guidelines recommend dual antiplatelet therapy to be continued for three to 12 months following new-generation drug-eluting stent placement and becomes preferable for 1 year after a PCI performed for acute coronary event, unless the risk of life-threatening surgical bleeding is unacceptably high [24] (Class 2a level of evidence C). The major recommendations are summarized in Table 5.2.

To sum up, the decision to continue dual antiplatelet therapy in the perioperative period depends on many factors, including the time from PCI, the type of cardiac stent, the pathology that led to the PCI, the risk of surgical bleeding, and the risk for thrombosis. Since multiple factors are involved, it is important to establish a proper collaboration between the anesthesiologist, the cardiologist, and the surgeon in order to make an informed decision concerning the management of dual antiplatelet therapy in the perioperative period.

Patients on Chronic Anticoagulation Therapy

Patients with atrial fibrillation, mechanical heart valves, history of deep vein thrombosis, or pulmonary embolism require treatment with oral anticoagulation, whether warfarin or novel anticoagulation. The risk of bleeding must be weighed against the benefit of maintaining anticoagulants on a case-by-case basis. Whenever the risk of bleeding is minimal or mild, such as cataract surgery or minor dermatologic procedures, it may be reasonable to continue anticoagulation preoperatively [27, 29]. However, for surgeries with a high risk of bleeding, the decision becomes more challenging, as one needs to keep the patient anticoagulated for the longest period possible, without significantly increasing the risk of excessive surgical bleeding.

Patients at low risk for thromboembolism should not create a dilemma, as the oral anticoagulation can be comfortably withheld [27, 29]. Bridging therapy is

Table 5.2 Summary of the recommendations concerning the management of patients with recent cardiac stents on dual antiplatelet therapy [23, 24, 28]

Type of surgery	Bare metal stents	Drug-eluting stents
Elective surgery	Postpone surgery 30 days from PCI	Postpone surgery 360 days from PCI if first-generation drug-eluting stent Postpone surgery 180 days if second-generation drug-eluting stent Postpone surgery 360 days if stent placement performed for acute coronary event
Urgent or lifesaving surgery 4–6 weeks after PCI	Proceed with surgery without stopping dual antiplatelet	Proceed with surgery without stopping dual antiplatelet
Surgery more than 30 days but less than 360 days from PCI and risk of delaying surgery is higher than risk of stent thrombosis	Proceed with surgery	Proceed with surgery 180 days after PCI with first-generation stents, and 90–180 days after PCI with second-generation stents
Surgery more than 30 days but less than 360 days from PCI and risk of thrombosis higher than risk of delaying surgery	Proceed with the surgery	Postpone surgery 360 days after PCI with first-generation stents Postpone surgery 180 days after PCI with second-generation stents

Proceeding with the surgery usually requires the discontinuation of the $P2Y_{12}$ platelet receptor inhibitors and maintaining aspirin if risk of bleeding is acceptable
PCI percutaneous coronary intervention

considered for patients with a high risk for thromboembolism without excessive risk of bleeding [27, 29]. The concept of bridging consists of replacing warfarin with intravenous unfractionated heparin (UFH) or LMWH during the perioperative period since these medications have a shorter duration of action than warfarin and can be stopped at a shorter interval from surgery. This is particularly useful for patients at high risk of thromboembolism. Warfarin is usually stopped at least 5 days prior to an elective surgery to achieve a normal INR prior to surgery. An INR more than 1.5 justifies vitamin K administration, in order to reverse the effect of warfarin. If immediate reversal of warfarin's effect needs to be done, fresh frozen plasma should be administered [27]. The preferred bridging therapy is usually subcutaneous LMWH or intravenous UFH. The last dose of LMWH should be halved and should be given 24 h before surgery. UFH should be 4–6 h before surgery [27]. Antithrombic therapy should be resumed 24 h post-surgery for patients at low risk of bleeding and 48–72 h for patients at high risk for bleeding [27, 30, 31].

Patients with intermediate risk of thromboembolism should be managed on a case-by-case basis. The landmark BRIDGE trial showed that bridging in moderate-risk atrial fibrillation population may cause harm without benefits. This study showed that in this population, no bridging does not increase the risk of thromboembolism; however, it decreases the risk of bleeding [32].

Concerning novel anticoagulation agents like direct thrombin inhibitors and direct factor X inhibitors, multiple studies have investigated perioperative interruption of these drugs among patients with atrial fibrillation [33–37]. None of these studies found an increased risk of thromboembolism or bleeding preoperatively regardless of bridging therapy, or the type of surgery [34, 35]. However, experience with these novel agents is still limited, and there are no answers yet as to whether the continuation of novel anticoagulation agents increases the risk for surgical bleeding. In addition, the exact safe timing for resuming these agents postoperatively is still unclear [35]. Further studies are required to devise safe perioperative regimens for these medications. So far, a conservative approach of no bridging is usually adopted in order to reduce the risk of perioperative bleeding as much as possible, in the absence of evidence [38].

Perioperative Management of Patients on Antihypertensive Medications

Beta Blockers

Surgical stress is usually associated with physiological responses that may adversely affect patients' outcomes. Beta blockers are usually used to alleviate the stress response, mainly tachycardia, with a proven benefit in the intensive care unit or in burned patients [39]. However, perioperative management of beta blockers is still unclear. The numerous trials addressing preoperative beta blockers resulted in conflicting results. For many years, beta blockers were stopped before surgery because of concerns about negative inotropic effects. This is until Mangano et al. demonstrated a beneficial role of beta blockers (atenolol) started 30 min in the preoperative period for non-cardiac surgery and continued 7 days postoperatively. The study proposed that beta blocker use could reduce cardiac adverse events and improve recovery outcomes [40]. This was followed by the Decrease I trial by Poldermans et al. that revealed significant decrease in serious cardiac events and nonfatal myocardial infarction (MI) with bisoprolol [41]. These studies showed promising results concerning the use of beta blockers in the perioperative period. Moreover, the POISE study, with around 9000 participants, demonstrated that perioperative beta blocker use (metoprolol) started 2–4 h before surgery until 30 days postoperatively decreases nonfatal MI. However, this study also showed a significant increase in the number of deaths because of a higher incidence of hypotension, bradycardia, and stroke [42]. Despite those alarming results, the Decrease IV trial demonstrated a beneficial role of bisoprolol in the reduction of nonfatal MI and risk of cardiac death in intermediate-risk patients undergoing non-cardiac surgery [43]. It is noteworthy to mention that most of the trials studied the effect of beta blockers started within 1 day or less before non-cardiac surgery. The Decrease trials were the only studies that assessed beta blocker use 2 or more days before surgery, and thus their results differed significantly from other trials [44]. However, the Decrease trials had their integrity questioned [45] and the POISE trial was criticized for the use of high-dose, long-acting beta blockers and for initiation of the dose immediately before non-cardiac surgery. Other studies that used a lower starting dose showed no harm nor benefit [46–48].

In the presence of conflicting results, the ACC/AHA published guidelines on beta blockers use in the perioperative period in 2009. The main message was that patients already on beta blockers prior to surgery should keep taking them perioperatively (class IC) [49]. Patients with known ischemic heart disease or MI and those undergoing high-risk surgery including vascular surgeries should start beta blockers in the perioperative period (class II) [49]. Titration of beta blockers in naïve patients was also stressed (class III recommendations) [49].

In 2014, the perioperative guidelines were revised by the ESC and ACC/AHA. Most of the recommendations that required revision were not supported by evidence; the systematic reviews did not yield to confirmative results because of insufficient data on beta blockade start and controversial results regarding the effects on all-cause and cardiovascular death among studies. Also the exclusion of the decrease trials and POISE trial leaves few data to draw solid conclusions. The guidelines were based mainly on expert opinion and pharmacological properties of the drug.

Multiple parameters should be considered when perioperative beta blocker therapy is being evaluated. The discrepancy in the effects of beta blockers is attributed to different variables. These include age, gender, comorbidities, type of surgery, beta blocker type, dose, titration, administration (initiated/continued/withdrawn) and the endpoint in question (mortality, stroke, MI). Treatment should be individualized for every single patient. Bradycardia and hypotension should be avoided, thus the importance of drug titration to appropriate heart rate (60–70 bpm) and blood pressure (SBP > 100 mmHg and MAP > 55 mmHg) targets. Strategies for the use of beta blockers before surgery have been changing and evolving over time. Very few studies have emerged within recent years; therefore, the 2014 guidelines included most of the available studies.

Continuing beta blockers in patients taking them for symptomatic cardiovascular disease remains unchallenged (class I) [23, 24]. Initiation of beta blockers before non-cardiac surgery is controversial. A cardiac benefit is present at the expense of increased death and stroke, whereas in patients with three or more revised cardiac risk index (RCRI) risk factors, it may be reasonable to start beta blockers before surgery (class IIB) [23, 24]. Treatment effects of perioperative beta blockade vary across patients, with benefits confined to high-risk individuals (ASA equal or more than 3). It is not recommended to start beta blockade on low-risk surgery (class III) [23, 24].

Beta blocker initiation should ideally begin 1 week and up to 30 days before surgery and should never be started on the same morning. Atenolol or bisoprolol are considered as first-choice oral beta blockers (class IIb) in ESC [24] but not ACC/AHA recommendations. The lack of evidence of systematic differences in perioperative risks with specific beta blockers subtype makes this current recommendation questionable.

In 2018, a meta-analysis of 88 randomized controlled trials (53 trials of cardiac surgeries and 35 trials of non-cardiac surgeries) included around 20,000 participants. The main findings were as follows [50]. The role of beta blockers in cardiac surgery is essential for supraventricular and ventricular arrhythmias reduction, whereas their role with respect to mortality, MI, stroke, congestive heart failure, hypotension, and bradycardia is still unclear. In those taking beta blockers, the length of hospital stay after heart surgery was reduced by half a day. In cardiac surgery, there seems to be an overall benefit in the use of beta blockade, as it is protective against postoperative rhythm disturbances. Current evidence recommends that patients should continue beta blockers before elective and non-elective heart surgery (class IIa level B). One should consider switching to short-acting agents, and careful up-titration is recommended to limit adverse events. Beta blockers are most beneficial in patients with a recent MI. Preoperative beta blockers use among patients who didn't have a recent MI was not associated with improved perioperative outcomes. It is still unclear if patients with low ventricular ejection fraction (LVEF) but without a recent MI should be started preoperatively on beta blockers. It is crucial to continue beta blockers in patients with a recent MI or low LVEF in the perioperative period, as it significantly reduces the 30-days' mortality (class I level A). Metoprolol succinate, bisoprolol, nebivolol, and carvedilol are accepted beta blockers choices. In non-cardiac surgery, the above review showed that the reduction in rhythm disturbances and non-fatal MI is offset by the potential increase in mortality, stroke, hypotension, bradycardia, and sepsis [50].

In conclusion, the only available class I recommendation is to continue beta blockers in patients chronically treated. The remaining recommendations are weak (class IIb) [50]. The quality of evidence is still low to moderate. As a result, more research is needed before stronger recommendations can be issued.

Angiotensin-Converting Enzyme Inhibitors and Angiotensin-Receptor Blockers

High-risk surgical patients are frequently on angiotensin-converting enzyme inhibitors and angiotensin-receptor blockers (ACEi and ARB). Their role in hypertension, heart failure, ischemic heart diseases, diabetes mellitus, and renal disease is well recognized. However, there is conflicting data about their perioperative management. Theoretically, ACEi/ARBs blunt the renin-angiotensin system during surgery and result in profound hypotension. Preoperative treatment with this class of medications was associated with an increased incidence of intraoperative hypotension [51, 52] and with major perioperative morbidity [53]. Conversely, continuation of the ACEi/ARB therapy may have improved outcome in patients undergoing vascular surgery who have sustained a perioperative myocardial infarction [54]. In a study including 79,000 patients, Turan et al. did not find any association between the use of ACEi and in-hospital complications or increased 30-day mortality [55]. An observational cohort study of almost 15,000 patients concluded that withholding ACEi/ARBs 24 h before major non-cardiac surgery was associated with a lower

30-day all cause death, stroke, myocardial injury, and intraoperative hypotension [53]. Vaquero Roncero et al. concluded that withholding AECI/ARBs on the morning prior to surgery could be recommended with a low level of evidence in order to reduce hypotension in the perioperative period of non-cardiac surgery [56]. A meta-analysis of more than 6000 patients undergoing non-cardiac surgery did not find an association between perioperative administration of ACEi/ARBs and mortality or major cardiac events. However, withholding these medications preoperatively is associated with significant decrease in intraoperative hypotension [57]. Shiffermiller et al. demonstrated that transient preoperative interruption of ACEI therapy in patients undergoing non-cardiac surgery is associated with a decreased risk of intraoperative hypotension. However, postoperative hypertensive events were more frequent [58].

There are various conflicting recommendations regarding perioperative management of ACEi/ARBs in patients undergoing non-cardiac surgery. The ESC/ESA 2014 guidelines are all of class IIa. They recommend continuing ACEi or ARB therapy in stable patients with heart failure undergoing non-cardiac surgery under close monitoring, whereas their transient discontinuation in hypertensive patients should be considered [24]. The ACC/AHA guidelines in 2014 are of class IIa as well and recommend the continuation of ACEi/ARBs in the perioperative period and, if withheld before surgery, it is reasonable to restart as soon as clinically feasible [23]. The French Society of Anesthesiologists guidelines in 2012 recommends discontinuation of ACEi/ARBs administered for hypotension >12 h before surgery, but no discontinuation in case of heart failure [59].

Additional studies evaluated the effect of ACEi/ARBs in patients undergoing cardiac surgery. Benedetto et al. and Drenger et al. suggested a possible myocardial protective effect of ACEi in patients undergoing coronary artery bypass grafting (CABG) surgery [60, 61]. Multiple studies showed conflicting results concerning the effect of ACEi on acute kidney injury after CABG [62–64]. It has been debated whether ACEi should be discontinued before CABG. The exact timing of discontinuation and reinstitution is poorly studied. It is believed that ACEi/ARBs increase the risk of perioperative hypotension and vasodilatory shock, thus requiring the use of inotropes and vasopressors, which will lead to extended intensive care unit stay and ventilator-dependent time [65]. Van Diepen et al. concluded that the routine continuation or discontinuation of ACEi/ARBs before cardiac surgery was not associated with differences in the postoperative physiological or clinical outcomes [65].

The European Association for Cardio-Thoracic Surgery (EACTS) 2017 guidelines recommend discontinuing ACEi/ARB's perioperatively in patients undergoing cardiac surgery (Class I) [66]. Whereas in patients with uncontrolled hypertension, it is reasonable to switch long-acting ACEi or ARB treatment to short-acting ACEi (Class IIa) [66]. In the postoperative period, ACEi/ARBs have protective effects in patients with reduced LVEF and impaired kidney function post CABG [66]. In those patients, it should be considered to start short-acting ACEi no earlier than 48 h (Class IIa) [66]. In ACEi-intolerant patients, an ARB is recommended (Class I) [66]. For other patients without hypertension or reduced LVEF, the routine use of ACEi is not recommended, as it may increase potential adverse events [66].

Table 5.3 Summary of the recommendations concerning the management of antihypertensive medications in the perioperative period [23, 24, 50, 66]

Medication	Non-cardiac surgery	Cardiac surgery
Beta blockers	Maintain beta blockers for patient already on beta blockers for symptomatic cardiovascular disease Initiation of beta blockers is controversial	Maintain beta blockers before elective and non-elective heart surgery Continuing beta blockers is crucial in patients with recent MI or low LVEF; initiation of beta blockers preoperatively is reasonable in these patients
ACEi/ARB	Maintain ACEi/ARB therapy in patients with heart failure Withholding ACEi/ARB therapy in hypertensive patients is reasonable	Maintain ACEi/ARB therapy in patients with uncontrolled hypertension, reduced LVEF and impaired kidney function Withhold therapy in patients with controlled blood pressure and normal LVEF

MI myocardial infarction, *LVEF* left ventricular ejection fraction, *ACEi/ARB* angiotensin-converting enzyme inhibitor/angiotensin-receptor blocker

Most findings suggest that continuing ACEi/ARB therapy in the perioperative period increases the incidence of perioperative hypotension. For the majority of patients, it is usually recommended to withhold them on the day of surgery. However, it is reasonable to continue them in patients with heart failure or in patients with uncontrolled hypertension. Resuming ACEi/ARB treatment is recommended within 48 h in the postoperative period.

In conclusion, the decision to continue or withhold ACEi/ARB should be individualized, taking into consideration the indications of the drug, the patient hemodynamics and cardiac status, as well as the type of surgery and anesthesia planned. Thus, a one-size-fits-all approach for perioperative ACEi/ARB management is not recommended. A summary of the management of patients on antihypertensive medications is presented in Table 5.3.

Conclusion

Many areas of controversy remain regarding the optimal perioperative management of medications such as antiplatelets, anticoagulants, beta blockers, and ACEi/ARBs. International guidelines are regularly revised and updated to incorporate the most recent and relevant data. They are a practical and evidence-based framework that is helpful in guiding the clinician's decisions and help him navigate through the many challenges of the high-risk patient.

References

1. Abbott TEF, Pearse RM, Archbold RA, Wragg A, Kam E, Ahmad T, et al. Association between preoperative pulse pressure and perioperative myocardial injury: an international observational cohort study of patients undergoing non-cardiac surgery. Br J Anaesth. 2017;119(1):78–86.

2. Venkatesan S, Myles PR, Manning HJ, Mozid AM, Andersson C, Jørgensen ME, et al. Cohort study of preoperative blood pressure and risk of 30-day mortality after elective non-cardiac surgery. Br J Anesth. 2017;119(1):65–77.
3. Tryba M. [Epidural regional anesthesia and low molecular heparin: pro]. Anasthesiol Intensivmed Notfallmed Schmerzther. 1993;28(3):179–81. [German].
4. Moen V, Dahlgren N, Irestedt L. Severe neurological complications after central neuraxial blockades in Sweden 1990-1999. Anesthesiology. 2004;101(4):950–9.
5. Vandermeulen EP, Van Aken H, Vermylen J. Anticoagulants and spinal-epidural anesthesia. Anesth Analg. 1994;79(6):1165–77.
6. Lee LA, Posner KL, Domino KB, Caplan RA, Cheney FW. Injuries associated with regional anesthesia in the 1980s and 1990s: a closed claims analysis. Anesthesiology. 2004;101(1):143–52.
7. Wiegel M, Gottschaldt U, Hennebach R, Hirschberg T, Reske A. Complications and adverse effects associated with continuous peripheral nerve blocks in orthopedic patients. Anesth Analg. 2007;104(6):1578–82.
8. Mariano ER, Loland VJ, Bellars RH, Sandhu NS, Bishop ML, Abrams RA, et al. Ultrasound guidance versus electrical stimulation for infraclavicular brachial plexus perineural catheter insertion. J Ultrasound Med. 2009;28(9):1211–8.
9. Bergman BD, Hebl JR, Kent J, Horlocker TT. Neurologic complications of 405 consecutive continuous axillary catheters. Anesth Analg. 2003;96(1):247–52.
10. Weller RS, Gerancher JC, Crews JC, Wade KL. Extensive retroperitoneal hematoma without neurologic deficit in two patients who underwent lumbar plexus block and were later anticoagulated. Anesthesiology. 2003;98(2):581–5.
11. Bickler P, Brandes J, Lee M, Bozic K, Chesbro B, Claassen J. Bleeding complications from femoral and sciatic nerve catheters in patients receiving low molecular weight heparin. Anesth Analg. 2006;103(4):1036–7.
12. Ozturk B, Johnsen SP, Rock ND, Pedersen L, Pedersen AB. Impact of comorbidity on the association between surgery delay and mortality in hip fracture patients: a Danish nationwide cohort study. Injury. 2019;50(2):424–31.
13. Quinlan J, Cox F. Acute pain management in patients with drug dependence syndrome. Pain Rep. 2017;2(4):e611.
14. Hopkins PM. Does regional anaesthesia improve outcome? Br J Anaesth. 2015;115(Suppl 2):ii26–33.
15. Smith LM, Cozowicz C, Uda Y, Memtsoudis SG, Barrington MJ. Neuraxial and combined neuraxial/general anesthesia compared to general anesthesia for major truncal and lower limb surgery: a systematic review and meta-analysis. Anesth Analg. 2017;125(6):1931–45.
16. Andreae MH, Andreae DA. Regional anaesthesia to prevent chronic pain after surgery: a cochrane systematic review and meta-analysis. Br J Anaesth. 2013;111(5):711–20.
17. Gan TJ, Diemunsch P, Habib AS, Kovac A, Kranke P, Meyer TA, et al. Consensus guidelines for the management of postoperative nausea and vomiting. Anesth Analg. 2014;118(1):85–113.
18. Hutton M, Brull R, Macfarlane AJR. Regional anaesthesia and outcomes. BJA Educ. 2018;18(2):52–6.
19. Horlocker TT, Vandermeulen E, Kopp SL, Gogarten W, Leffert LR, Benzon HT. Regional anesthesia in the patient receiving antithrombotic or thrombolytic therapy: American Society of Regional Anesthesia and Pain Medicine evidence-based guidelines (fourth edition). Reg Anesth Pain Med. 2018;43(3):263–309.
20. Bouma BN, Mosnier LO. Thrombin activatable fibrinolysis inhibitor (TAFI)—how does thrombin regulate fibrinolysis? Ann Med. 2006;38(6):378–88.
21. Rosencher N, Bonnet MP, Sessler DI. Selected new antithrombotic agents and neuraxial anaesthesia for major orthopaedic surgery: management strategies. Anaesthesia. 2007;62(11):1154–60.
22. Hawn MT, Graham LA, Richman JS, Itani KM, Henderson WG, Maddox TM. Risk of major adverse cardiac events following noncardiac surgery in patients with coronary stents. JAMA. 2013;310(14):1462–72.

23. Fleisher LA, Fleischmann KE, Auerbach AD, Barnason SA, Beckman JA, Bozkurt B, et al. 2014 ACC/AHA guideline on perioperative cardiovascular evaluation and management of patients undergoing noncardiac surgery: a report of the American College of Cardiology/American Heart Association task force on practice guidelines. Circulation. 2014;130(24):e278–333.
24. Kristensen SD, Knuuti J, Saraste A, Anker S, Botker HE, Hert SD, et al. 2014 ESC/ESA guidelines on non-cardiac surgery: cardiovascular assessment and management: the joint task force on non-cardiac surgery: cardiovascular assessment and management of the European Society of Cardiology (ESC) and the European Society of Anaesthesiology (ESA). Eur Heart J. 2014;35(35):2383–431.
25. Lee DH, de la Torre Hernandez JM. The newest generation of drug-eluting stents and beyond. Eur Cardiol. 2018;13(1):54–9.
26. Rabbitts JA, Nuttall GA, Brown MJ, Hanson AC, Oliver WC, Holmes DR, et al. Cardiac risk of noncardiac surgery after percutaneous coronary intervention with drug-eluting stents. Anesthesiology. 2008;109(4):596–604.
27. Douketis JD, Spyropoulos AC, Spencer FA, Mayr M, Jaffer AK, Eckman MH, et al. Perioperative management of antithrombotic therapy: antithrombotic therapy and prevention of thrombosis, 9th ed: American College of Chest Physicians evidence-based clinical practice guidelines. Chest. 2012;141(2 Suppl):e326S–50S.
28. Levine GN, Bates ER, Bittl JA, Brindis RG, Fihn SD, Fleisher LA, et al. 2016 ACC/AHA guideline focused update on duration of dual antiplatelet therapy in patients with coronary artery disease: a report of the American College of Cardiology/American Heart Association task force on clinical practice guidelines: an update of the 2011 ACCF/AHA/SCAI guideline for percutaneous coronary intervention, 2011 ACCF/AHA guideline for coronary artery bypass graft surgery, 2012 ACC/AHA/ACP/AATS/PCNA/SCAI/STS guideline for the diagnosis and management of patients with stable ischemic heart disease, 2013 ACCF/AHA guideline for the management of ST-elevation myocardial infarction, 2014 AHA/ACC guideline for the management of patients with non-ST-elevation acute coronary syndromes, and 2014 ACC/AHA guideline on perioperative cardiovascular evaluation and management of patients undergoing noncardiac surgery. Circulation. 2016;134(10):e123–55.
29. January CT, Wann LS, Alpert JS, Calkins H, Cigarroa JE, Cleveland JC Jr, et al. 2014 AHA/ACC/HRS guideline for the management of patients with atrial fibrillation: executive summary: a report of the American College of Cardiology/American Heart Association task force on practice guidelines and the Heart Rhythm Society. Circulation. 2014;130(23):2071–104.
30. Dowling NF, Beckman MG, Manco-Johnson M, Hassell K, Philipp CS, Michaels LA, et al. The U.S. thrombosis and hemostasis centers pilot sites program. J Thromb Thrombolysis. 2007;23(1):1–7.
31. Liew A, Douketis J. Perioperative management of patients who are receiving a novel oral anticoagulant. Intern Emerg Med. 2013;8(6):477–84.
32. Douketis JD, Spyropoulos AC, Kaatz S, Becker RC, Caprini JA, Dunn AS, et al. Perioperative bridging anticoagulation in patients with atrial fibrillation. N Engl J Med. 2015;373(9):823–33.
33. Patel MR, Hellkamp AS, Lokhnygina Y, Piccini JP, Zhang Z, Mohanty S, et al. Outcomes of discontinuing rivaroxaban compared with warfarin in patients with nonvalvular atrial fibrillation: analysis from the ROCKET AF trial (Rivaroxaban once-daily, oral, direct factor Xa inhibition compared with vitamin K antagonism for prevention of stroke and embolism trial in atrial fibrillation). J Am Coll Cardiol. 2013;61(6):651–8.
34. Douketis JD, Healey JS, Brueckmann M, Eikelboom JW, Ezekowitz MD, Fraessdorf M, et al. Perioperative bridging anticoagulation during dabigatran or warfarin interruption among patients who had an elective surgery or procedure. Substudy of the RE-LY trial. Thromb Haemost. 2015;113(3):625–32.
35. Healey JS, Brambatti M. Periprocedural management of oral anticoagulation in patients with atrial fibrillation: approach in the era of new oral anticoagulants. Can J Cardiol. 2013;29(7 Suppl):S54–9.
36. Healey JS, Eikelboom J, Douketis J, Wallentin L, Oldgren J, Yang S, et al. Periprocedural bleeding and thromboembolic events with dabigatran compared with warfarin: results from

the randomized evaluation of long-term anticoagulation therapy (RE-LY) randomized trial. Circulation. 2012;126(3):343–8.
37. Granger CB, Lopes RD, Hanna M, Ansell J, Hylek EM, Alexander JH, et al. Clinical events after transitioning from apixaban versus warfarin to warfarin at the end of the apixaban for reduction in stroke and other thromboembolic events in atrial fibrillation (ARISTOTLE) trial. Am Heart J. 2015;169(1):25–30.
38. Rechenmacher SJ, Fang JC. Bridging anticoagulation: primum non nocere. J Am Coll Cardiol. 2015;66(12):1392–403.
39. Finnerty CC, Mabvuure NT, Ali A, Kozar RA, Herndon DN. The surgically induced stress response. JPEN J Parenter Enteral Nutr. 2013;37(5 Suppl):21S–9S.
40. Mangano DT, Layug EL, Wallace A, Tateo I. Effect of atenolol on mortality and cardiovascular morbidity after noncardiac surgery. Multicenter study of perioperative ischemia research group. N Engl J Med. 1996;335(23):1713–20.
41. Poldermans D, Boersma E, Bax JJ, Thomson IR, van de Ven LL, Blankensteijn JD, et al. The effect of bisoprolol on perioperative mortality and myocardial infarction in high-risk patients undergoing vascular surgery. Dutch echocardiographic cardiac risk evaluation applying stress echocardiography study group. N Engl J Med. 1999;341(24):1789–94.
42. Devereaux PJ, Yang H, Yusuf S, Guyatt G, Leslie K, Villar JC, et al. Effects of extended-release metoprolol succinate in patients undergoing non-cardiac surgery (POISE trial): a randomised controlled trial. Lancet. 2008;371(9627):1839–47.
43. Schouten O, Poldermans D, Visser L, Kertai MD, Klein J, van Urk H, et al. Fluvastatin and bisoprolol for the reduction of perioperative cardiac mortality and morbidity in high-risk patients undergoing non-cardiac surgery: rationale and design of the DECREASE-IV study. Am Heart J. 2004;148(6):1047–52.
44. Poldermans D, Schouten O, Bax J, Winkel TA. Reducing cardiac risk in non-cardiac surgery: evidence from the DECREASE studies. Eur Heart J Suppl. 2009;11(suppl_A):A9–A14.
45. Erasmus MC Follow-up Investigation Committee. Report on the 2012 follow-up investigation of possible breaches of academic integrity. 2012.
46. Brady AR, Gibbs JS, Greenhalgh RM, Powell JT, Sydes MR. Perioperative beta-blockade (POBBLE) for patients undergoing infrarenal vascular surgery: results of a randomized double-blind controlled trial. J Vasc Surg. 2005;41(4):602–9.
47. Yang H, Raymer K, Butler R, Parlow J, Roberts R. The effects of perioperative beta-blockade: results of the metoprolol after vascular surgery (MaVS) study, a randomized controlled trial. Am Heart J. 2006;152(5):983–90.
48. Juul AB, Wetterslev J, Kofoed-Enevoldsen A, Callesen T, Jensen G, Gluud C. The diabetic postoperative mortality and morbidity (DIPOM) trial: rationale and design of a multicenter, randomized, placebo-controlled, clinical trial of metoprolol for patients with diabetes mellitus who are undergoing major noncardiac surgery. Am Heart J. 2004;147(4):677–83.
49. Fleisher LA, Beckman JA, Brown KA, Calkins H, Chaikof EL, Fleischmann KE, et al. 2009 ACCF/AHA focused update on perioperative beta blockade incorporated into the ACC/AHA 2007 guidelines on perioperative cardiovascular evaluation and care for noncardiac surgery. J Am Coll Cardiol. 2009;54(22):e13–e118.
50. Blessberger H, Kammler J, Domanovits H, Schlager O, Wildner B, Azar D, et al. Perioperative beta-blockers for preventing surgery-related mortality and morbidity. Cochrane Database Syst Rev. 2018;3(3):CD004476.
51. Coriat P, Richer C, Douraki T, Gomez C, Hendricks K, Giudicelli JF, et al. Influence of chronic angiotensin-converting enzyme inhibition on anesthetic induction. Anesthesiology. 1994;81(2):299–307.
52. Bertrand M, Godet G, Meersschaert K, Brun L, Salcedo E, Coriat P. Should the angiotensin II antagonists be discontinued before surgery? Anesth Analg. 2001;92(1):26–30.
53. Roshanov PS, Rochwerg B, Patel A, Salehian O, Duceppe E, Belley-Cote EP, et al. Withholding versus continuing angiotensin-converting enzyme inhibitors or angiotensin II receptor blockers before noncardiac surgery: an analysis of the vascular events in noncardiac surgery patients cohort evaluation prospective cohort. Anesthesiology. 2017;126(1):16–27.

54. Foucrier A, Rodseth R, Aissaoui M, Ibanes C, Goarin JP, Landais P, et al. The long-term impact of early cardiovascular therapy intensification for postoperative troponin elevation after major vascular surgery. Anesth Analg. 2014;119(5):1053–63.
55. Turan A, You J, Shiba A, Kurz A, Saager L, Sessler DI. Angiotensin converting enzyme inhibitors are not associated with respiratory complications or mortality after noncardiac surgery. Anesth Analg. 2012;114(3):552–60.
56. Vaquero Roncero LM, Sanchez Poveda D, Valdunciel Garcia JJ, Sanchez Barrado ME, Calvo Vecino JM. Perioperative use of angiotensin-converting-enzyme inhibitors and angiotensin receptor antagonists. J Clin Anesth. 2017;40:91–8.
57. Hollmann C, Fernandes NL, Biccard BM. A systematic review of outcomes associated with withholding or continuing angiotensin-converting enzyme inhibitors and angiotensin receptor blockers before noncardiac surgery. Anesth Analg. 2018;127(3):678–87.
58. Shiffermiller JF, Monson BJ, Vokoun CW, Beachy MW, Smith MP, Sullivan JN, et al. Prospective randomized evaluation of preoperative angiotensin-converting enzyme inhibition (PREOP-ACEI). J Hosp Med. 2018;13(10):661–7.
59. Bogebjerg MK. No consensus on withholding angiotensin-converting enzyme inhibitors and angiotensin receptor blockers before spinal anaesthesia. Danish Med J. 2012;59(12):A4543.
60. Benedetto U, Sciarretta S, Roscitano A, Fiorani B, Refice S, Angeloni E, et al. Preoperative angiotensin-converting enzyme inhibitors and acute kidney injury after coronary artery bypass grafting. Ann Thorac Surg. 2008;86(4):1160–5.
61. Drenger B, Fontes ML, Miao Y, Mathew JP, Gozal Y, Aronson S, et al. Patterns of use of perioperative angiotensin-converting enzyme inhibitors in coronary artery bypass graft surgery with cardiopulmonary bypass: effects on in-hospital morbidity and mortality. Circulation. 2012;126(3):261–9.
62. Mann JF, Gerstein HC, Yi QL, Lonn EM, Hoogwerf BJ, Rashkow A, et al. Development of renal disease in people at high cardiovascular risk: results of the HOPE randomized study. J Am Soc Nephrol. 2003;14(3):641–7.
63. Marre M, Lievre M, Chatellier G, Mann JF, Passa P, Menard J. Effects of low dose ramipril on cardiovascular and renal outcomes in patients with type 2 diabetes and raised excretion of urinary albumin: randomised, double blind, placebo controlled trial (the DIABHYCAR study). BMJ. 2004;328(7438):495.
64. Filion KB, Pilote L, Rahme E, Eisenberg MJ. Perioperative use of cardiac medical therapy among patients undergoing coronary artery bypass graft surgery: a systematic review. Am Heart J. 2007;154(3):407–14.
65. van Diepen S, Norris CM, Zheng Y, Nagendran J, Graham MM, Gaete Ortega D, et al. Comparison of angiotensin-converting enzyme inhibitor and angiotensin receptor blocker management strategies before cardiac surgery: a pilot randomized controlled registry trial. J Am Heart Assoc. 2018;7(20):e009917.
66. Sousa-Uva M, Head SJ, Milojevic M, Collet JP, Landoni G, Castella M, et al. 2017 EACTS guidelines on perioperative medication in adult cardiac surgery. Eur J Cardiothorac Surg. 2018;53(1):5–33.

Reducing Surgical Site Infections

6

Kamal M. F. Itani and Gentian Kristo

Introduction

Surgical site infections (SSIs) occur at or near the incision site and/or deeper underlying tissue spaces and organs within 30 days of a surgical procedure (or up to 90 days when a prosthetic implant is used). They are the most common healthcare-associated infections among surgical patients [1] and are associated with substantial morbidity.

SSIs are associated with approximately 8205 deaths each year in the United States and account for an estimated 11% of all deaths in intensive care units [2]. They increase the hospital stay by 11 days per patient [3] and are the most frequent cause (20%) of unplanned readmissions after surgery [4]. The financial burden of SSIs is significant, with overall US cost estimates of $3.5 to $10 billion annually, approximately $12,000 to $35,000 per patient [5]. Given that about 60% of SSIs are considered preventable [6], SSI has become an important quality improvement and pay-for-performance metric.

In order to standardize SSI data collection, the Centers for Disease Control and Prevention (CDC) has defined SSI based on depth and tissue space involved [7]. In the criteria put forth by the CDC, SSIs are classified as either incisional or organ/space, with incisional SSIs being further subclassified as superficial (involving only skin and subcutaneous tissue) versus deep (involving underlying fascia and muscle).

Table 6.1 describes the criteria used by the CDC to classify SSI into its various categories [8]. These criteria are used for surveillance purposes and allow for

K. M. F. Itani (✉)
Department of Surgery, Veterans Affairs Boston Healthcare System, West Roxbury, MA, USA

Department of Surgery, Boston University, Boston, USA

Harvard Medical School, Boston, MA, USA
e-mail: Kamal.Itani@va.gov

G. Kristo
Department of Surgery, Veterans Affairs Boston Healthcare System, West Roxbury, MA, USA

Harvard Medical School, Boston, MA, USA

J. J. Hoballah et al. (eds.), *Principles of Perioperative Safety and Efficiency*,
https://doi.org/10.1007/978-3-031-41089-5_6

Table 6.1 CDC surgical site infection (SSI) classification (adapted from Mangram et al. [8])

Superficial Incisional SSI
Infection occurs within 30 days after the operation *and* infection involves only skin or subcutaneous tissue of the incision *and* at least *one* of the following:
1. Purulent drainage, with or without laboratory confirmation, from the superficial incision
2. Organisms isolated from an aseptically obtained culture of fluid or tissue from the superficial incision
3. At least one of the following indicators of infection: pain or tenderness, localized swelling, redness, or *heat* and superficial incision is deliberately opened by surgeon, *unless* incision is culture-negative
4. Diagnosis of superficial incisional SSI by the surgeon or attending physician
Do *not* report the following conditions as SSI:
1. Stitch abscess (minimal inflammation and discharge confined to the points of suture penetration)
2. Infection of an episiotomy or newborn circumcision site
3. Infected burn wound
4. Incisional SSI that extends into the fascial and muscle layers (see deep incisional SSI)
Note: Specific criteria are used for identifying infected episiotomy and circumcision sites and burn wounds
Deep Incisional SSI
Infection occurs within 30 days after the operation if no prosthetic implant is left in place or within one year if implant is in place and the infection appears to be related to the operation *and* infection involves deep soft tissues (e.g., fascial and muscle layers) of the incision *and* at least *one* of the following:
1. Purulent drainage from the deep incision but not from the organ/space component of the surgical site
2. A deep incision spontaneously dehisces or is deliberately opened by a surgeon when the patient has at least one of the following signs or symptoms: fever (>38 °C), localized pain, or tenderness, unless site is culture-negative
3. An abscess or other evidence of infection involving the deep incision is found on direct examination, during reoperation, or by histopathologic or radiologic examination
4. Diagnosis of a deep incisional SSI by a surgeon or attending physician
Notes:
1. Report infection that involves both superficial and deep incision sites as deep incisional SSI
2. Report an organ/space SSI that drains through the incision as a deep incisional SSI
Organ/Space SSI
Infection occurs within 30 days after the operation if no prosthetic implant is left in place or within one year if implant is in place and the infection appears to be related to the operation and infection involves any part of the anatomy (e.g., organs or spaces), other than the incision, which was opened or manipulated during an operation *and* at least *one* of the following:
1. Purulent drainage from a drain that is placed through a stab wound[a] into the organ/space
2. Organisms isolated from an aseptically obtained culture of fluid or tissue in the organ/space
3. An abscess or other evidence of infection involving the organ/space that is found on direct examination, during reoperation, or by histopathologic or radiologic examination
4. Diagnosis of an organ/space SSI by a surgeon or attending physician

[a] If the area around a stab wound becomes infected, it is not an SSI. It is considered a skin or soft tissue infection, depending on its depth

objective definitions in quality improvement, public reporting, *pay-for-performance and research.*

Microbiology of SSIs

In most SSIs, the responsible pathogens originate from the patient's endogenous flora. Overall, the most commonly involved organisms are *Staphylococcus aureus*, coagulase-negative *staphylococci*, *Enterococcus* spp., and *Escherichia coli* [8]. However, the specific pathogens isolated depend primarily on the type of surgical procedure performed. In clean surgical procedures, in which the gastrointestinal, genito-urinary, and respiratory tracts have not been entered, endogenous *Staphylococcus aureus* from the patient's skin flora is the usual cause of infection. Entry into hollow viscera exposes surrounding tissue to Gram-negative bacilli such as *Escherichia coli*, Gram-positive organisms such as *Enterococcus* spp., anaerobes such as *Bacillus fragilis*, and, occasionally, yeast species [8]. Pathogens may also originate from preoperative infections at sites remote from the operative site, particularly in patients undergoing insertion of prosthetic implants.

In addition to the patient's endogenous flora, SSI pathogens may originate from exogenous sources such as colonized surgical team personnel, operating room environment, and instruments and materials used during the surgical procedure. Such pathogens are predominantly aerobes, particularly Gram-positive organisms such as staphylococci and streptococci.

The risk of SSI caused by resistant bacteria has become a major healthcare concern. In particular, there is concern about the rise in SSIs due to methicillin-resistant *S. aureus* (MRSA), vancomycin-resistant *Enterococci* (VRE), third-generation cephalosporin-resistant *Escherichia coli*, and imipenem- and quinolone-resistant *Pseudomonas aeruginosa.* Antimicrobial resistance among nosocomial pathogens often results in prolonged periods of antimicrobial therapy and increased treatment costs, prolonged hospital stays, and higher mortality [9]. For adequate antimicrobial stewardship, antibiotic prophylaxis for surgical interventions should consider the expected flora, bacterial resistance patterns, drug pharmacokinetics and recommended duration not to exceed 24 h.

Table 6.2 further expands upon the most likely pathogens encountered in different surgical procedures.

Table 6.2 Pathogens commonly associated with different surgical procedures (adapted from Mangram et al. [8])

Type of surgery	Common pathogens
Placement of all grafts, prostheses, or implants	*S. aureus*; coagulase-negative staphylococci
Cardiac	*S. aureus*; coagulase-negative staphylococci
Thoracic	*S. aureus*; coagulase-negative staphylococci, *Streptococcus pneumoniae*, Gram-negative bacilli
Breast	*S. aureus*; coagulase-negative staphylococci
Ophthalmic	*S. aureus*; coagulase-negative staphylococci; streptococci; Gram-negative bacilli
Orthopedic	*S. aureus*; coagulase-negative staphylococci; streptococci; Gram-negative bacilli
Vascular	*S. aureus*; coagulase-negative staphylococci
Appendectomy	Gram-negative bacilli; anaerobes
Biliary tract	Gram-negative bacilli; anaerobes
Colorectal	Gram-negative bacilli; anaerobes
Gastroduodenal	Gram-negative bacilli; streptococci; oropharyngeal anaerobes (e.g., peptostreptococci)
Head and neck	*S. aureus*; streptococci; oropharyngeal anaerobes (e.g., peptostreptococci)
Obstetric and gynecological	Gram-negative bacilli; enterococci; Group B streptococci; anaerobes
Urological	Gram-negative bacilli

Risk Factors

Several modifiable and non-modifiable patient (intrinsic) risk factors have been identified for the development of SSIs. Potentially modifiable patient risk factors include diabetes, obesity, dyspnea, alcoholism, smoking, preoperative albumin <3.5 mg/dL, total bilirubin >1.0 mg/dL, and immunosuppression [10]. Non-modifiable patient factors include increasing age, recent radiotherapy, and history of skin or soft tissue infection.

In addition to intrinsic factors, the role of extrinsic risk factors in the pathogenesis of SSI is well recognized [8]. Extrinsic risk factors include emergency and more complex surgeries; higher wound classification; inadequate operating room (OR) ventilation; increased OR traffic; improper sterilization of surgical instruments; presence of a pre-existing infection; inadequate skin preparation; hair removal; inadequate prophylactic antibiotic choice, administration, and duration; prolonged duration of surgery; intraoperative blood transfusion; improper surgical hand scrubbing and gloving; and intraoperative hypothermia and poor glycemic control [10]. Table 6.3 further expands upon the risk factors for developing SSI.

Table 6.3 Risk factors for surgical site infections (adapted from Ban et al. [10])

Intrinsic (Patient) risk factors		Extrinsic (Procedural) risk factors			
Modifiable	Non-modifiable	Procedure	Facility	Pre-operative	Intra-operative
Diabetes Obesity Alcoholism Current smoker Preoperative albumin <3.5 mg/dL Total bilirubin >1.0 mg/dL Immunosuppression	Increased age Recent radiotherapy History of skin or soft tissue infection	Emergency Increasing complexity Higher wound classification	Inadequate ventilation Increased operating room traffic Contaminated environmental surfaces Non-sterile equipment	Pre-existing infection Inadequate skin preparation Inappropriate antibiotic choice, timing, and weight-based Dosing Hair removal method Poor glycemic control	Longer procedure duration Blood transfusion Breach in asepsis Inappropriate antibiotic re-dosing Inadequate gloving Inappropriate surgical scrub Poor glycemic control

Guidelines for Prevention

Various national and international organizations have developed guidelines for the prevention of SSI. In 1999, the CDC released expert-opinion based guidelines for preventing SSIs [8]. The World Health Organization (WHO) published their SSI prevention guidelines in 2016 [11] and the American College of Surgeons and the Surgical Infection Society (ACS/SIS) published theirs in 2017 [10]. The CDC updated its SSI prevention guidelines in 2017, based on a systematic review and grading of the medical literature [12].

These guidelines agree on most preventative measures. Each guideline also addresses additional measures based on the level and quality of evidence established for the guideline as well as the target audiences and priorities for each organization. Their summarized recommendations are discussed in detail below.

Prehospital Interventions

Prehospital interventions for reducing SSI include preoperative bathing, smoking cessation, glucose control, MRSA screening, and bowel preparation (Table 6.4).

Table 6.4 Guidelines for prehospital interventions as endorsed by specific guidelines (adapted from Ban [10], Allegranzi [11], and Berrios-Torres [12])

Guideline (Organization)	Recommendation
Preoperative bathing (CDC; ACS/SIS; WHO)	Routine preoperative bathing with chlorhexidine reduces the bacterial colonization of the skin but has not been shown to reduce SSI
Smoking cessation (CDC; ACS/SIS)	Smoking cessation 4–6 weeks before surgery reduces SSI and is recommended for all current smokers, especially those undergoing procedures with implanted materials. There is no literature to support cessation of marijuana and electronic cigarette use to prevent SSI
Glucose control (CDC; ACS/SIS; WHO)	Optimal blood glucose control should be encouraged for all diabetic patients; however, there is no evidence that improved Hgb A1C decreases SSI risk
MRSA screening (ACS/SIS; WHO)	MRSA bundles (screening, decolonization, contact precautions, hand hygiene) are highly effective if adhered to, otherwise there is no benefit No standard decolonization protocol supported by literature; consider nasal mupirocin alone vs nasal mupirocin plus chlorhexidine gluconate bathing Decolonization protocols should be completed close to date of surgery to be effective Vancomycin should not be administered as prophylaxis to MRSA-negative patients
Bowel preparation (ACS/SIS; WHO)	Combination mechanical and antibiotic oral preparation is recommended for all elective colectomies

CDC Centers for Disease Control and Prevention, *ACS/SIS* American College of Surgeons and the Surgical Infection Society, *WHO* World Health Organization

Preoperative Bathing

Routine preoperative bathing with chlorhexidine decreases skin surface pathogen concentrations but has not been shown to reduce SSI [10].

Smoking Cessation

Smoking cessation 4–6 weeks before surgery reduces SSI [10, 12] and is recommended for all current smokers, especially those undergoing procedures with implanted materials. There is no literature to support cessation of marijuana and electronic cigarette use to prevent SSI. There is no evidence suggesting that alternative nicotine-containing substances (e.g., gum, patch, and lozenges) are linked to SSI [10]. As such, their use is supported as smoking-cessation aids before surgery.

Glucose Control

Optimal blood glucose control should be encouraged for all diabetic patients; however, there is no definitive evidence that improved Hgb A1C decreases SSI risk [10].

MRSA Screening

MRSA colonization is associated with worse outcomes and a higher risk for both MRSA SSI and SSI overall [13–15]. MRSA bundles include screening, decolonization, contact precautions, hand hygiene, and vancomycin-containing antibiotic prophylaxis. They are highly effective in reducing rates of SSI if adhered to; otherwise, there is no benefit [10]. Decolonization protocols should be completed close to the date of surgery to be effective.

Typical preoperative decolonization protocols include the use of nasal mupirocin alone vs. nasal mupirocin plus chlorhexidine gluconate bathing, although no standard decolonization protocol is supported by literature [10].

For antibiotic prophylaxis, use of vancomycin alone in MRSA-negative patients is associated with a higher risk of methicillin-sensitive *S. aureus* SSI [16] and an increased risk of conversion to MRSA-positive status and development of SSI [17]. As such, routine administration of vancomycin antibiotic prophylaxis in MRSA-negative patients is not recommended [10].

Bowel Preparation

Mechanical bowel preparation alone or oral antibiotics alone do not decrease SSIs [18–20]. The combination of mechanical and oral antibiotic bowel preparations is associated with lower rates of SSI, anastomotic leak, *Clostridium difficile* infection, postoperative ileus, reduced length of stay, and lower readmission rates [18–23].

For these reasons, combination mechanical and antibiotic oral preparation is increasingly recommended for all elective colorectal surgeries [10, 18, 19]. Routine intravenous prophylactic antibiotics in the immediate preoperative period should also be given.

Hospital Interventions

Hospital interventions for reducing SSI include perioperative glucose control, hair removal, preoperative skin preparation, surgical hand scrub, surgical attire, prophylactic antibiotics, maintaining normothermia, maintaining euvolemia, wound protectors, antibiotic sutures, gloves/instruments, adhesive incise drapes, incisional wound irrigation, operating room ventilation, and wound care (Table 6.5).

Table 6.5 Guidelines for hospital interventions (adapted from Ban [10], Allegranzi [11], and Berrios-Torres [12])

Guideline (Organization)	Recommendation
Perioperative glucose control (CDC; ACS/SIS; WHO)	Perioperative hyperglycemia increases the risk of SSI in both diabetics and nondiabetics. As such, implementation of perioperative glycemic control protocols is strongly recommended, with blood glucose target levels less than 200 mg/dL in patients with and without diabetes There is no evidence to recommend an optimal hemoglobin A1C target level for the prevention of SSI
Hair removal (CDC; ACS/SIS; WHO)	Hair removal should be avoided unless hair interferes with surgery. If hair removal is necessary, clippers should be used instead of a razor
Preoperative skin preparation (CDC; ACS/SIS; WHO)	The use of prophylactic antibiotics is strongly recommended with the choice of prophylactic: Alcohol-containing preparations are more effective in reducing SSI than aqueous preparations and should be used unless contraindications exist. When comparing chlorhexidine- to iodine-based alcohol solutions, there is no clear superior agent to reduce SSI. In the absence of alcohol, chlorhexidine gluconate may be superior to povidone-iodine
Surgical hand scrub (CDC; ACS/SIS; WHO)	Use of a waterless chlorhexidine scrub is as effective as traditional water scrub and requires less time, but there is no superior agent if used according to manufacturer's instructions
Surgical attire (CDC; ACS/SIS; WHO)	In the operating room, wear a surgical mask that fully covers the mouth and nose, and use a skull cap if minimal hair is exposed Remove or cover all jewelry on the head and neck, and professional attire when outside the operating room (no scrubs or clean scrubs covered with a white coat)
Prophylactic antibiotics (CDC; ACS/SIS; WHO)	The use of prophylactic antibiotics is strongly recommended with the choice of prophylactic antibiotic dictated by the type of the surgical procedure and pathogens most likely to cause SSI Administration of antibiotics should be completed within 1 h prior to incision (2 h for vancomycin or fluoroquinolone) Antibiotics should be redosed based on agent half-life or for every 1500 mL blood loss There is no evidence that prophylactic antibiotic administration after incision closure decreases SSI risk The presence of a wound drain does not require prophylactic antibiotic
Perioperative oxygenation (CDC; ACS/SIS; WHO)	Adult patients with normal pulmonary function undergoing general anesthesia with endotracheal intubation for surgical procedures should receive 80% fraction of inspired oxygen intraoperatively and, if feasible, in the immediate postoperative period for 2–6 h. There is no evidence to recommend an optimal oxygen delivery method or a target oxygenation level
Maintaining normothermia (CDC; ACS/SIS; WHO)	Perioperative maintenance of normothermia is strongly recommended. There is no evidence to recommend optimal strategies to achieve and maintain normothermia, the lower limit of normothermia, or the optimal timing and duration of normothermia for the prevention of SSI
Maintaining normovolemia (WHO)	Intraoperative goal-directed fluid therapy is suggested for preventing SSI

Table 6.5 (continued)

Guideline (Organization)	Recommendation
Wound protectors (ACS/SIS; WHO)	Use of an impervious plastic wound protector can prevent SSI in open abdominal surgery. Evidence is strongest for elective colorectal and biliary tract procedures
Antibiotic sutures (CDC; ACS/SIS; WHO)	Triclosan antibacterial suture use is recommended for wound closure in any type of surgery when available
Gloves/Instruments (ACS/SIS)	The use of double gloves is recommended Changing gloves before closure in colorectal cases is recommended; however, rescrubbing before closure in colorectal cases is not recommended The use of new instruments for closure in colorectal cases is recommended
Adhesive drapes (CDC; ACS/SIS; WHO)	Plastic adhesive incise drapes with or without antimicrobial properties are not necessary for the prevention of SSI and should not be used. Application of microbial sealant immediately after skin preparation is not needed
Incisional wound irrigation (CDC; WHO)	Consider the use of irrigation of the incisional wound with an aqueous povidone-iodine solution before closure, particularly in clean and clean-contaminated wounds Intraperitoneal lavage with aqueous iodophor solution in contaminated or dirty abdominal procedures is not necessary Antibiotic incisional wound irrigation before closure should not be used
Operating room ventilation (CDC; WHO)	Maintain positive pressure ventilation in the operating room and adjoining spaces Laminar airflow ventilation systems should not be used for patients undergoing total arthroplasty surgery
Wound care (CDC; ACS/SIS; WHO)	No type of advanced dressing should be used over a standard dressing on primarily closed surgical wounds Use of wound vacuum therapy over stapled skin can reduce SSI in open colorectal (abdominal incision) and vascular (groin incision) cases Mupirocin topic antibiotic application can decrease SSI compared with a standard dressing While close incisions are usually covered with a sterile dressing for 24–48 h postoperatively, there is no evidence in the literature that timing of dressing removal increases SSI risk Early showering (12 h postoperative) does not increase the risk of SSI Daily wound probing can decrease SSI in contaminated wounds

CDC Centers for Disease Control and Prevention, *ACS/SIS* American College of Surgeons and the Surgical Infection Society, *WHO* World Health Organization

Perioperative Glucose Control

Perioperative hyperglycemia increases the risk of SSI in both diabetics and nondiabetics [24–26]. As such, implementation of perioperative glycemic control protocols is strongly recommended, [10–12] with blood glucose target levels less than 200 mg/dL in patients with and without diabetes. There is no evidence to recommend an optimal hemoglobin A1C target levels for the prevention of SSI. Furthermore, short-term glucose control can be more impactful in decreasing SSIs than long-term control of hemoglobin A1C [10].

Close monitoring of blood glucose levels is very important, as hypoglycemia can occur with perioperative glycemic control protocols.

Hair Removal

Hair removal should be avoided unless hair interferes with surgery. If hair removal is necessary, clippers should be used instead of a razor [10, 12].

Preoperative Skin Preparation

The use of alcohol-based skin scrubs is strongly recommended and has been shown to be more effective in reducing SSI than aqueous preparations and should be used unless contraindications exist [10, 12]. When comparing chlorhexidine- to iodine-based alcohol solutions, there is no clear superior agent to reduce SSI [10, 12]. In the absence of alcohol, chlorhexidine gluconate may be superior to povidone-iodine.

Surgical Hand Scrub

Use of a waterless chlorhexidine scrub is as effective as traditional water scrub and requires less time, but there is no superior agent if used according to manufacturer's recommendations [10, 12]. Water-based scrub for first cases is recommended. Hand hygiene with soap and water is also recommended prior to waterless scrub for subsequent cases.

Surgical Attire

In the operating room, surgical mask that fully covers the mouth and nose should be worn. All scalp and facial hair should be properly covered [10, 12]. Skull cap is now accepted in addition to the bouffant cap.

All jewelry on the head and neck should be removed. Operating room scrubs should not be worn outside the sterile area, or should be properly covered when leaving the operating room areas [10].

Prophylactic Antibiotics

The use of prophylactic antibiotics is strongly recommended, with the choice of prophylactic antibiotic dictated by the type of the surgical procedure and pathogens most likely to cause SSI. To achieve bactericidal concentration at time of the surgical incision, administration of weight-adjusted antibiotics should be completed within 1 h prior to incision (2 h for vancomycin or fluoroquinolone) [10–12]. To maintain adequate tissue levels, antibiotics should be redosed based on agent half-life or for every 1500 mL blood loss [10].

There is no evidence that prophylactic antibiotic administration after incision closure decreases SSI risk. As such, in clean and clean-contaminated procedures, additional prophylactic antibiotics should not be administered after incision closure, even in the presence of a drain (possible exceptions include implant-based breast reconstruction, joint arthroplasty, and cardiac procedures where optimal duration of antibiotic therapy remains unknown) [10–12].

Although there is no evidence to recommend an optimal time for removal of wound drains, they should be removed as soon as clinically indicated [10–12].

Perioperative Supplemental Oxygenation

Adequate surgical-site tissue oxygenation is thought to have a role in preventing SSIs. Infected tissue has a lower oxygen tension than non-infected tissue [27]. Administration of high-concentration oxygen (80% FiO_2) provides more adequate oxygenation at the surgical incision and might enhance oxidative killing by neutrophils [28].

Adult patients with normal pulmonary function undergoing general anesthesia with endotracheal intubation for surgical procedures should receive 80% fraction of inspired oxygen intraoperatively [10–12] and, if feasible, in the immediate postoperative period for 2–6 h [10, 11].There is no evidence to recommend an optimal oxygen delivery method or a target oxygenation level.

Maintaining Normothermia

Hypothermia (core temperature < 36 °C) commonly occurs during and after surgical procedures because of the impairment of thermoregulation by anesthetic agents and the exposure to a cold operating room environment. Given evidence that hypothermia is associated with an increased risk of SSI [29], perioperative maintenance of normothermia is strongly recommended [10–12]. There is insufficient evidence to recommend specific strategies to achieve and maintain normothermia, the lower limit of normothermia, or the optimal timing and duration of normothermia for the prevention of SSI.

Maintaining Euvolemia

Fluid imbalance (hypovolemia and hypervolemia) can affect tissue perfusion, leading to decreased tissue oxygenation that might increase the risk of SSI [30]. As such, intraoperative goal-directed fluid therapy is suggested for preventing SSI [11]. There is no evidence to suggest the optimal type of fluid to be administered.

Wound Protectors

Use of an impervious plastic wound protector can prevent SSI in open abdominal surgery [10, 11]. Evidence is strongest for elective colorectal and biliary tract procedures [10].

Antibiotic Sutures

Given evidence of decreased risk of SSI with use of triclosan antibiotic sutures [31], their use is recommended for wound closure [10–12] in any type of surgery [11].

Gloves/Instruments

Double gloving decreases the risk of holes to the inner glove, and so routine double gloving is recommended to protect the surgeon and reduce surgical cross-contamination [32].

Although there is no evidence to support the practice of changing gloves before closure and the use of new instruments, these practices are recommended for colorectal cases, based on expert consensus and evidence supporting bundles that incorporate these practices [33]. Rescrubbing before closure in colorectal cases is not recommended [10].

Adhesive Drapes

Plastic adhesive incise drapes, with or without antimicrobial properties, are not necessary for the prevention of SSI and should not be used [10–12]. Application of microbial sealant immediately after intraoperative skin preparation is not needed.

Incisional Wound Irrigation

Incisional wound irrigation with an aqueous povidone-iodine solution before closure can be considered, as it might have a benefit in reducing SSI, particularly in clean and clean-contaminated wounds [11, 12]. Intraperitoneal lavage with antibacterial solution in contaminated or dirty abdominal procedures is not necessary [12]. Antibiotic incisional wound irrigation before closure should not be used because it is associated with an unnecessary risk of antimicrobial resistance. [11]

Operating Room Ventilation

The air in operating room should be kept at a higher pressure than in corridors and adjacent areas [12]. This positive pressure prevents the flow of air from less sterile areas into the operating room and can help prevent SSI [34].

Laminar (unidirectional) airflow ventilation systems have shown no benefits in reducing SSI and should not be used for patients undergoing total arthroplasty surgery. [11]

Wound Care

No type of advanced dressing should be used over a standard dressing on primarily closed surgical wounds [10]. Use of wound vacuum therapy over stapled skin can reduce SSI in open colorectal (abdominal incision) and vascular (groin incision) cases [10, 11].

It has been common practice to protect closed incisions with a sterile dressing for 24–48 h postoperatively [8, 12] in order to protect the wound from microorganisms and subsequent infection. However, there is no evidence that timing of dressing removal increases SSI risk. Furthermore, early showering (12 h postoperative) does not increase the risk of SSI [10].

Daily probing of closed wounds after contaminated surgery can decrease SSI [10].

Post-hospital Interventions

Adequate SSI surveillance after discharge is very important, as a substantial number of SSIs occur after patients leave the hospital. However, currently there is insufficient research exploring post-hospital discharge interventions to prevent SSI.

Conclusion

Sustained efforts from all healthcare providers and organizational leaders are crucial to prevent SSIs. Guidelines for SSI prevention are important, but their success depends on sound implementation and compliance. Structuring available guidelines in simple bundles of care by multidisciplinary teams, based on institution characteristics and resources, has been shown to improve standardization, automation, and education of staff and patients, ultimately decreasing the rate of SSI.

References

1. Weigelt JA, Lipsky BA, Tabak YP, Derby KG, Kim M, Gupta V. Surgical site infections: causative pathogens and associated outcomes. Am J Infect Control. 2010;38(2):112–20.

2. Klevens RM, Edwards JR, Richards CL Jr, Horan TC, Gaynes RP, Pollock DA, et al. Estimating healthcare-associated infections and deaths in U.S. hospitals, 2002. Public Health Rep. 2007;122:160–6.
3. Zimlichman E, Henderson D, Tamir O, Franz C, Song P, Yamin CK, et al. Health care-associated infections: a meta-analysis of costs and financial impact on the US health care system. JAMA Intern Med. 2013;173(22):2039–46.
4. Merkow RP, Ju MH, Chung JW, Hall BL, Cohen ME, Williams MV, et al. Underlying reasons associated with hospital readmission following surgery in the United States. JAMA. 2015;313(5):483–95.
5. Scott RD. The direct medical costs of healthcare-associated infections in us hospitals and the benefits of prevention. Atlanta: Centers for Disease Control and Prevention; 2009. www.cdc.gov/HAI/pdfs/hai/Scott_CostPaper.pdf. Accessed 12 June 2019.
6. Anderson DJ, Podgorny K, Berríos-Torres SI, Bratzler DW, Dellinger EP, Greene L, et al. Strategies to prevent surgical site infections in acute care hospitals: 2014 update. Infect Control Hosp Epidemiol. 2014;35(6):605–27.
7. Horan TC, Gaynes RP, Martone WJ, Jarvis WR, Emori TG. CDC definitions of nosocomial surgical site infections, 1992: a modification of CDC definitions of surgical wound infections. Infect Control Hosp Epidemiol. 1992;13(10):606–8.
8. Mangram AJ, Horan TC, Pearson ML, Silver LC, Jarvis WR. Guideline for prevention of surgical site infection, 1999. Hospital Infection Control Practices Advisory Committee. Infect Control Hosp Epidemiol. 1999;20:247–78.
9. Howard DH, Scott RD, Packard R, Jones D. The global impact of antibiotic resistance. Clin Infect Dis. 2003;36:S4–S10.
10. Ban KA, Minei JP, Laronga C, Harbrecht BG, Jensen EH, Fry DE, et al. American College of Surgeons and Surgical Infection Society: surgical site infection guidelines, 2016 update. J Am Coll Surg. 2017;224(1):59–74.
11. Allegranzi B, Zayed B, Bischoff P, Kubilay NZ, de Jonge S, de Vries F, et al. New WHO recommendations on intraoperative and postoperative measures for surgical site infection prevention: an evidence-based global perspective. Lancet Infect Dis. 2016;16(12):e288–303.
12. Berrios-Torres SI, Umscheid CA, Bratzler DW, Leas B, Stone EC, Kelz RR, et al. Centers for Disease Control and Prevention guideline for the prevention of surgical site infection, 2017. JAMA Surg. 2017;152(8):784–91.
13. Gupta K, Strymish J, Abi-Haidar Y, Williams SA, Itani KM. Preoperative nasal methicillin-resistant Staphylococcus aureus status, surgical prophylaxis, and risk-adjusted postoperative outcomes in veterans. Infect Control Hosp Epidemiol. 2011;32:791–6.
14. Allareddy V, Das A, Lee MK, Nalliah RP, Rampa S, Allareddy V, et al. Prevalence, predictors, and outcomes of methicillin-resistant Staphylococcus aureus infections in patients undergoing major surgical procedures in the United States: a population-based study. Am J Surg. 2015;210:59–67.
15. Kalra L, Camacho F, Whitener CJ, Du P, Miller M, Zalonis C, et al. Risk of methicillin-resistant *Staphylococcus aureus* surgical site infection in patients with nasal MRSA colonization. Am J Infect Control. 2013;41:1253–7.
16. Bull AL, Worth LJ, Richards MJ. Impact of vancomycin surgical antibiotic prophylaxis on the development of methicillin-sensitive staphylococcus aureus surgical site infections: report from Australian Surveillance Data (VICNISS). Ann Surg. 2012;256:1089–92.
17. Abi-Haidar Y, Gupta K, Strymish J, Williams SA, Itani KM. Factors associated with post-operative conversion to MRSA positivity or infection in initially MRSA-negative patients. Surg Infect. 2011;12:435–42.
18. Toh JWT, Phan K, Hitos K, Pathma-Nathan N, El-Khoury T, Richardson AJ, et al. Association of mechanical bowel preparation and oral antibiotics before elective colorectal surgery with surgical site infection: a network meta-analysis. JAMA Netw Open. 2018;1(6):e183226.

19. Battersby CLF, Battersby NJ, Slade DAJ, Soop M, Walsh CJ. Preoperative mechanical and oral antibiotic bowel preparation to reduce infectious complications of colorectal surgery—the need for updated guidelines. J Hosp Infect. 2019;101(3):295–9.
20. Kiran RP, Murray AC, Chiuzan C, Estrada D, Forde K. Combined preoperative mechanical bowel preparation with oral antibiotics significantly reduces surgical site infection, anastomotic leak, and ileus after colorectal surgery. Ann Surg. 2015;262:416–25.
21. Chen M, Song X, Chen LZ, Lin ZD, Zhang XL. Comparing mechanical bowel preparation with both oral and systemic antibiotics versus mechanical bowel preparation and systemic antibiotics alone for the prevention of surgical site infection after elective colorectal surgery: a meta-analysis of randomized controlled clinical trials. Dis Colon Rectum. 2016;59:70–8.
22. Nelson RL, Gladman E, Barbateskovic M. Antimicrobial prophylaxis for colorectal surgery. Cochrane Database Syst Rev. 2014;5:CD001181.
23. Morris MS, Graham LA, Chu DI, Cannon JA, Hawn MT. Oral antibiotic bowel preparation significantly reduces surgical site infection rates and readmission rates in elective colorectal surgery. Ann Surg. 2015;261:1034–40.
24. Ata A, Lee J, Bestle SL, Desemone J, Stain SC. Postoperative hyperglycemia and surgical site infection in general surgery patients. Arch Surg. 2010;145:858–64.
25. Kao LS, Phatak UR. Glycemic control and prevention of surgical site infection. Surg Infect. 2013;14:437–44.
26. Kotagal M, Symons RG, Hirsch IB, Umpierrez GE, Dellinger EP, Farrokhi ET, et al. Perioperative hyperglycemia and risk of adverse events among patients with and without diabetes. Ann Surg. 2015;261:97–103.
27. Hays RC, Mandell GL. PO2, pH, and redox potential of experimental abscesses. Proc Soc Exp Biol Med. 1974;147:29–30.
28. Allen DB, Maguire JJ, Mahdavian M, Wicke C, Marcocci L, Scheuenstuhl H, et al. Wound hypoxia and acidosis limit neutrophil bacterial killing mechanisms. Arch Surg. 1997;132:991–6.
29. Seamon MJ, Wobb J, Gaughan JP, Kulp H, Kamel I, Dempsey DT. The effects of intraoperative hypothermia on surgical site infection: an analysis of 524 trauma laparotomies. Ann Surg. 2012;255(4):789–95.
30. Silva JM, de Oliveira AM, Nogueira FA, Vianna PM, Pereira Filho MC, Dias LF, et al. The effect of excess fluid balance on the mortality rate of surgical patients: a multicenter prospective study. Crit Care. 2013;17:R288.
31. Nakamura T, Kashimura N, Noji T, Suzuki O, Ambo Y, Nakamura F, et al. Triclosan-coated sutures reduce the incidence of wound infections and the costs after colorectal surgery: a randomized controlled trial. Surgery. 2013;153:576–83.
32. Tanner J, Parkinson H. Double gloving to reduce surgical cross-infection. Cochrane Database Syst Rev. 2006;2006:CD003087.
33. Cima R, Dankbar E, Lovely J, Pendlimari R, Aronhalt K, Nehring S, et al. Colorectal surgery surgical site infection reduction program: a National Surgical Quality Improvement Program-driven multidisciplinary single-institution experience. J Am Coll Surg. 2013;216:23–33.
34. Wenzel RP. Minimizing surgical-site infections. N Engl J Med. 2010;362:75–7.

Perioperative Deep Vein Thrombosis Prophylaxis

7

Mohammad Rachad Wehbe, Charbel F. Matar, Ali Taher, and Jamal J. Hoballah

Introduction

Venous thromboembolism (VTE) is a serious medical pathology associated with significant morbidity and mortality. VTE usually comprises both deep vein thrombosis (DVT) and pulmonary emboli (PE).

DVT can form in the deep veins of upper/lower extremities, the pelvis and, less frequently, in the renal veins, vena cava, and the heart. These thrombi might break down and dislodge to travel within the blood stream as emboli to occlude the pulmonary artery, forming a PE that might be fatal or cause a cryptogenic stroke in the presence of a patent foramen ovale (PFO) [1].

Perioperative prophylaxis against VTE is of utmost importance and is considered a patient-safety measure in most mandates and quality initiatives. Any patient undergoing major surgical intervention with greater than minimal risk should be placed on thromboprophylaxis. This prophylaxis can be achieved using mechanical and/or pharmacological interventions.

M. R. Wehbe
Division of Vascular Surgery, Department of Surgery, University of Rochester, Rochester, NY, USA

C. F. Matar
Department of Internal Medicine, University of Connecticut, Farmington, CT, USA

A. Taher
Division of Hematology and Oncology, Department of Internal Medicine, American University of Beirut Medical Center, Beirut, Lebanon

J. J. Hoballah (✉)
Department of Surgery, American University of Beirut Medical Center, Beirut, Lebanon
e-mail: jh34@aub.edu.lb

J. J. Hoballah et al. (eds.), *Principles of Perioperative Safety and Efficiency*,
https://doi.org/10.1007/978-3-031-41089-5_7

Risk Factors for VTE

As VTE became the third cause of death from cardiovascular origin, identification of the population at risk is one of the most important elements in VTE prophylaxis [2].

Preexisting risk factors for developing VTE include any previous history of VTE, heart failure, COPD, lower limb venous insufficiency, body mass index I > 30 kg/m^2, limb immobility, complete rest over 72 h, nephrotic syndrome, myeloproliferative disorder, pregnancy, inflammatory bowel disease, increasing age, higher American Society of Anesthesiologists (ASA) classification, multiple trauma, and cerebrovascular accidents (ischemic or hemorrhagic). Moreover, having active cancer is considered to be among the highest risk factor, increasing the risk by six-fold compared to non-cancer patients. The risk is particularly high in cancer patients on active treatment (chemotherapy, radiotherapy, hormonal or angiogenesis inhibitors) or those with disease progression [3].

In addition, congenital and acquired thrombophilia alterations as protein C, S, anti-thrombin III deficiencies, hyperhomocysteinemia, elevated antiphospholipid antibodies, factor V Leiden, and prothrombin mutations all place patients at a higher risk for VTE [4].

Although VTE is a common cause of death in surgical patients, it remains a preventable one. The risk of VTE in surgical subpopulations ranges widely from 0.4 to 80%, attributed to variations in the anatomic site of the veins involved, type of operation, and patient comorbidities [5].

Neurosurgical patients are among those in whom the VTE risk is among the highest, at 25%, with the risk of PE specifically reaching 3% and being associated with mortality rates as high as 50%. The expected incidence in moderate-risk neurosurgical patients of distal and proximal DVT is 10%–40% and 2%–8%, respectively, with 1%–8% and 0.1%–4% being for symptomatic and fatal PE, respectively. These figures are increased by a factor of two in high-risk patients [1].

A study by Rogers et al. that evaluated 183,069 patients with vascular or general surgical procedures identified 15 independent variables associated with higher VTE risk [5]. These included patient-related factors (e.g., female gender, higher ASA class, ventilator dependence, preoperative dyspnea, disseminated cancer, chemotherapy within 30 days, and >4 units of packed red blood cell transfusion in the 72 h before operation); preoperative laboratory values (e.g., albumin <3.5 mg/dL, bilirubin >1 mg/dL, sodium >145 mmol/L, and hematocrit <38%); and operative characteristics, for example, (type of surgical procedure, emergency operation, work relative value units, and infected/contaminated wounds). An assessment risk index in general and vascular surgical patients was created based on these factors.

Cancer and venous thromboembolic disease are interrelated. Armand Trosseau was the first to describe the relationship between visceral malignancy and thrombophlebitis as its presenting sign more than 150 years ago. Since then, blood coagulation (bleeding, disseminated intravascular coagulation, and thrombosis) and cancer have been a multidisciplinary challenge for physicians.

DVT in the postoperative period is frequently more in patients treated for malignancy than that in benign disease [6].

Liem et al. studied 372 patients with prior history of DVT who underwent subsequent surgeries. They concluded that perioperative symptomatic recurrence is frequent and related to high-risk procedures (Tables 7.1, 7.2, 7.3, 7.4, and 7.5). They also found that the more time elapsed between a DVT episode and a subsequent surgery, the less was the risk of recurrence [7].

Table 7.1 Surgical procedures classified into lower risk vs higher risk for venous thromboembolism

	Low VTE risk	High VTE risk
Orthopedic	Arthroscopy and arthroscopic surgery	Hip arthroplasty
	Hardware removal	Knee arthroplasty
	Elective spine surgery	Hip fracture surgery
	Lower extremity injuries below knee	Pelvic reconstruction
Neurosurgical	Elective spine surgery	Procedures requiring craniotomy
	Transphenoidal procedures	Surgery for central nervous malignancy
	Shunt procedures	
	Biopsics	
General surgical	Laparoscopic procedures	Open procedures for benign disease >45 min
	Open procedures for benign disease <45 min	Open procedures for malignancy
		Bariatric surgery
Urologic	Cystoscopy	Open surgery for malignancy
	Transurethral surgery	Open prostectomy
	Laparoscopic procedures	Renal surgery/transplantation
		Radical cystectomy
		Pelvic surgery
		Urethral reconstruction
Gynecologic	Laparoscopic procedures	Open surgery for benign disease >30 min
	Open procedures <30 min	Open surgery for malignancy
Head and neck surgical	Open procedures for benign disease <45 min	Open procedures for benign disease >45 min
		Open procedures for malignancy
Other	Aortic and lower extremity arterial reconstruction	Major lower extremity amputations
	Plastic and reconstructive surgery	Open thoracic surgery
		Coronary bypass surgery

VTE Venous thromboembolism

Table 7.2 Risk stratification for VTE in general gastrointestinal and abdominal-pelvic surgery

Risk category	Rogers score	Caprini score	Observed risk of VTE (%)	Estimated baseline risk without prophylaxis (%)
Very low	<7	0	0	<0.5
Low	7–10	1–2	0.7	1.5
Moderate	>10	3–4	1	3
High	NA	5 or >5	1.9	6

NA not applicable, *VTE* venous thromboembolism

Table 7.3 Caprini risk assessment model

One point	Two points	Three points	Five points
Age 41–60 years	Age 61–74 years	Age >75 years	Stroke (<1 month)
Minor surgery	Arthroscopic surgery	History of VTE	Elective arthroplasty
BMI > 25 kg/m^3	Major open surgery (>45 min)	Factor V Leiden	Hip, pelvis, or leg fracture
Swollen legs	Laparoscopic surgery (>45 min)	Lupus anticoagulant	Acute spinal cord injury (<1 month)
Varicose veins	Malignancy	Anticardiolipin antibodies	
Pregnancy or postpartum	Confined to bed (>72 h)	Elevated serum homocysteine	
History of spontaneous abortion	Immobilizing cast	Heparin-induced thrombocytopenia	
Oral contraceptives	Central venous access	Other congenital or acquired thrombophilia	
Sepsis (<1 month)			
COPD, pneumonia (<1 month)			
Abnormal PFTs			
Acute myocardial infarction			
Congestive heart failure			
Inflammatory bowel disease			
Bed rest			

BMI body mass index, *COPD* chronic obstructive pulmonary disease, *PFTs* pulmonary function tests, *VTE* venous thromboembolism

Table 7.4 Risk assessment model from the patient safety in surgery study: Rogers score

General risk factor	Specific risk factor	Risk score points
Operation type	Respiratory	9
	Thoracoabdominal aneurysm	7
	Abdominal aneurysm	4
	Mouth, palate	4
	Stomach, small/large intestine	4
	Integument	3
	Hernia	2
ASA	3, 4, 5	2
	2	1
Female sex		
Work RVU	>17	3
	10–17	2
2 point conditions	Disseminated cancer	2
	Chemotherapy within 30 days	2
	Preoperative serum sodium >145 mmol/L	2
	Transfusion >4 units packed RBCs in 72 h within operation	2
	Ventilator dependent	2
One point conditions	Wound class 3 or 4	1
	Preoperative Hct <38	1
	Preoperative bili >1.0	1
	Dyspnea	1
	Albumin <3.5	1
	Emergency	1
Zero point conditions	ASA class 1	0
	Work RVU <10	0
	Male sex	0

Table 7.5 Types of surgery

Type of surgery	Recommendations		
General surgery	Low-risk bleeding: Pharmacological prophylaxis LMWH/ LDUH	High-risk bleeding: Mechanical thromboprophylaxis (ICD > GCS)	Very high risk for VTE: Combined pharmacological and mechanical prophylaxis
Orthopedic surgery	Total hip or Total knee: preferable DOAC (if not ASA or LMWH)		
Laparoscopic cholecystectomy	If no other VTE risk factors: no prophylaxis		
Neurological surgery	Low risk for VTE: no prophylaxis	High risk for VTE and high risk of bleeding: Mechanical prophylaxis	High risk for VTE and low risk of bleeding: Pharmacological prophylaxis (LMWH)
TURP or radical prostatectomy	If no other VTE risk factors: no prophylaxis		
Vascular surgery	If no other VTE risk factors: no prophylaxis		
Trauma	High risk of bleeding: Mechanical prophylaxis	Low risk of bleeding: Pharmacological prophylaxis (LMWH)	

Basis for VTE Prophylaxis

Most hospitalized patients present with a minimum of one risk factor for VTE, while around 40% of them have three risk factors or more. Without an appropriate prevention, the risk of DVT prevalence ranges from 10 to 80% among medical and surgical patients [8]. Based on the American College of Chest Physicians (ACCP) guidelines, the DVT prevalence among hospitalized patients varies according to their hospitalization: medical patients 10–20%, general surgery 15–40%, major gynecologic surgery 15–40%, neurosurgery 15–40%, stroke 20–50%, hip or knee arthroplasty 40–60%, major trauma 40–80%, spinal cord injury patients 60–80%, and critical care patients 10–80%.

A study done by Zhan et al. looking into 7.45 million American hospital discharges covering 944 acute care hospitals found the VTE (DVT + PE) was among the top five safety indicators causing excess charges, length of stay, and mortality [9].

Moreover, the adverse consequences of unprevented VTE (symptomatic DVT, symptomatic/fatal PE, cost of investigating symptomatic patients, risk and cost of treating unprevented VTE, increased future risk of recurrent VTE and post-thrombotic syndrome) all highlight the importance of thromboprophylaxis in hospitalized patients [10].

The literature over 30 years sums up with concrete evidence that primary VTE prophylaxis is effective and has become a must since PE is regarded as the most common cause of preventable inpatient deaths, causing around 200,000 deaths yearly in the United States alone [11].

Regular use of thromboprophylaxis has been highly effective at preventing VTE and fatal PE, while at the same time has been repeatedly shown to be cost effective [12]. On the other hand, the complications of thromboprophylaxis tend to set minimal or no increase on clinically major bleeding with the use of chemical thromboprophylaxis (LMWH, low-dose UH, warfarin) supported by several meta-analyses and randomized controlled trials (RCTs) [13]. To sum up, VTE prophylaxis has more benefits than risks and is more cost effective when compared to the burden of developing DVT or PE [14].

Risk Category

VTE prophylaxis is one of the key factors of patient safety in the perioperative period. The VTE prophylaxis should be proportionate to the patient's risk. The cause of the patient's admission to medical/surgical and his risk factors will determine his risk category for further prophylaxis. There are numerous VTE risk scores published in the literature. The differences between them are mainly related to efficacy, safety, cost, and ease of implementation. The recent ACCP guidelines assess risk category scores based on two proven methods: the Caprini score and the Rogers score. The Caprini score assigns numerical points for risk factors (1 point to 5 points) and the sum of these points is categorized with the risk as very low (0–1 point), low (2 points), moderate (3–4 points), and high (5 or more points). This scoring system was also validated and recommended support to the use of individual patient VTE risk assessment up to 30 days postoperatively [15]. From this retrospective validation study, the ACCP investigators concluded estimates of the baseline risk of VTE. These estimated risks were as follows: 0.5%—very low, 1.5%—low, 3%—moderate, and 6%—high risk.

On the other hand, the Rogers score was developed after studying data of more than 183,000 patients who underwent vascular, general, or thoracic procedures. From this data, points were assigned to variables that were found to be independent predictors of VTE risk. The Rogers score was then calculated from these points and the estimated risk of VTE was categorized into the following: 0.1%—very low, 0.5%—low, and 1.5% for the moderate score group [5].

Venous Thromboembolism Prophylaxis

Thromboprophylaxis is essential in reducing morbidity and mortality of VTE. VTE pathogenesis depends on three main factors: (1) venous stasis, (2) hypercoagulability, and (3) endothelial damage, which were demonstrated by Rudolph Virchow as "Virchow's triad." Upon closer inspection of this triad, we find that "hypercoagulability" and "stasis" were first described by Richard Weisman, a surgeon to King Charles II around 200 years prior to Virchow, while the third factor "inflammation of the endothelium" was described in 1830 by the founder of hematology, Gabriel Andaral [16].

Based on these findings, preoperative VTE should target factors affecting venous stasis, hypercoagulability, and endothelial damage. Venous stasis disrupts the normal balance of procoagulants and anticoagulants, leading to intravascular thrombus formation. Venous stasis is encountered during bed rest/hospitalization, periods of immobility, and having orthopedic casts. On the other hand, hypercoagulability is a major occurrence after surgery, with extensive hemostatic system alterations beginning 2 days postoperatively—especially in patients with malignancy, inherited and acquired thrombophilia, sepsis, and trauma [17]. Moreover, a damaged endothelium might contribute to Virchow's triad by the inability to provide its anticoagulant and antiplatelet surface diverting hemostasis toward coagulation [18]. This endothelial damage might be due to several factors: direct trauma to major deep veins, iatrogenic injury, encircling tumors, and major orthopedic surgeries.

For all of the above-mentioned factors, VTE prophylaxis is a treatment directed against the Virchow's triad. This prophylaxis can be mechanical or pharmacologic, and used as a single or combined treatment, depending on the patient's risk factors.

Mechanical Methods of Thromboprophylaxis

Adequate but not excessive anesthesia, regional anesthesia, and hydration with early ambulation are the oldest and simplest methods of thromboprophylaxis.

Methods of mechanical thromboprophylaxis include graduated compression stockings (GCS), intermittent pneumatic compression (IPC) of the lower and upper limbs, and foot compression devices. These methods tackle venous stasis by displacing blood from the distal to a more proximal venous system, hence increasing the blood flow (volume and speed) in the deep venous system [19].

These methods, although not studied as extensively as chemoprophylaxis, are acceptable alternatives to anticoagulants in patients with serious bleeding contraindications. They should also be used as adjuncts to chemoprophylaxis in high-VTE risk patients.

These mechanical methods have several advantages and limitations. They might decrease leg swelling and enhance the efficacy of chemoprophylaxis. One drawback is that these mechanical methods were not adequately studied with respect to standards of use (e.g., size, pressure, and physiologic features), and the trials reporting on them were mostly unblinded. They are also not as effective in high-VTE risk groups and their effect on pulmonary emboli and death is still unknown. Finally, the compliance of use by the patients and medical staff is often poor.

Graduated Compression Stockings (GCS)

GCS exert the highest compression pressure at the level of the ankle, which gradually decreases up the stocking. In a systematic review of 18 randomized controlled trials (RCTs) assessing the role of GCS in the prevention of DVT where GCS were used alone or in addition to chemoprophylaxis, DVT developed in 13% with GCS with chemoprophylaxis vs. 26% of those with GCS alone. In the remaining trials where GCS were used in addition to chemoprophylaxis, DVT was found in 4% of those with GCS combined with another method vs. 16% of those given the other method alone. Other reviews stated an incidence reduction of DVT reaching 57% with GCS. These studies prove the efficacy of GCS in low- and moderate-risk patients, but don't prove correct for high-risk patients undergoing malignancy and major orthopedic surgeries.

Nevertheless, several restraints and contraindications of GCS use remain pertinent. These stockings are difficult to wear, especially in large sizes, unusual leg shapes, and dermatitis, thus decreasing patients compliance. They are prohibited from use in patients with peripheral arterial disease and ABIs of <0.8 [20].

Intermittent Pneumatic Compression (IPC)

IPC is the most studied and effective method of mechanical thromboprophylaxis. This method consists of applying a selected pressure through sequential intermittent air insufflation using garments or a specific boot connected to a compressor, thus preventing venous stasis. IPC also works on the coagulation cascade by increasing several factors as prostacyclin, tissue factor pathway inhibitor, and tissue plasminogen activator.

RCTs of a variety of surgical patients (neurosurgical, orthopedic, urologic, and general) show that IPC is more effective as a prophylaxis versus no prophylaxis at all or GCS only. One of the largest stratified meta-analysis of IPC devices looking into data from 16,164 hospitalized patients showed that IPC was more efficient in reducing VTE, with an absolute DVT risk reduction of 9.4%, and PE absolute risk reduction of 1.6%. Additionally, IPC combined with chemical thromboprophylaxis was found to be more efficient than IPC alone.

Similar to GCS, IPC use also has problems with compliance and size fit. They are also contraindicated in patients with peripheral arterial disease. Aside from its contraindications, there are concerns regarding dislodging newly formed venous thrombi in immobilized patients of >72 h after application of IPC. Ultrasound examination prior to application may have a role in this dislodgment prevention, but more studies are required in this aspect.

Recommendations in Surgical Procedures

General Surgery

Recent general surgical procedures' risk without thromboprophylaxis is unknown, due to the lack of such protocols in the present literature. The risk of such procedures is based on older data that reports up to 30% risk of asymptomatic DVT and up to 0.9% risk of a fatal pulmonary embolus in the absence of thromboprophylaxis [21]. Such risk must have decreased in the present general surgical patients due to several factors: earlier mobilization, abidance by thromboprophylaxis protocols, and increase in the number of surgeries done under regional anesthesia. On the other hand, a few factors increase the current risk of general surgical procedures' VTE such as: older patients requiring complicated surgeries, surgeries requiring intraoperative chemotherapy, and earlier discharges lacking accurate postoperative thromboprophylaxis. The type of surgery done remains the most important predictive value for VTE risk. Same-day surgeries are among those with the lowest risk [22]. For example, a study done in Denmark concluded that a day-case hernia surgery doesn't require thromboprophylaxis after looking into the 30-day follow-up data of 2281 patients. In another study, it was found that in the absence of thromboprophylaxis, epidural anesthesia is safer than general anesthesia with respect to postoperative DVT [23].

Major general surgical procedures require routine postoperative thromboprophylaxis, according to data from different RCTs. The routine use of low-dose unfractionated heparin (LDUH) or low molecular weight heparin (LMWH) decreases the risk of VTE by up to 60%. In several trials, LDUH is used as 5000 IU up to 2 h prior to surgery and continued as TID (three times a day) doses for a week postoperatively. Based on indirect comparisons, most literature stated the TID dose was more beneficial than the BID (twice a day) dose. In an overview of results of 46 general surgery randomized trials, the rate of DVT was significantly reduced when using LDUH as thromboprophylaxis versus none, with a decrease from 22 to 9%; odds ratio (OR) 0.3, as were the rates of symptomatic PE from 2 to 1.3%; OR 0.5. But this, on the other hand, was associated with a slight increase in mostly non-major bleeding events' rate from 3.8 to 5.9%; OR 1.6. The rate of major bleeding was stable at 0.3% in both groups [24].

LMWH thromboprophylaxis in general surgical procedures was also studied thoroughly in the literature. Similar to LDUH, LMWH was found to reduce asymptomatic and symptomatic DVT by more than 60% [25]. When it comes to comparing both agents LDUH and LMWH, results in the literature didn't show a significant difference in the rate of symptomatic VTE [26].

Vascular Surgery

The majority of vascular patients are treated intraoperatively with anticoagulants such as heparin or dextran at clamping time to achieve ACT >250. In addition, antiplatelet agents (aspirin and clopidogrel) are used in these patients pre- and postoperatively. These factors play a major role in thromboprophylaxis in this surgical category [27]. Up to 25% of patients suffer from asymptomatic DVT after vascular surgery if the appropriate prophylaxis wasn't given [8]. A study done with 142 consecutive vascular patients for aortic aneurysm repair with pre- and 7- to-10-day postoperative duplex ultrasound after receiving appropriate LDUH prophylaxis and intraoperative sequential compressive device found that 9.8% had postoperative DVT, with a single patient diagnosed with pulmonary embolus. In another study, symptomatic DVT was <1% in a follow-up of up to 30 days' post-abdominal aortic aneurysm repair or lower extremity bypass [28].

Thromboembolic risk appears to be higher in aortic aneurysm repair and aorto-femoral bypass surgeries versus femoro-distal bypass surgery [29]. Moreover, increased age, limb ischemia, and operative time were found to enhance thromboembolic risks in vascular surgery. Few RCTs discussed VTE prophylaxis after arterial surgery. Belch, et al. terminated their randomized double-blind control trial after having bleeding risk outweighing their VTE prophylaxis benefit. In their study, they compared LDUH twice daily vs. placebo in elective aortic bifurcation surgery of 45 patients. Their risk of DVT was higher in the placebo group, 24% vs. 4% [30]. Another study showed no benefit of thromboprophylaxis in 24 vascular surgery patients compared to 25 patients with no prophylaxis [31]. In the last study, 100 vascular patients undergoing aortic surgery were randomized into a group with LDUH and graduated compression stockings versus another with no prophylaxis. In this study, there was no differences between both groups, with each having 2% risk of proximal DVT [32].

Urologic Surgery

VTE is a major concern after major urologic surgical procedures, with symptomatic VTE risks reaching 5%. Increase in patients' risk is seen with open procedures, pelvic surgery, increase in age, lithotomy position intraoperatively, and malignant pathologies. Most of this data in urologic procedures was withdrawn from open prostatectomies. Moreover, several urologic procedures pose a risk of VTE, such as major renal procedures, radical cystectomies, urethral reconstructions, and transplant surgeries that require prophylaxis. The literature poorly addressed VTE in urology patients, with an unknown best practice. Based on this, most patients are being given their prophylaxis according to general and gynecologic surgery prophylaxis guidelines. Low-risk urologic procedures, such as transurethral ones, are advised to provide early postoperative ambulation rather than anticoagulation prophylaxis, due to the higher risk of bleeding. Similarly, laparoscopic urologic procedures face higher risk of bleeding, with thromboprophylaxis data scarce in the literature to give recommendations. Conversely, the group of urologic surgeries with high risk of bleeding is advised to use non-pharmacologic prophylaxis preoperatively, with the addition of LDUH or LMWH postoperatively, once the bleeding risk declines [33].

Bariatric Surgery

Nowadays the number of yearly bariatric operations has increased tremendously for morbidly obese patients. These procedures range from sleeve gastrectomy, biliopancreatic diversion, and Roux-en-Y gastric bypass. The majority of these procedures are done laparoscopically with a minimal postoperative hospital stay. Several studies report thromboembolism complications after bariatric procedures. VTE was reported over an 11-year period for more than 14,000 patients to be less than 0.2% in the National Bariatric Surgery Registry. A different study showed only one PE was found in 2000 consecutive patients undergoing Roux-en-Y gastric bypass in the first month postoperatively [34]. Similarly, a PE rate of 1% among 2011 bariatric surgery patients was shown in 2002, when 69,072 patients underwent morbid obesity surgery, among which 0.34% had VTE after surgical discharge. Deadly PE was detected in 0.2% within 1 month postoperatively after studying more than 5000 patients during a 24-year period [35]. VTE post bariatric surgery is increased in those complicated by a leak, older population, and history of VTE [36]. VTE criteria for bariatric surgery patients are not well known.

There is a single published RCT for VTE prophylaxis in morbid obesity surgery. Sixty consecutive patients undergoing Roux-en-Y gastric bypass were randomized to receive either 0.6 mL or 1.0 mL of nadroparin started pre-operatively and then given once daily postoperatively until discharge. They concluded that 0.6 mL of nadroparin once daily is safe and as effective in prophylaxis of VTE as the higher dose of 1 mL.

In another RCT, 164 patients scheduled for gastric bypass were divided into three groups depending on the dose of enoxaparin received: 4000, 6000, or twice the 4000 IU. The objective was to determine the best regimen of enoxaparin providing an antifactor Xa peak activity between 0.3 and 0.5 IU/mL and to evaluate the course of procoagulant microparticles (MPs). At the end of this study, they concluded that a once-daily dose of 6000 IU/day allowed the majority of the patients to sustain the target range of antifactor Xa activity without increasing the bleeding risk [37].

Due to the small number of studies tackling VTE in bariatric surgery, some studies came across a regimen of low-dose continuous intravenous heparin as VTE prophylaxis with an outcome of low VTE and bleeding. This practice still lacks any randomized controlled trials. Due to the scarcity of data among VTE prophylaxis in bariatric surgery patients, their guidelines are also extrapolated from high-risk general surgery patients.

Thoracic Surgery

Undervalued VTE risk in thoracic surgery is attributed to the low number of RCTs reporting this issue. The majority of thoracic surgery patients have multiple VTE risk factors such as old age, cancer, or decreased postoperative mobility. The risk of PE after major thoracic operations is up to 5.2%, with a risk of mortality post major thoracic surgery reaching 1.3% [38]. The rate of DVT could be as high as 14% if screening duplex ultrasounds are used. The National Surgical Quality Improvement Program diagnosed 1.6% of 13,000 patients undergoing lung resection with symptomatic DVT [28]. Pneumonectomy for malignancy with appropriate VTE prophylaxis of IPC and LDUH reported 7.4% symptomatic VTE in a retrospective review. In an RCT comparing the common dose of heparin prophylaxis 5000 U twice daily versus a higher dose of 7500 U twice daily in 100 consecutive patients having thoracotomies for lung or esophageal cancer, it was found that the 7500 U heparin doesn't significantly provide more prophylaxis compared to the lower 5000 U dose (22% versus 33% total DVT), but had significant less extensive DVT (0% versus 4% for popliteal DVT). Moreover, no postoperative excessive bleeding was noted in either treatment group. In another RCT, 150 lung cancer resection patients were allocated to two groups and followed up with routine duplex US at postoperative day eight. The first group received a fixed low dose of Fraxiparine while the second group received two higher doses in accordance with weight. This study concluded no significant difference of prophylaxis safety between the two groups; however, there was a non-significant higher bleeding risk with the higher dose of Fraxiparine.

VTE prophylaxis in thoracic surgery also lacks major definitive studies. According to the ACCP guidelines, patients undergoing major thoracic surgery require routine thromboprophylaxis with LMWH, LDUH, or fondaparinux, while those with high risk of bleeding are recommended to have mechanical thromboprophylaxis only.

Coronary Artery Bypass Graft (CABG) Surgery

All cardiac bypass surgeries are done under systemic anticoagulation with heparin, which almost eliminates the risk of thrombus formation intraoperatively. Furthermore, these patients are prescribed postoperative antiplatelet therapy (aspirin and/or clopidogrel) with possible oral anticoagulation, which makes the need for VTE prophylaxis debatable [39]. Data in this group of patients lacks RCTs and most of the guidelines are extrapolated from retrospective studies that lack VTE prophylaxis accuracy of dosage, results, and duration and entirety of patient-pool follow-up. Routine follow-up duplex ultrasound (US) post-CABG show that asymptomatic DVT can be diagnosed in up to 48% of cases [40]. In a RCT comparing two mechanical thromboprophylaxis methods, asymptomatic DVT among 330 patients was found in 19% in patients assigned IPC with GCS versus 22% assigned stockings alone [41]. Another study looked into serial leg venous ultrasounds of 270 CABG patients from 19 cardiac surgery units upon admission to three rehabilitative centers. The rate of proximal DVT was found to be 2.6%, while that of isolated distal DVT was 14.8%. Half of these DVT cases were found in the leg contralateral to the saphenous vein harvest site, leading to the conclusion that the use of unilateral GCS post-CABG is of limited efficacy.

These incidences are less for symptomatic DVT <0.5%, symptomatic PE <3.9%, and <0.7% for fatal PE. When a retrospective cohort of 10,638 patients was studied post open-heart surgery, only 0.7% had symptomatic DVT within 10 days postoperatively [42]. Similarly, this number remains low for a PE risk that was found in 0.6% of 5694 patients within 60 days post open-heart surgery. Predictors of PE included prolonged hospital stay, cardiac catheterization within 15 days of surgery, and congestive heart failure. In another retrospective cohort, 500 off-pump coronary artery operations were done with no prophylaxis, and resulted in 1% thromboembolic complications, which caused death of one patient. This study concluded that VTE complications in off-pump CABG operations are comparable to those with cardiopulmonary bypass [43].

With all previous study conclusions, it remains unclear whether VTE routine prophylaxis is required for all CABG patients. Patients at high risk of late mobility and prolonged length of stay should likely receive pharmacologic thromboprophylaxis with LMWH, LDUH, or bilateral mechanical thromboprophylaxis. LMWH is preferred in coronary artery bypass surgery over LDUH as a pharmacologic VTE prophylaxis. This holds true due to the fact the coronary artery bypass surgery is associated with higher risk of heparin-induced thrombocytopenia (HIT) and so is LDUH.

Neurosurgery

Major neurosurgical procedures are also associated with a DVT risk, which requires a form of VTE prophylaxis. Several characteristics pose a higher risk for VTE, including: longer time procedures, intracerebral procedures, lower extremity weakness, cancer, and older patients. Patients with cancerous brain tumors are especially at a higher risk of VTE both perioperatively and after discharge [44]. In a retrospective review of 264 malignant glioma patients who did not receive any form of thromboprophylaxis, 36% of patients developed DVT within 6 weeks of craniotomy [45]. An RCT of neurosurgical patients indicated that mechanical thromboprophylaxis from GCS by itself or in conjunction with IPC can decrease the risk from 20 to 9% [46]. In another RCT, a statistically significant decrease in DVT incidence from 34 to 6% was detected in 110 elective neurosurgical patients with the use of heparin prophylaxis [47]. Another RCT of 485 patients that studied the efficacy of

LMWH and GCS started in the postoperative period versus GCS as thromboprophylaxis in neurosurgical patients. This study showed a relative risk reduction of 28.9% of VTE between the two groups, concluding that LMWH added to GCS postoperatively leads to a significant decrease in VTE rates versus GCS alone, and with no significant increase of major intracranial bleed [48]. Goldhaber et al. in a RCT studied 150 patients undergoing craniotomy for malignancy randomized to either enoxaparin, 40 mg/day, or LDUH 5000 U bid in addition to GCS, IPC, and venous US to lower extremities pre-discharge. Their study resulted in no symptomatic DVT or PE, an asymptomatic VTE rate of 9.3%, and no statistically significant difference between the different types of pharmacologic prophylaxis [49]. Hamilton et al. conducted a systematic review evaluating six RCTs for VTE prophylaxis in neurosurgical craniotomy patients. A statistically significant reduction was identified in five of six RCTs of symptomatic and asymptomatic VTE with heparin prophylaxis. They also concluded that heparin prophylaxis decreases the risk of VTE but may also increase bleeding risks with a ratio of major or symptomatic thromboembolism relative to serious bleeding, which is only slightly favorable [50]. Recently, the American Society of Hematology (ASH) published their VTE recommendations where the panel agreed against the use of pharmacological thromboprophylaxis due to the high major bleeding risk. However, they also added that anticoagulation may be considered for a special subset of patients, especially those who have prolonged immobility after surgery or have lower risk of major bleeding.

To summarize, mechanical thromboprophylaxis, mainly IPC, is recommended in elective craniotomies. IPC in conjunction with thromboprophylaxis appears to be highly efficacious if feasible. In most practices, IPC is started solely perioperatively to be followed by a pharmacologic thromboprophylaxis postoperatively, provided that postoperative imaging is negative for bleeding [51].

Trauma

The incidence of VTE post major trauma is the highest among inpatients. In the absence of prophylaxis, it can be as high as 80%. Delay of thromboprophylaxis is usually attributed to injury-associated bleeding risks. In a multicenter prospective cohort of 315 patients, a delay of prophylaxis start was associated with three-fold increase of VTE risk [52]. The risk of DVT in trauma patients is increased due to several factors: spinal cord trauma, spinal injuries, increased age, pelvic trauma, requirement of surgical operation, delay in thromboprophylaxis initiation, and restoration of major veins [51].

In a prospective trial of 400 patients, sequential gradient pneumatic leg compression (SCD) was found to be more effective than control as DVT thromboprophylaxis [53]. On the contrary, compliance issues limit SCD use in trauma patients, with an inability to use in up to 30% of patients due to leg trauma and improper use by both the nursing staff and patients [54]. Mechanical thromboprophylaxis can still be recommended in bleeding trauma patients with a therapeutic anticoagulation contraindication, as they were shown to significantly decrease the risk of asymptomatic DVT in patients with acute bleeds [55].

In a meta-analysis by Velmahos et al. there was no evidence that LDUH, LMWH was better than the other or even to no prophylaxis [51]. In a double-blinded RCT of 344 trauma patients with injury severity score of at least nine, and in the absence of intracranial bleed, patients were randomly assigned to LMWH versus LDUH subcutaneously every 12 h. In this study, Geerts et al. concluded that LMWH was significantly more effective than LDUH in VTE prophylaxis post vital trauma. Both interventions were similarly safe, with a bleeding risk of less than 2% [56]. In another RCT of 442 trauma patients receiving either IPC device or LMWH as thromboprophylaxis, proximal DVT and PE were seen in 3% of the IPC group and 1% of the LMWH group upon weekly follow-up with duplex US. In this study, the rate of major bleeding was again less than 2% [57]. In a prospective randomized comparison of 200 patients, Stannard et al. found significantly less VTE among trauma patients who were treated on admission with foot pumps with the addition of LMWH on a delayed basis versus those treated with LMWH alone within 24–48 h of admission [58]. In a review study of 2169 patients, Bandle et al. concluded that venous duplex surveillance of DVT is warranted in highest risk groups versus moderate-risk trauma patients [59]. In addition, a study by Allen et al. of 1218 trauma patients showed that venous duplex ultrasound surveillance with early DVT management had decreased rates of PE [60]. While the best duration of thromboprophylaxis in trauma patients is not clear, the recommended VTE prophylaxis should usually continue until hospital or rehabilitation discharge. If this period takes longer than 14 days, then the preferred method should be with an LMWH [61].

Orthopedic Surgery

Postoperative risk of deep vein thrombosis in orthopedic surgery remains one of the highest among other surgical fields. Similar to any surgical field, the risk of DVT in orthopedic surgical patients varies according to the risk of the procedure itself, be it total hip arthroplasty (THA), total knee arthroplasty (TKA), or pelvic surgery, which are considered higher risk than upper extremity (hand, elbow, and shoulder surgery) or lower extremity (foot, ankle, and tibial surgery). The higher risk surgery is mainly due to the venous stasis caused by immobility, reflected by positioning of these patients and the risk of endothelial venous injury. There is paucity of data tackling thromboprophylaxis in minor-risk orthopedic surgery, and most of the guidelines and literature are derived from major orthopedic surgery in higher risk older patient population groups undergoing TKA and THA. Both the American College of Chest Physicians and the American Academy of Orthopedic Surgeons support prophylaxis recommendation in the high-risk orthopedic surgery patient population.

A retrospective database review by Bawa et al. of 239,949 patients with anticoagulant prescription medications undergoing THA and TKA between 2004 and 2013, found that patients with a hypercoagulable diagnosis had statistically significant higher DVT rates within 6 months of major orthopedic TKA or THA surgeries [62].

In another review by Hirsh et al. aspirin was found to be more effective than placebo and less effective than LMWH in preventing VTE, especially pulmonary emboli, in high-risk orthopedic surgery patients [63].

Fondaparinux was found to be more effective in VTE prophylaxis vs. LMWH, but it was associated with a higher risk of bleeding; this was demonstrated by a Cochrane study by Zhu et al. that reviewed 21,004 patients [64].

On the other hand, unfractionated heparin in high-risk orthopedic surgery (typically given as 5000 IU subcutaneously twice daily) vs. LMWH was found to be less effective in VTE prophylaxis with a similar risk of bleeding. Hill et al. illustrated this in a meta-analysis with a study population of more than 3000 patients [65].

In the ninth edition of the Chest guidelines, several ranging from grade IB to 2C were published. The use of antithrombotic agent prophylaxis was recommended in high-risk THA or TKA, but not in hip fracture surgery (HFS) for a minimum of 10–14 days. The agents that can be used include LMWH, fondaparinux, dabigatran, apixaban, rivaroxaban, LDUH, adjusted-dose vitamin K antagonist, and aspirin. All of those were grade IB evidence vs. IC evidence for IPC devices. LMWH was preferred over other agents with grade 2C/2B evidence. VTE prophylaxis extension up to 35 days postoperatively was suggested as a grade 2B recommendation. The guidelines recommended against the use of IVC filter placement as a modality of primary prevention in patients with contraindication to mechanical and pharmacologic thromboprophylaxis graded 2C, and against the use of non-invasive duplex studies as a screening tool before hospital discharge, with a grade IB evidence [66].

Conclusion

In conclusion, VTE is a potentially devastating and life-threatening complication seen in patients undergoing surgeries. Thromboprophylaxis should be considered in all patients undergoing surgeries that carry higher than minimal risk. The type of thromboprophylaxis and its duration should be addressed based on the type of the surgical procedure as well as the risk of associated bleeding.

References

1. Chibbaro S, Cebula H, Todeschi J, Fricia M, Vigouroux D, Abid H, et al. Evolution of prophylaxis protocols for venous thromboembolism in neurosurgery: results from a prospective comparative study on low-molecular-weight heparin, elastic stockings, and intermittent pneumatic compression devices. World Neurosurg. 2018;109:e510–6.
2. Bottaro FJ, Ceresetto JM, Emery J, Bruetman J, Emery N, Pellegrini D, et al. Cross-sectional study of adherence to venous thromboembolism prophylaxis guidelines in hospitalized patients. The Trombo-Brit study. Thromb J. 2012;10(1):7.
3. Donellan E, Kevane B, Healey Bird BR, Ni Ailne F. Cancer and venous thromboembolic disease: from molecular mechanisms to clinical management. Curr Oncol. 2014;21(3):134–43.
4. Cosmi B, Legnani C, Tosetto A, Pengo V, Ghirarduzzi A, Testa S, et al. Usefulness of repeated D-dimer testing after stopping anticoagulation for a first episode of unprovoked venous thromboembolism: the PROLONG II prospective study. Blood. 2010;115(3):481–8.

5. Rogers SO Jr, Kilaru RK, Hosokawa P, Henderson WG, Zinner MJ, Khuri SF. Multivariable predictors of postoperative venous thromboembolic events after general and vascular surgery: results from the patient safety in surgery study. J Am Coll Surg. 2007;204(6):1211–21.
6. Donati MB. Cancer and thrombosis. Haemostasis. 1994;24(2):128–31.
7. Liem TK, Huynh TM, Moseley SE, Minjarez RC, Landry GJ, Mitchell EL, et al. Symptomatic perioperative venous thromboembolism is a frequent complication in patients with a history of deep vein thrombosis. J Vasc Surg. 2010;52(3):651–7.
8. Geerts WH, Pineo GF, Heit JA, Bergqvist D, Lassen MR, Colwell CW, et al. Prevention of venous thromboembolism: the seventh ACCP conference on antithrombotic and thrombolytic therapy. Chest. 2004;126(3 Suppl):338S–400S.
9. Zhan C, Miller MR. Excess length of stay, charges, and mortality attributable to medical injuries during hospitalization. JAMA. 2003;290(14):1868–74.
10. Geerts WH, Bergqvist D, Pineo GF, Heit JA, Samama CM, Lassen MR, et al. Prevention of venous thromboembolism: American College of Chest Physicians evidence-based clinical practice guidelines (8th edition). Chest. 2008;133(6 Suppl):381S–453S.
11. Laryea J, Champagne B. Venous thromboembolism prophylaxis. Clin Colon Rectal Surg. 2013;26(3):153–9.
12. Sullivan SD, Kahn SR, Davidson BL, Borris L, Bossuyt P, Raskob G. Measuring the outcomes and pharmacoeconomic consequences of venous thromboembolism prophylaxis in major orthopaedic surgery. Pharmacoeconomics. 2003;21(7):477–96.
13. Koch A, Ziegler S, Breitschwerdt H, Victor N. Low molecular weight heparin and unfractionated heparin in thrombosis prophylaxis: meta-analysis based on original patient data. Thromb Res. 2001;102(4):295–309.
14. Nicolaides AN, Fareed J, Kakkar AK, Comerota AJ, Goldhaber SZ, Hull R, et al. Prevention and treatment of venous thromboembolism—International Consensus Statement. Int Angiol. 2013;32(2):111–260.
15. Bahl V, Hu HM, Henke PK, Wakefield TW, Campbell DA Jr, Caprini JA. A validation study of a retrospective venous thromboembolism risk scoring method. Ann Surg. 2010;251(2):344–50.
16. Kumar DR, Hanlin E, Glurich I, Mazza JJ, Yale SH. Virchow's contribution to the understanding of thrombosis and cellular biology. Clin Med Res. 2010;8(3–4):168–72.
17. Lison S, Weiss G, Spannagl M, Heindl B. Postoperative changes in procoagulant factors after surgery. Blood Coagul Fibrinolysis. 2011;22(3):190–6.
18. Blann AD. How a damaged blood vessel wall contributes to thrombosis and hypertension. Pathophysiol Haemost Thromb. 2003–2004;33(5–6):445–8.
19. Tamowicz B, Mikstacki A, Urbanek T, Zawilska K. Mechanical methods of venous thromboembolism prevention: from guidelines to clinical practice. Pol Arch Intern Med. 2019;129(5):335–41.
20. Sachdeva A, Dalton M, Lees T. Graduated compression stockings for prevention of deep venous thrombosis. Cochrane Database Syst Rev. 2018;11(11):CD001484.
21. Clagett GP, Reisch JS. Prevention of venous thromboembolism in general surgical patients. Results of meta-analysis. Ann Surg. 1988;208(2):227–40.
22. Enoch S, Woon E, Blair SD. Thromboprophylaxis can be omitted in selected patients undergoing varicose vein surgery and hernia repair. Br J Surg. 2003;90(7):818–20.
23. Riber C, Alstrup N, Nymann T, Bogstad JW, Wille-Jørgensen P, Tønnesen H. Postoperative thromboembolism after day-case herniorrhaphy. Br J Surg. 1996;83(3):420–1.
24. Collins R, Scrimgeour A, Yusuf S, Peto R. Reduction in fatal pulmonary embolism and venous thrombosis by perioperative administration of subcutaneous heparin. Overview of results of randomized trials in general, orthopedic, and urologic surgery. N Engl J Med. 1988;318(18):1162–73.
25. Mismetti P, Laporte S, Darmon JY, Buchmüller A, Decousus H. Meta-analysis of low molecular weight heparin in the prevention of venous thromboembolism in general surgery. Br J Surg. 2001;88(7):913–30.
26. Bergqvist D. Low molecular weight heparin for the prevention of venous thromboembolism after abdominal surgery. Br J Surg. 2004;91(8):965–74.

27. Collins TC, Souchek J, Beyth RJ. Benefits of antithrombotic therapy after infrainguinal bypass grafting: a meta-analysis. Am J Med. 2004;117(2):93–9.
28. Gangireddy C, Rectenwald JR, Upchurch GR, Wakefield TW, Khuri S, Henderson WG, et al. Risk factors and clinical impact of postoperative symptomatic venous thromboembolism. J Vasc Surg. 2007;45(2):335–41; discussion 341–2.
29. Hollyoak M, Woodruff P, Muller M, Daunt N, Weir P. Deep venous thrombosis in post-operative vascular surgical patients: a frequent finding without prophylaxis. J Vasc Surg. 2001;34(4):656–60.
30. Belch JJ, Lowe GD, Pollock JG, Forbes CD, Prentice CR. Low dose heparin in the prevention of deep-vein thrombosis after aortic bifurcation graft surgery. Thromb Haemost. 1980;42(5):1429–33.
31. Spebar MJ, Collins GJ Jr, Rich NM, Kang IY, Clagett GP, Salander JM. Perioperative heparin prophylaxis of deep venous thrombosis in patients with peripheral vascular disease. Am J Surg. 1981;142(6):649–50.
32. Killewich LA, Aswad MA, Sandager GP, Lilly MP, Flinn WR. A randomized, prospective trial of deep venous thrombosis prophylaxis in aortic surgery. Arch Surg. 1997;132(5):499–504.
33. Ljungström KG. Is there a need for antithromboembolic prophylaxis during laparoscopic surgery? Not always. J Thromb Haemost. 2005;3(2):212–3.
34. Prystowsky JB, Morasch MD, Eskandari MK, Hungness ES, Nagle AP. Prospective analysis of the incidence of deep venous thrombosis in bariatric surgery patients. Surgery. 2005;138(4):759–63; discussion 763–5.
35. Sapala JA, Wood MH, Schuhknecht MP, Sapala MA. Fatal pulmonary embolism after bariatric operations for morbid obesity: a 24-year retrospective analysis. Obes Surg. 2003;13(6):819–25.
36. Gonzalez R, Haines K, Nelson LG, Gallagher SF, Murr MM. Predictive factors of thromboembolic events in patients undergoing Roux-en-Y gastric bypass. Surg Obes Relat Dis. 2006;2(1):30–5; discussion 35–6.
37. Steib A, Degirmenci S-E, Junke E, Asehnoune K, Figier M, Pericard C, et al. Once versus twice daily injection of enoxaparin for thromboprophylaxis in bariatric surgery: effects on antifactor Xa activity and procoagulant microparticles. A randomized controlled study. Surg Obes Relat Dis. 2016;12(3):613–21.
38. Ziomek S, Read RC, Tobler HG, Harrell JE Jr, Gocio JC, Fink LM, et al. Thromboembolism in patients undergoing thoracotomy. Ann Thorac Surg. 1993;56(2):223–6; discussion 227.
39. Goldhaber SZ, Schoepf UJ. Pulmonary embolism after coronary artery bypass grafting. Circulation. 2004;109(22):2712–5.
40. Ambrosetti M, Salerno M, Zambelli M, Mastropasqua F, Tramarin R, Pedretti RFE. Deep vein thrombosis among patients entering cardiac rehabilitation after coronary artery bypass surgery. Chest. 2004;125(1):191–6.
41. Goldhaber SZ, Hirsch DR, MacDougall RC, Polak JF, Creager MA, Cohn LH. Prevention of venous thrombosis after coronary artery bypass surgery (a randomized trial comparing two mechanical prophylaxis strategies). Am J Cardiol. 1995;76(14):993–6.
42. DeLaria GA, Hunter JA. Deep venous thrombosis. Implications after open heart surgery. Chest. 1991;99(2):284–8.
43. Cartier R, Robitaille D. Thrombotic complications in beating heart operations. J Thorac Cardiovasc Surg. 2001;121(5):920–2.
44. Simanek R, Vormittag R, Hassler M, Roessler K, Schwarz M, Zielinski C, et al. Venous thromboembolism and survival in patients with high-grade glioma. Neuro Oncol. 2007;9(2):89–95.
45. Ruff RL, Posner JB. Incidence and treatment of peripheral venous thrombosis in patients with glioma. Ann Neurol. 1983;13(3):334–6.
46. Turpie AG, Hirsh J, Gent M, Julian D, Johnson J. Prevention of deep vein thrombosis in potential neurosurgical patients: a randomized trial comparing graduated compression stockings alone or graduated compression stockings plus intermittent pneumatic compression with control. Arch Intern Med. 1989;149(3):679–81.
47. Cerrato D, Ariano C, Fiacchino F. Deep vein thrombosis and low-dose heparin prophylaxis in neurosurgical patients. J Neurosurg. 1978;49(3):378–81.

48. Nurmohamed MT, van Riel AM, Henkens CM, Koopman MM, Que GT, d'Azemar P, et al. Low molecular weight heparin and compression stockings in the prevention of venous thromboembolism in neurosurgery. Thromb Haemost. 1996;75(2):233–8.
49. Goldhaber SZ, Dunn K, Gerhard-Herman M, Park JK, McL Black P. Low rate of venous thromboembolism after craniotomy for brain tumor using multimodality prophylaxis. Chest. 2002;122(6):1933–7.
50. Hamilton MG, Yee WH, Hull RD, Ghali WA. Venous thromboembolism prophylaxis in patients undergoing cranial neurosurgery: a systematic review and meta-analysis. Neurosurgery. 2011;68(3):571–81.
51. Velmahos GC, Kern J, Chan LS, Murray JA, Shekelle P. Prevention of venous thromboembolism after injury: an evidence-based report—part II: analysis of risk factors and evaluation of the role of vena cava filters. J Trauma. 2000;49(1):140–4.
52. Nathens AB, McMurray MK, Cuschieri J, Durr EA, Moore EE, Bankey PE, et al. The practice of venous thromboembolism prophylaxis in the major trauma patient. J Trauma. 2007;62(3):557–62; discussion 562–3.
53. Knudson MM, Lewis FR, Clinton A, Atkinson K, Megerman J. Prevention of venous thromboembolism in trauma patients. J Trauma. 1994;37(3):480–7.
54. Murakami M, McDill TL, Cindrick-Pounds L, Loran DB, Woodside KJ, Mileski WJ, et al. Deep venous thrombosis prophylaxis in trauma: improved compliance with a novel miniaturized pneumatic compression device. J Vasc Surg. 2003;38(5):923–7.
55. Lacut K, Bressollette L, Le Gal G, Etienne E, De Tinteniac A, Renault A, et al. Prevention of venous thrombosis in patients with acute intracerebral hemorrhage. Neurology. 2005;65(6):865–9.
56. Geerts WH, Jay RM, Code KI, Chen E, Szalai JP, Saibil EA, et al. A comparison of low-dose heparin with low-molecular-weight heparin as prophylaxis against venous thromboembolism after major trauma. N Engl J Med. 1996;335(10):701–7.
57. Ginzburg E, Cohn SM, Lopez J, Jackowski J, Brown M, Hameed SM, et al. Randomized clinical trial of intermittent pneumatic compression and low molecular weight heparin in trauma. Br J Surg. 2003;90(11):1338–44.
58. Stannard JP, Lopez-Ben RR, Volgas DA, Anderson ER, Busbee M, Karr DK, et al. Prophylaxis against deep-vein thrombosis following trauma: a prospective, randomized comparison of mechanical and pharmacologic prophylaxis. J Bone Joint Surg Am. 2006;88(2):261–6.
59. Bandle J, Shackford SR, Kahl JE, Sise CB, Calvo RY, Shackford MC, et al. The value of lower-extremity duplex surveillance to detect deep vein thrombosis in trauma patients. J Trauma Acute Care Surg. 2013;74(2):575–80.
60. Allen CJ, Murray CR, Meizoso JP, Ginzburg E, Schulman CI, Lineen EB, et al. Surveillance and early management of deep vein thrombosis decreases the rate of pulmonary embolism in high-risk trauma patients. J Am Coll Surg. 2016;222(1):65–72.
61. Bridges GG, Lee MD, Jenkins JK, Stephens MA, Croce MA, Fabian TC. Expedited discharge in trauma patients requiring anticoagulation for deep venous thrombosis prophylaxis: the LEAP program. J Trauma. 2003;54(2):232–5.
62. Bawa H, Weick JW, Dirschl DR, Luu HH. Trends in deep vein thrombosis prophylaxis and deep vein thrombosis rates after total hip and knee arthroplasty. J Am Acad Orthop Surg. 2018;26:698–705.
63. Karthikeyan G, Eikelboom JW, Turpie AGG, Hirsh J. Does acetyl salicylic acid (ASA) have a role in prevention of venous thromboembolism? Br J Haematol. 2009;146(2):142–9.
64. Dong K, Song Y, Li X, Ding J, Gao Z, Lu D, et al. Pentasaccharides for the prevention of venous thromboembolism. Cochrane Database Syst Rev. 2016;10(10):CD005134.
65. Hill J, Treasure T. National Clinical Guideline Centre for Acute and Chronic Conditions. Reducing the risk of venous thromboembolism in patients admitted to hospital: summary of NICE guidance. BMJ. 2010;340:c95.
66. Bates SM, Jaeschke R, Stevens SM, Goodacre S, Wells PS, Stevenson MD, et al. Diagnosis of DVT: antithrombotic therapy and prevention of thrombosis, 9th ed: American College of Chest Physicians evidence-based clinical practice guidelines. Chest. 2012;141(2 Suppl):e351S–418S.

8 Handling Pacemakers and Implantable Cardioverter Defibrillators in the Operating Room

Mohammad Sabra and Marwan M. Refaat

Introduction

The current estimated prevalence of conventional pacemakers in the United States is estimated at three million, with more than 30,000 patients having implantable cardioverter defibrillator (ICD) with pacing abilities [1, 2]. The increased use of cardiac implantable electronic devices (CIEDs) raises the importance of perioperative safety and management of those devices when patients present for any procedure. The establishment of perioperative care algorithms for patients with CIEDs is complex due to several factors that include: different programming abilities of currently manufactured devices, presence of older devices in some patients, continuing advancements in CIED technology (such as the leadless pacing and subcutaneous defibrillation technology), and confusion concerning the difference between pacemakers and ICDs, including their various response to magnetic fields [3].

Guidelines for the perioperative management of CIEDs have been established by several professional societies, such as Heart Rhythm Society, American Society of Anesthesiologists, and British Heart Rhythm Society. Those recommendations are being universally used in the management of CIED in patients at risk for interference during their procedures.

M. Sabra
Department of Internal Medicine/Division of Cardiology, Henry Ford Health, Detroit, MI, USA

M. M. Refaat (✉)
Department of Internal Medicine/ Division of Cardiology, American University of Beirut, Faculty of Medicine and Medical Center (AUBMC), Beirut, Lebanon

Department of Biochemistry and Molecular Genetics, American University of Beirut Faculty of Medicine, Beirut, Lebanon
e-mail: mr48@aub.edu.lb; marwanrefaat@alumni.harvard.edu

J. J. Hoballah et al. (eds.), *Principles of Perioperative Safety and Efficiency*,
https://doi.org/10.1007/978-3-031-41089-5_8

Sources of Interference

There are two major sources of interference of CIEDs: electromagnetic and mechanical.

Electromagnetic Interference

Electromagnetic interference (EMI) refers to the potential disruption of the operation of an electronic device when it is near an electromagnetic field generated by an external source. EMI is likely when there is planned use of an electrosurgery unit (ESU) superior to the umbilicus and is potentially problematic in patients with an ICD and in patients who are pacing-dependent. In addition, CIEDs with unipolar pacing are more vulnerable to EMI than those with bipolar pacing [4].

The function of CIED can be affected by EMI. The clinical responses depend on the device (pacemaker or ICD) and the patient (pacemaker-dependent or not). These responses include:

- Inappropriate inhibition of pacing in a pacing-dependent patient leading to asystole. All CIEDs sense ventricular intracardiac activity through electrodes. EMI in the ventricular channel of an electrode can be sensed and misinterpreted as "intrinsic" ventricular activity (oversensing), which causes an inhibition of pacing. This could lead to asystole in a pacing-dependent patient [5].
- Delivery of inappropriate anti-tachycardia therapy (pacing or shock) by an ICD due to misinterpretation of EMI as tachyarrhythmia.
- Direct damage to the CIED, causing malfunction and inability to deliver appropriate shocks.
- Misinterpretation of EMI as atrial signals, leading to maximum ventricular pacing (inappropriate tracking) in a dual chamber pacemaker.
- Switching of the device to the "power-on reset" mode due to large amount of EMI identified by the device. This can be thought of as the basic, manufacturer-set functions of the device similar to "reset to factory settings" on electronic devices.
- Total device failure may occur in older devices. When there is a possibility of device failure in a pacing-dependent patient, an alternate pacing modality should be used.
- Triggering an active sensor for rate-responsive pacing, causing pacing in an upper desirable rate and an unfavorable tachycardia.

EMI Caused by ESUs

EMI is most commonly generated from ESU during a surgical procedure. For example, monopolar electrosurgery causes more EMI than bipolar electrosurgery, and coagulation (high-voltage) generates more EMI than the non-blended cutting (low-voltage). The probability of EMI by ESU is correlated to the distance from the pulse generator or the electrodes of the CIED. As the distance increases, the risk of EMI decreases. The risk is highest when performing surgical procedures superior to the umbilicus [6].

EMI Caused by Other Surgical or Anesthetic Equipment

In addition to the surgical equipment, other sources of EMI can be: transcutaneous electrical nerve stimulation units, lithotripsy, radiofrequency ablation devices, and nerve stimulators for nerve blocks.

Mechanical Interference

Mechanical interference refers to the potential disruption of the operation of an electronic device by external mechanical operations.

Guidewires During Central Venous Catheter Insertion

During the insertion of a central venous catheter, mechanical interference through the guidewires can lead to adverse outcomes. For example, ventricular oversensing may occur, leading to the delivery of inappropriate shock or the inhibition of pacing in a pacing-dependent patient. Physical contact between the guidewire and the right ventricular pacing electrode may cause electrical short circuit with irreversible damage to the CIED [7].

Bone Saws

Bone saws can cause mechanical interference with CIED through vibration.

Preoperative Assessment

Before an elective procedure, a multidisciplinary team that includes the cardiac or cardiac electrophysiology team, the anesthesiology team, and the surgical team is required in the preoperative assessment. The goal of the assessment is to determine the type of CIED, manufacturer, model number, current settings, and proper functioning of the device. Typically, the CIED has the manufacturer's identification card carried by the patient, which helps understand some of those factors.

Pre-anesthesia Consultation

Communication with the CIED care team should provide important information about the type of device—pacemaker (PM), implantable cardioverter defibrillator (ICD), cardiac resynchronization therapy (CRT), implantable loop recorder (ILR)—adequacy of function, current settings, specific recommendations for reprogramming with a programming machine or magnet application, and clinical implications of the expected response. It is important to assess the regularity of the pulse and location of the device generator during physical examination. A recent electrocardiogram (ECG) should be available. If appropriate CIED function has been confirmed, no other special laboratory tests are needed. If a chest radiograph (CXR) is available, the CIED location is noted. A CIED is typically in a pectoral position, with leads from the device following the superior vena cava into the heart and terminating in the right ventricle, right atrium, or coronary sinus (depending on the device type). However, the pulse generator of newer ICDs might be implanted subcutaneously in the left mid-axillary line, with subcutaneous lead(s) positioned over the heart.

Device Interrogation

In the preoperative period, appropriate device interrogation by the CIED team is performed to determine the patient's underlying rhythm, appropriate function, and programming of the CIED. The Heart Rhythm Society (HRS) recommends device interrogation prior to scheduled surgery as follows [7]:

- Within 6 months for an implantable cardioverter defibrillator (ICD)
- Within 12 months for a conventional pacemaker (PM)
- Within 3–6 months for any cardiac resynchronization therapy (CRT) device

This is a very important step in the subsequent intraoperative management of devices in case of malfunction.

Preoperatively, decision-making by the CIED care team should consider issues that include:

- Determine whether a CIED is present and the functionality of the device (Pacemaker or ICD, for example).
- Determine if a significant EMI will be present during the surgical procedure that may affect the function of the CIED and act accordingly.
  - When EMI is likely, there is a risk of inappropriate shocks or anti-tachycardia pacing in the presence of ICD. Hence, the pacing function of the ICD is disabled. In addition, the ICD or PM should be switched to asynchronous pacing mode to avoid oversensing in patients who are pacing-dependent.
- Establish if the patient is pacing-dependent on anti-bradycardia pacing and whether reprogramming of the pacemaker is required.
- Decide the ways in which anti-tachyarrhythmia therapy in the case of ICD shall be suspended (reprogramming or magnet application).
- Make sure that the CIED is functioning as intended.

If unwanted patient movement can occur due to ICD shock, causing injury to the patient or surgical team, the anti-tachyarrhythmias function of the ICD should be disabled. Moreover, some CIED have mechanical or physiologic sensors that should be disabled during a surgery to prevent undesirable tachycardia. Table 8.1 summarizes the perioperative CIED—loop recorder, pacemaker (transvenous and

Table 8.1 Perioperative CIED—loop recorder, Pacemaker (transvenous and leadless), ICD (transvenous and subcutaneous), cardiac resynchronization therapy—management recommendations

Elective surgery	Emergency surgery
Check if the surgery is superior to the umbilicus	Where possible, follow elective surgery guidance
Check if the device is an ICD and the device manufacturer from the patient-held card or by the radiological appearance of the generator	If the device can't be switched to monitor mode preoperatively: • Restrict diathermy usage and where possible use bipolar diathermy • Ensure that cardiopulmonary resuscitation facilities are available
Arrange interrogation of the CIED, if not performed within the last 3–6 months for any cardiac resynchronization therapy device, 6 months for ICD, and 12 months for a conventional pacemaker	If an appropriate CIED shock occurs, correct any reversible causes
Determine the need for asynchronous pacing if the patient is pacing-dependent and the pacing rate needed	If recurrent CIED shocks occur, follow standard CPR guidelines
Position transcutaneous pacing/defibrillator pads on the patient and continuous monitoring with both ECG and pulse oximetry plethysmography	Arrange for ICD interrogation postoperatively
If diathermy will be required, the diathermy cables and the grounding electrode should be remote from the ICD	–
If reprogramming is necessary, reprogram the CIED preoperatively to monitor mode and determine whether CIED reprogramming with a programming machine or magnet application is necessary (a magnet does not produce asynchronous pacing in an ICD)	–
Position the current dispersion pad of the electrosurgical unit (ESU) so the current path does not cross the CIED	–
Bipolar diathermy is preferred and low-energy short bursts are desirable	–
If monopolar diathermy is essential, low-energy, short intermittent and irregular bursts are preferred	–
Arrange for ICD interrogation postoperatively	–

leadless), ICD (transvenous and subcutaneous), cardiac resynchronization therapy—management recommendations for elective and emergent surgeries.

Reprogramming of the CIED

Formal reprogramming of a CIED is necessary and performed when the patient is pacing-dependent and there is a significant EMI exposure [8]. An ICD is usually reprogrammed to suspend the anti-tachyarrhythmia function by using a programming machine or a magnet. Meanwhile, defibrillator pads/transcutaneous pacing are placed on the patient while the anti-tachyarrhythmia functions are disabled.

Programming Machine

The importance of a programming machine is with ICDs. Several functions such as switching to asynchronous mode or disabling a rate-responsive sensor can be done by this machine [9]. Regarding pacemakers, a programming machine promises versatile options not found with the use of magnets, which might prove useful in a patient with suboptimal cardiac function. The use of programming machines requires the presence of specialized personnel before and after the procedure. Furthermore, the changes made with a programming machine are not as fast as those done by a magnet, and the reprogramming process takes several minutes as well. Defibrillator pads/transcutaneous pacing are always placed on the patient and ready as a backup therapy [10].

Magnet Application

Magnet application is considered an alternative to the programming machine to suspend anti-tachyarrhythmia function in ICD. Preoperatively, the response of the CIED to the magnet should be tested by the CIED care team. There are several scenarios where the magnet function on the CIED might be disabled or the CIED is on "power on reset" mode where the magnet function is disabled [11].

Magnet application on pacemakers will initiate asynchronous pacing at a fixed rate as well as a fixed AV delay. Magnet application on ICDs will suspend tachyarrhythmia detection and therapy, but has no effect on the pacing mode.

In pacing-dependent patient with ICDs, magnet application does not cause asynchronous pacing. If pacing is inhibited by EMI, profound bradycardia or asystole may occur. Also, it may be difficult to maintain the magnet over the pulse generator if the patient is in prone or lateral position. Magnet application may risk the field sterility if the incision is near the magnet location. In addition, magnet-induced asynchronous pacing in patients with pacemakers may compromise cardiac function, causing morbidity [12].

Intraoperative Management

Intraoperatively, the management of patients with CIED requires careful monitoring and continuous assessment since this patient population is at risk of life-threatening arrhythmias. Continuous monitoring of the cardiac rhythm and rate (through ECG) and the peripheral pulse is required. Providers should be alert to any electrical changes observed on the ECG and hemodynamic instability due to EMI and act accordingly though stopping the ESU. Furthermore, providers within the operating room should be aware of any changes in pacing (adverse pacing behavior or inhibition of pacing) and apply magnet on pulse generator to switch to asynchronous mode of the ICD [8]. Surgical and anesthesia teams should always consider the possibility of cardioversion and defibrillation during a surgical procedure, and thus should always be prepared in patients with CIEDs.

Transcutaneous pacing/defibrillator pads are placed on the patient before reprogramming/ magnet application and before surgical prepping and draping. It is important to consider the positioning of the defibrillator pads to avoid any damage to the CIED. Generally, an anteroposterior pad position is preferred for patients with left-sided CIED. Anterolateral pad position is used when the anteroposterior position is not feasible [3].

During the surgical procedure for patients with CIED, it is imperative to have continuous monitoring of both ECG and arterial pulse. Continuous ECG monitoring requires reconfiguration to clearly display pacing pulses. In addition, it is important to distinguish pacing artifacts from "true" QRS complexes by the clinicians [13]. Continuous monitoring of arterial pulse through pulse oximetry plethysmography or invasive intra-arterial pressure monitoring to detect a mechanical systole by the heart [14].

During central venous catheterization insertion for patients with CIED, special precautions should be taken. Guidewires insertion may alter the CIED function through inhibition of pacing or inappropriate shock delivery. In addition to continuous ECG and pulse oximetry monitoring, anti-tachycardia functions must be suspended for patients with ICD. In the first 3 months of CIED insertion, there is a significant risk of lead dislodgement during a central line insertion. Caution must be taken through performing a CXR before the line insertion to locate the position of the coronary sinus since that lead is predisposed to dislodgement [7].

Anesthetic agents do not in general affect CIED. In patients with bradycardia, drugs that may cause decreased heart rate should be avoided (fentanyl, dexamethasone) to prevent pacing dependence [15, 16]. Moreover, agents that prolong the QT interval should be avoided in patients with CIED due to long QT syndrome.

When there is a need for emergency external defibrillation or cardioversion during a surgery, several measures should be taken. The magnet should be removed from the ICD to allow the anti-tachyarrhythmia function. In addition, all sources of EMI should be removed to allow correct interpretation of rhythm. Sometimes, the magnet cannot be immediately removed and, in that case, external defibrillators should be used via the transcutaneous pacing/defibrillator pads that were placed before the procedure.

When such events happen, there is a need for proper recording of ECG on the bedside monitor to allow future interrogation of the cardiac rhythm and the presence of ventricular tachycardia. It is important to record the ventricular rate since it may be lower than the minimum threshold of the anti-tachyarrhythmia function of the CIED. In that case, future reprogramming is needed.

Even when older CIEDs are used, intraoperative failure of those devices is rare when exposed to EMI. When it happens, failure can manifest as absence of any response or as inappropriate therapy, such as repeated shock delivery or "runaway" high-rate pacing (typically 180–200 beats/min) [6]. Discovery or even suspicion of cessation of inappropriate therapy requires prompt or immediate termination of the surgery, removal of all EMI sources, and investigation of the CIED.

Emergent Surgery

For emergency surgery with potential for EMI superior to the umbilicus, a magnet is placed over a pacemaker in a pacing-dependent patient to initiate asynchronous pacing, or over an ICD to disable anti-tachyarrhythmia therapy. However, a magnet will not result in asynchronous pacing in an ICD, and profound bradycardia or asystole may still occur due to EMI-induced pacing inhibition. Thus, it may be necessary to minimize EMI by use of bipolar instead of monopolar ESU, or use monopolar ESU in short, intermittent, and irregular bursts at the lowest feasible energy levels.

Evaluation

During physical examination, the presence of a scar may indicate the presence of a CIED. Further history taking from the patient or family member may reveal the manufacturer's identification card that contains the type of device, model, and current settings. A 12-lead ECG should be obtained from the patient. In the case where an ECG was not obtained, the anesthesia monitoring equipment may be used to generate a paced rhythm strip at multiple leads. Next, the ECG needs to be examined to determine the presence of atrial and/or ventricular pacing. When identifiable pacing artifacts are absent, a consistently regular rhythm at 60, 65, or 70 bpm usually indicates pacing [17].

When a chest radiograph is obtained, the type of the device (ICD versus pacemaker) can be identified. If the time allows before the emergency surgery, a magnet should be applied to the CIED to determine if it will produce the desired effect. This can be performed in the operating room after continuous monitoring of ECG and pulse oximeter plethysmography has been established. After the magnet is applied, the ECG response and the intra-arterial waveform are compared to the expected response from magnet application to the device (PM or ICD) [18]. However, magnet response does not always occur, due to the previous disabling of the magnet switch from the device. When this happens, future interrogation of the CIED is indicated to determine if it is functioning properly.

Management

In the case of an emergency surgery where there is no time for adequate preoperative device interrogation and reprogramming and EMI is likely, transcutaneous pacing/defibrillator pads should be placed. Also, continuous ECG monitoring and pulse oximeter plethysmography are indicated. Furthermore, a magnet should be applied prior to the use of ESU or EMI-producing device. If necessary, the nonsterile magnet can be placed in a plastic sterile bag and placed over the CIED.

For patients with a pacemaker, magnet application will almost always initiate asynchronous pacing at a fixed rate with a fixed atrioventricular (AV) delay. It is important to observe the ECG rhythm to ensure that the asynchronous pacing is not competing with the patient's intrinsic rhythm [19].

For patients with an ICD, magnet application will cause suspension of the tachyarrhythmia detection and the anti-tachyarrhythmia function. Nonetheless, EMI may still cause ventricular oversensing and pacing inhibition. It is important to keep observing the ECG rhythm to ensure that profound bradycardia or asystole occur [19].

Postoperative Management

CIEDs that were reprogrammed preoperatively require the reactivation of the previous settings before the patient leaves the recovery unit where they are closely monitored. Sometimes, changes in the patient's condition, such as hemodynamic instability, may necessitate changes in the CIED function. For example, the use of more optimal atrioventricular delay or the use of higher paced rate in patients with hemodynamic instability.

Until the CIED original settings are restored, the patient should be continuously monitored with continuous ECG monitoring and pulse oximetry plethysmography. In addition, the transcutaneous/defibrillator pads should not be removed with the presence of an external defibrillator with pacing capabilities.

There are several recommendations regarding the postoperative management of patients with CIED. The Heart Rhythm Society recommends immediate postoperative interrogation is needed only for hemodynamically unstable patients or when a CIED is exposed to significant EMI (e.g., monopolar electrosurgery superior to the umbilicus) [7]. The Canadian Anesthesiologists' Society and Canadian Cardiovascular Society guidelines recommend monitoring the patient until hemodynamic stability is assured, and suggest that postoperative device interrogation is routinely required only after thoracotomy [20]. The British Medicines and Healthcare products Regulatory Agency recommends contacting the patient's CIED clinic for support in order to confirm device functionality shortly after surgery (timeframe unspecified) [18].

Postoperative interrogation of CIED is preferred when the patient underwent an emergent surgery without appropriate preoperative CIED evaluation.

Conclusion

The high prevalence of cardiac implantable electronic devices (CIEDs), along with their increased use in patients who have cardiac indications, make the understanding of CIED's preoperative, intraoperative, and postoperative management of high importance.

References

1. Kremers MS, Hammill SC, Berul CI, Koutras C, Curtis JS, Wang Y, et al. The national ICD registry report: version 2.1 including leads and pediatrics for years 2010 and 2011. Heart Rhythm. 2013;10(4):e59–65.
2. Pokorney SD, Miller AL, Chen AY, Thomas L, Fonarow GC, De Lemos JA, et al. Implantable cardioverter-defibrillator use among Medicare patients with low ejection fraction after acute myocardial infarction. JAMA. 2015;313(24):2433–40.
3. Rooke GA, Bowdle TA. Perioperative management of pacemakers and implantable cardioverter defibrillators: it's not just about the magnet. Anesth Analg. 2013;117(2):292–4.
4. Schulman PM, Rozner MA, Sera V, Stecker EC. Patients with pacemaker or implantable cardioverter-defibrillator. Med Clin. 2013;97(6):1051–75.
5. Misiri J, Kusumoto F, Goldschlager N. Electromagnetic interference and implanted cardiac devices: the nonmedical environment (part I). Clin Cardiol. 2012;35(5):276–80.
6. Lau W, Corcoran SJ, Mond HG. Pacemaker tachycardia in a minute ventilation rate-adaptive pacemaker induced by electrocardiographic monitoring. Pacing Clin Electrophysiol. 2006;29(4):438–40.
7. Crossley GH, Poole JE, Rozner MA, Asirvatham SJ, Cheng A, Chung MK, et al. The Heart Rhythm Society (HRS)/American Society of Anesthesiologists (ASA) expert consensus statement on the perioperative management of patients with implantable defibrillators, pacemakers and arrhythmia monitors: facilities and patient management. Heart Rhythm. 2011;8(7):1114–54.
8. Stone ME, Salter B, Fischer A. Perioperative management of patients with cardiac implantable electronic devices. Br J Anaesth. 2011;107(suppl_1):i16–26.
9. Schulman PM, Rozner MA. Case report: use caution when applying magnets to pacemakers or defibrillators for surgery. Anesth Analg. 2013;117(2):422–7.
10. Carlson T, Andrell P, Ekre O, Edvardsson N, Holmgren C, Jacobsson F, et al. Interference of transcutaneous electrical nerve stimulation with permanent ventricular stimulation: a new clinical problem? Europace. 2008;11(3):364–9.
11. Plakke MJ, Maisonave Y, Daley SM. Radiofrequency scanning for retained surgical items can cause electromagnetic interference and pacing inhibition if an asynchronous pacing mode is not applied. A A Case Rep. 2016;6(6):143–5.
12. Miller RD, Eriksson LI, Fleisher LA, Wiener-Kronish JP, Cohen NH, Young WL, editors. Miller's anesthesia. Philadelphia: Elsevier Health Sciences; 2014.
13. Reddy VY, Exner DV, Cantillon DJ, Doshi R, Bunch TJ, Tomassoni GF, et al. Percutaneous implantation of an entirely intracardiac leadless pacemaker. N Engl J Med. 2015;373(12):1125–35.
14. American Society of Anesthesiologists. Practice advisory for the perioperative management of patients with cardiac implantable electronic devices: pacemakers and implantable cardioverter-defibrillators: an updated report by the American Society of Anesthesiologists task force on perioperative management of patients with cardiac implantable electronic devices. Anesthesiology. 2011;114(2):247–61.
15. Badrinath SS, Bhaskaran S, Sundararaj I, Rao BS, Mukesh BN. Mortality and morbidity associated with ophthalmic surgery. Ophthalmic Surg Lasers. 1995;26(6):535–41.
16. Pili-Floury S, Farah E, Samain E, Schauvliege F, Marty J. Perioperative outcome of pacemaker patients undergoing non-cardiac surgery. Eur J Anaesthesiol. 2008;25(6):514–6.
17. Mark JB. Atlas of cardiovascular monitoring. London: Churchill Livingstone; 1998.
18. Donnelly P, Pal N, Herity NA. Perioperative management of patients with implantable cardioverter defibrillators. Ulster Med J. 2007;76(2):66.
19. Miller RD, Eriksson LI, Fleisher LA, Wiener-Kronish JP, Young WL, editors. Miller's anesthesia. Philadelphia: Elsevier Health Sciences; 2010.
20. Healey JS, Merchant R, Simpson C, Tang T, Beardsall M, Tung S, et al. Canadian Cardiovascular Society/Canadian Anesthesiologists' Society/Canadian Heart Rhythm Society joint position statement on the perioperative management of patients with implanted pacemakers, defibrillators, and neurostimulating devices. Can J Cardiol. 2012;28(2):141–51.

Traffic, Attire, and Distractions in the Operating Room

9

Chrysanthos D. Christou, Jamal J. Hoballah, and Georgios Tsoulfas

Introduction

The operating room (OR) is undeniably among the most challenging workplaces. It is a resource-dense environment that requires advanced infrastructure, utilizes new technologies, and employs specialized, multidisciplinary human resources. Communication in the OR can be challenging since most surgical teams are ad hoc teams whose members have no previous experience working together and are assembled for the task on hand [1]. Nowadays, failure to coordinate care and lack of effective communication are the leading causes of medical errors [2]. Even though reports support surgical teams' consistency since it increases their efficiency through cumulative team experience, this concept has not yet been widely embraced [3, 4].

The modern OR is a unique workplace with specific, often conflicting, environmental requirements for its inhabitants. Even minor fluctuations of its internal environment could substantially impact patient care and the surgical team members' safety and comfort. Therefore, in the OR lurk various potential hazards. These hazards include surgical smoke, infectious materials, hazardous drugs with carcinogenic and teratogenic toxicity, hazardous disinfecting chemicals and waste, waste anesthesia gases, aerosols, radiation, ergonomic hazards, work-related injuries, noise, and electrical and fire hazards [5–9].

C. D. Christou · G. Tsoulfas (✉)
Center for Research and Innovation in Solid Organ Transplantation, Department of Transplantation Surgery, Aristotle University School of Medicine, Thessaloniki, Greece

J. J. Hoballah
Department of Surgery, American University of Beirut Medical Center, Beirut, Lebanon

J. J. Hoballah et al. (eds.), *Principles of Perioperative Safety and Efficiency*,
https://doi.org/10.1007/978-3-031-41089-5_9

Studies have reported that surgical smoke from 1 g of cauterized tissue has the mutagenic and toxic effects of six cigarettes, while the total exposure in a day is the mutagenic equivalent of 27–30 cigarettes [10, 11] Even though most of the OR personnel acknowledge adverse symptoms from surgical smoke, only a few were adequate personal protective equipment (PPE), and only 14% always use local exhaust ventilation during electrosurgery [12, 13]. In surgery ergonomics, 19% of surgeons report a work-related injury [14], 84% consider their working posture as uncomfortable and painful [6], and up to 73% had at a point suffered from musculoskeletal conditions [15] that could even lead to early retirement [16].

Ensuring a safe, comfortable, and efficient working environment for all OR team members can be challenging. Traffic, attire, and distractions are all an integral part of the OR and play a crucial role in addressing all the above challenges. This chapter aims to provide insight into their role in creating a safe, efficient environment in the OR that is directly linked to the surgical outcome and the patient's well-being. Before discussing the role of traffic, attire, and distractions in the OR, we present the surgical suite's main features, particularly the different designated areas of movement and the OR's main ventilation features. The knowledge regarding these main aspects of the surgical suite facilitates an understating of how the surgical suite's design contributes to a safe, efficient environment. We then demonstrate how OR traffic affects the surgical outcome and, specifically, the development of surgical site infections (SSIs). Thirdly, we present the controversies surrounding our current practices regarding the appropriate attire in the OR and summarize the current recommendations. Finally, we demonstrate how distractions, particularly personal electronic devices, noise, and disruptive behavior, could compromise surgical care quality and jeopardize patient safety.

The Surgical Suite

The surgical suite is divided into three designated areas: the unrestricted, the semi-restricted, and the restricted. This classification is based on access to each area, the activities performed, and the appropriate attire and PPE required in each area. First, the unrestricted areas include a central control point where the designated personnel monitors patients, staff, and materials' traffic into the semi-restricted areas [17]. Unrestricted areas are isolated from the main hospital, and they include locker rooms, offices, break rooms, and waiting rooms [17]. Public access to these areas could be restricted based on each healthcare facility's protocols and regulations.

The semi-restricted areas provide peripheral support to the OR and are accessible from unrestricted areas and restricted areas. These include storages for clean and sterile materials, sterilization processing areas, scrub sink areas, corridors that connect unrestricted and restricted areas, and preoperative admission areas [17].

Lastly, restricted areas are designated areas confined within semi-restricted areas that are accessible only through semi-restricted areas. The restricted areas include the OR and other rooms where surgical or other invasive procedures are performed [17]. Typically, sterile and clean materials are introduced into the OR from a clean core corridor and are contained and transported, following decontamination, through peripheral corridors. In principle, as we progress from the unrestricted to the surgical suite's restricted areas, regulations regarding environmental control, attire policies, and personnel/material traffic become stricter.

Ventilation

The OR's ventilation is designed to provide a comfortable, safe environment for the patient and the surgical team by controlling the temperature, the humidity, and the circulation of various potential biological and chemical pollutants [18]. Also, it aims to prevent SSIs through sufficient air exchange [19]. Air exchange is commonly expressed as air exchanges per hour, and a standard recommendation is 20–25 air exchanges per hour with at least three to four air exchanges per hour from outdoor air [18, 20]. Positive pressure must be maintained regarding corridors and adjacent to the OR areas, while the OR doors should remain closed except from essential traffic [21]. The surgical suite utilizes either a conventional (turbulent) ventilation system or a laminar flow air (unidirectional–LAF) ventilation system or, finally, a combination of the above schemes [22].

Regarding the conventional system, the air is supplied from a high level and exhausted at a low level, typically on two sides [23]. On the other hand, LAF ventilation systems provide a uniform, directional airflow that aims to move floating particles from the areas that should remain contaminant-free toward the return ducts and filtration systems [24]. All of these airflow control systems are quite sensitive to introducing new air into the OR, which disrupts the ventilation patterns. As a result, these systems' ability to remove contaminants and skin scales away from the sterile field is compromised.

Traffic in the OR

Traffic in the OR regards the patterns of movement of materials and personnel among the surgical suite's three designated areas. Navigating these areas has several restrictions. While unrestricted areas could allow public access, unrestricted and restricted areas should strictly be accessible only to authorized personnel and patients accompanied by authorized personnel [17].

Door Openings

Door openings in the OR are surprisingly high. A study in orthopedics reported that during 100 primary total joint arthroplasty operations, with an average operation time of 111.9 min, 35–176 door openings were counted per case, with an average of

71.1 per case, or 0.64 door openings per minute [25]. A different study reported 33 and 54 average door swings per hour in general surgery and cardiac surgery, respectively [26]. The nursing staff contributes 23–52.2% of door openings [25, 26]. Reasons for door openings include informational reasons, breaks, and supply or equipment issues [26, 27]. Notably, informational reasons, such as asking a question, processing paperwork, and checking on the status of the case, account for 27–54% of all door openings [27].

The opening and closing of OR doors disrupt the ventilation patterns and impact air quality delivered to the sterile field and the patient incision [24]. LAF ventilation systems are purportedly superior to the conventional airflow systems in SSI prevention. However, their unidirectional airflow has been reported to be more sensitive to intraoperative activities [22, 28], such as door openings, room traffic, and forced air warmers [29, 30]. A study investigating environmental contamination caused by door openings in ORs within and outside LAF conditions reported that in LAF conditions, only the number of team members was associated with increased bacterial colony-forming units [31]. Increased number of door openings was associated with increased colony-forming unit counts outside LAF conditions [31]. A similar study reported that the positive correlation between the number of personnel and door openings per minute and particles' density in the OR is significantly reduced when the LAF ventilation system is on [32]. However, both of the above studies link LAF ventilation systems' utilization to potential pathogens' density rather than directly to SSI rates. Clinical trials that have investigated that correlation have failed to prove LAF ventilation systems' alleged superiority in decreasing SSI occurrence [33, 34]. A meta-analysis even supported that, if not correctly managed, an LAF ventilation system could act as a predisposing factor for severe SSIs [35]. Finally, the World Health Organization's (WHO) latest recommendations for preventing SSIs recommend that LAF systems are not implemented to reduce SSI risk for patients undergoing total arthroplasty surgery [36].

A study investigating the effect of door openings on airflow in the OR reported that depressurization followed by a single door opening did not reverse the positive pressure at any time [37]. The average time needed for re-pressurization at the baseline pressurization levels was between 14 and 15 s. However, two doors' simultaneous opening did generate a negative pressure gradient, allowing the inflow of potentially contaminated air into the OR [37]. In contrast, a different study reported that the positive pressure was defeated by a single door opening in 40.3% of the cases [38]. Regarding the correlation between opening doors and SSI rates, a prospective observational study reported a positive correlation with an adjusted hazard ratio per 5-unit increment of 1.49 [39]. In another study, a surgical team adopted several measures to limit OR door openings and reported a reduction in SSI rates from 2.8 to 2.1% [40]. Door openings threaten the positive pressure in the OR, jeopardizing the surgical field's sterility. Therefore, efficiently controlling the airflow patterns in the OR by minimizing door openings could lower the incidence of SSIs.

Foot Traffic

The primary source of particles in the OR's air is the personnel present. These particles originate at the surgical personnel's exposed skin. During a typical procedure, millions of skin scales are shed [41]. These squames are then aerosolized and settle on surfaces [42]. Between 5 and 10% of skin debris carries bacteria [43]; therefore, OR personnel's exposed skin is considered the primary source of pathogen transport in the OR. The activities that are linked with a large shed of airborne particles are unfolding the surgical gown, putting the arms through the sleeves, and removing gloves [44].

The number of personnel moving within the OR has been positively correlated with the room' s microbial count by multiple studies, both from air counts and wound sampling counts [31, 32, 45, 46]. However, all these studies use indirect metrics as surrogates for SSI risk, based on the assumption that high bacterial counts are directly linked with SSI rates. Up to date, there is no conclusive evidence for a direct cause-and-effect relation between increased OR foot traffic and SSI rates [47, 48].

Nevertheless, several indirect correlations advocate for OR foot traffic control. First, foot traffic is directly proportional to operative time [49], which positively correlates with SSI rates [50]. Again, this does not prove that OR foot traffic is an independent predisposing factor for SSIs [48]. Second, while door openings are directly proportional to surgery length, they have been found exponentially proportional to the number of personnel in the OR [27]. Therefore, increased OR foot traffic could compromise maintaining a positive pressure in the OR, endangering the inflow of contaminated air in the OR. Finally, increased foot traffic along with door openings could act as distractions in the OR. Therefore, limiting unnecessary traffic enhances team communication and concentration and eliminates one external factor that could affect SSI rates.

Despite the lack of conclusive evidence, the American College of Surgeons (ACS) has acknowledged increased traffic as a predisposing factor for SSI development [51], and the Centers for Disease Control and Prevention (CDC) recommends limiting the number of door openings and personnel in the OR to a minimum [52]. However, there is no recommendation on the amount of traffic that is necessary and justifiable. Eliminating unnecessary traffic can be challenging. A study reported that informing OR personnel about monitoring the traffic (Hawthorne Effect) [53] had no impact on the OR traffic flow [46]. A different study, which educated nurses regarding OR traffic, reported decreased nursing traffic and increased overall traffic, concluding that training is needed for all OR members [26]. Some measures that the surgical teams could adopt to limit traffic are storing necessary supplies and equipment in the OR, using pass-through windows, signage stating, and locking doors [26, 27, 54]. Most significantly, since the supply flow is the major constituter of traffic in the OR, interventions should aim to limit this traffic type. In a study, 65% of surgical case carts were found inadequately or inaccurately prepared [26]. Therefore, supply cupboards should be re-examined, modified, and standardized to minimize the traffic produced due to not having readily available instruments and equipment.

Attire

Attire is regulated among each of the three designated areas of the surgical suite. While unrestricted areas are accessible to personnel with street clothes, entering the semi-restricted and restricted surgical suite areas requires proper attire [51]. Surprisingly, most of our current practices regarding the OR's attire are intuitive and reflect historical methods rather than evidence-based practices.

Surgical Masks

Surgical masks are a physical barrier between the microbiome of nasopharyngeal and oropharyngeal origin and the patient's open wound. Surgical masks should cover the wearer's mouth and nose and be fitted in a manner that does not allow venting at the mask's sides [55]. Masks should be worn when entering restricted areas, especially in the presence of open sterile supplies or personnel who have completed the surgical scrub, and never be worn dangling [56, 57].

Wearing a surgical mask in the OR has been a standard practice for over a century as a means to reduce SSIs in the OR [58]. Nevertheless, there is no conclusive evidence as of yet that supports this. A review of the clinical effectiveness and guidelines regarding the use of surgical masks in the OR concluded that the current systematic reviews prove a lack of evidence to support any statistically significant correlation between wearing surgical masks and SSI rates [59]. However, the authors of these reviews agree that the included studies' quality, limitations, and findings could not justify any alteration of the current clinical practice [60, 61]. A randomized clinical trial evaluating the use of face masks by non-scrubbed personnel reported no increase in the SSI rates when non-scrubbed OR personnel did not wear a mask [62]. Finally, surgical masks could even act as a source of contamination, since it was found that they are contaminated from the surgeons' body surface [63]; thus, it is recommended that surgical masks be changed between operations, especially those that last more than 2 h [63].

Nevertheless, the role of surgical masks is not limited to protecting the patients' wounds from potential contamination from the OR personnel. Surgical masks protect the OR team members from potential splashes of the patients' bodily fluids, inhalable microparticulates, and blood aerosols [55]. However, many of these potential hazards, including acetylene, butadiene, and hydrogen cyanide found in surgical smoke, can circumvent the standard masks worn in the OR [64]. Therefore, it is essential when selecting a surgical mask for the OR that each mask's basic features—including fluid resistance, filtration efficiency, differential pressure, flammability, and filtration performance—are considered in choosing a mask of the appropriate performance classification [55].

Scrubs and Jackets

Regarding scrubs, the ACS Board of Regents statement regarding attire states that scrubs should be worn in both the semi-restricted and restricted areas of the surgical suite [57]. Scrubs should not be worn, under any circumstance, outside the hospital perimeter, and if worn outside the OR, they should be covered with a clean lab or appropriate cover-up [56, 57]. Also, scrubs, along with headgear, used in dirty or contaminated cases should be replaced before treating the following case, and at least once a day, even if not visibly spoiled [57]. As a sign of professionalism and respect, visibly spoiled scrubs should always be changed before speaking with the patient's family.

The scrubs should be tightly woven, low linting, durable, and stain-resistant [65]. Studies performed with scrubs made from fabrics with antimicrobials processed into the yarn reported significant microorganism reductions [66, 67]. Regarding laundering, the current Association of Perioperative Registered Nurses (AORN) guidelines recommend facility-laundered scrubs that should be changed daily or/ and when visibly soiled [65]. Even though there are no recommendations regarding wearing personal clothes under surgical scrubs, if those clothes become contaminated with potentially infectious materials such as blood or body fluids, they should remain at the facility for laundering [68]. Nevertheless, a clinical trial evaluating the bacterial burden regarding scrub laundering and the dressing site reported no statistical differences in total bacterial burden between home- and hospital-dressed cohorts when stratified by the site where scrubs where laundered [69]. The rationale behind facility laundering is that personnel cannot consistently monitor the required quality of laundering. Controlling the water temperature, agitation, and concentration of chemicals during home laundering is incredibly difficult [56]. Also, despite the rarity, there have been reports of contaminated home washing machines that caused wound infections [70].

Regarding long-sleeve jackets, a guideline implementation paper by AORN suggested in 2015 that all non-scrubbed personnel in restricted areas cover themselves with a long-sleeved scrub or jacket [65]. Since then, large retrospective cohort studies have been published, all concluding that there is no evidence that long-sleeve jackets help prevent SSIs [71–73], while they do present a significant financial burden. Specifically, a study that evaluated the ability of bouffants and jackets to prevent SSIs reported rates of SSI, mortality, postoperative sepsis, and wound dehiscence between the no bouffants or jackets group and the jackets-only group of 1.01%, 1.83%, 6.60%, and 1.07% vs. 0.99%, 2.05%, 6.24%, and 0.84%, respectively [74]. The authors have estimated the cost of supplying disposable long-sleeved jackets to all hospitals in the USA to comply with the recommendation of coverage of all exposed skin on the arm would be $540 million annually [74].

Finally, in a study funded by ACS, mock intraoperative skin preparations were performed by personnel who either wore long sleeves and gloves or performed the preparation with bare hands. Airborne particulate contamination and active/passive microbial assessment were assessed using particle counters and air samplers/settle plate analysis, respectively. The study's findings support the use of long sleeves and gloves when preparing the skin, as it was linked with significantly lower particulate and microbial shedding [42]. Specifically, the use of sleeves appeared to decrease the shed of *Micrococcus* [42].

Nevertheless, the latest recommendations acknowledge the lack of evidence to support the mandatory use of long-sleeve jackets for all personnel in the semi-restricted and restricted areas and suggest that each perioperative team evaluates and decides whether to implement this practice [56]. This does not apply to personnel performing intraoperative skin preparation, where the use of long sleeves is recommended [56].

Gloves

Wearing gloves is perhaps the most standard practice when operating. Introduced in the OR by Halsted [75], gloves play a vital role in preventing injuries by sharp items, bloodborne contamination, and SSIs. A reasonable dilemma regarding the use of gloves is double-gloving. A study investigating perforation rates in double latex gloves in a postmortem examination room reported 3.8% perforation of the outer-glove vs. 0.5% for the inner-glove [76]. Notably, 85.6% did not realize the perforation when it occurred [76]. A randomized, controlled study evaluated double-gloving efficacy in various surgical specialties and reported a 15.2% overall perforation rate in the single-glove group vs. a 14.4% in the double-glove group [77]. However, the percentage of a through-and-through puncture from the outer to the inner glove was 1.17%; thus, double gloves' protection was 98.83% [77]. Finally, a meta-analysis that compared single-gloving and double-gloving perforation rates reported 11% of perforated single gloves vs. 3% of innermost double gloves, with an estimated odds ratio of 4.14 [78].

Another issue is the changing of gloves. It is recommended that gloves be changed when a perforation is noticed [79]. However, there is no consensus on the justified frequency of changing gloves during long operations. A systematic review on glove change in orthopedics recommended that gloves be changed at least once per hour to decrease contamination rates, and always after draping and before handling implants [80]. In the field of general surgery, a meta-analysis reported that pre-closure change of gloves significantly decreased the SSI rates (56.9% vs. 28.5%) [58].

Another vital issue to address regarding gloves is the area where gloves and gowns are connected. The glove–gown interface is one of the weakest points of the PPE system, specifically during doffing. Several studies have investigated the effect of modifying the traditional glove–gown interface into ones with higher overlap between gowns and gloves; all reporting decreased contamination rates during doffing [81–83]. Double-gloving can decrease hand contamination during doffing by reducing the fluid leakages through the glove–gown-interface [84].

These findings extensively support double-gloving utilization in reducing both injuries and bloodborne contamination. As a result, the latest recommendations strongly recommend using double-gloving to prevent injury by sharp items and infections by bloodborne pathogens in the OR [2, 56, 57].

Headgear

In 2014, the AORN guidelines for surgical attire recommended "complete coverage of the ears, scalp, skin, sideburns, and nape of the neck" [85]. While never explicitly referring to a specific headgear, those familiar with the topic viewed this statement as an endorsement of bouffant caps over skull caps. As proof of the power of published guidelines, this recommendation soon became a benchmark, while hair exposure was shortly after seen as a poor infection control practice. As a response, the ACS Board of Regents task force published in 2016 their recommendations defending the use of skull caps by stating that "The skull cap is symbolic of the surgical profession. The skull cap may be worn when close to the totality of hair is covered by it and when only a limited amount of hair on the nape of the neck or modest sideburns remains uncovered" [57]. That sparked a heated debate [86–89], with reports even referring to the issue as a "scandal" [90]. In a joint statement, ACS and AORN, among many associations, acknowledged the need for collaboration in developing policies, and agreed that current scientific evidence does not demonstrate an association between the type of head covering and SSI rates [91].

Subsequently, several studies have been published evaluating bouffant caps and skull caps' efficacy in preventing SSIs. One study re-analyzed data from a prospective randomized control trial [92], based on the surgeons' preference for bouffant or skull cap. Their results report an overall 8% SSI rate in the bouffant group and 5% in the skull cap group, with a $p = 0.016$ [93]. However, no significant differences were observed between the two groups when adjusting for each type of operation, while in a study of porosity and permeability, it has been reported that a disposable bouffant cap is more permeable to bacteria than is a skull cap [94].

In a recent retrospective cohort study, bouffant caps and surgical jackets' effectiveness in preventing SSIs was evaluated [74]. The no bouffant or jacket group had 1.01% SSIs rate in the study, while the only bouffant group had 0.99%, a difference that did not reach statistical significance. Similarly, mortality, sepsis, and wound dehiscence rates were comparable between the two groups. Similarly, a study comparing SSI rates before and after the imposition of strict protocols regarding OR attire reported no evidence to support that such policies aid in SSI prevention [95]. Previous reviews have also concluded that there is little evidence that head coverings reduced SSIs rates [96, 97]. However, the idea that head coverings are neither efficient nor cost-effective in preventing SSIs remains controversial. As measured by the wound area sedimentation, the surgical wound's bacterial contamination is positively correlated with SSI rates, and it has been found to be 60 times greater when head coverings are omitted during a surgical procedure [94, 98]. Nevertheless, to date there is no conclusive evidence that supports a direct cause-and-effect relation.

In their latest recommendations, AORN guidelines state that "the available evidence does not show an association between the extent of hair coverage and SSI rates" [99], and they make no recommendation about the type of head covers to be worn in semi-restricted and restricted areas [100]. Therefore, the recommendation is to wear a head covering, of any kind, when entering the semi-restricted and restricted areas of the surgical suite. Those selecting a cloth skull cap should launder it daily since unlaundered cloth could lead to airborne contamination of the surgical suite [94]. Even though ears are among the exposed facial areas with the highest concentration of microbes [101], there is currently no documented association between SSI rates and covering the ears [56]. Finally, head coverings should be removed when leaving semi-restricted and restricted areas, and new ones should be worn when re-entering these areas.

Personal Belongings

Naturally, OR members usually need to bring personal belongings into the surgical suite's semi-restricted and restricted areas. These include backpacks, briefcases, cell phones, and jewelry. However, these items are typically highly contaminated with microorganisms, many of which are pathogenic [102, 103]. Each perioperative team should establish a protocol for preventing these items from contaminating the surgical suite. These protocols could include either disinfecting these items before bringing them along, or leaving them behind in designated unrestricted areas. Jewelry that cannot be confined within the scrubs or adequately covered should not be worn in the surgical suite's semi-restricted or restricted areas [57, 65].

Regarding cell phones, many studies have evaluated their role in OR contamination, with most studies concluding that they are a primary source of pathogen spreading [102, 104–106]. It has been reported that up to 83% of cell phones brought into the OR carry pathogens [102]. A week after disinfection, 75% of phones were found re-contaminated with pathogens. Therefore, electronic equipment such as cell phones and tablets should be cleaned with a low-level disinfectant, according to the manufacturer's instructions, before and after being brought into the perioperative setting [65]. The cleaning of electronic devices should be followed by hand hygiene.

Distractions

The OR is a fast-paced, stressful workplace where frequent interruptions occur, and personnel often face conflicting priorities. Most surgical teams are ad hoc teams assembled for the task on hand; thus, communication can be challenging [1]. Distractions such as phone calls and noisy background add complexity to an already challenging environment, making even simple exchanges difficult, and disrupt the OR members from their tasks [107, 108]. Other distractions include team communication failures, equipment problems, training-related distractions, traffic in and throughout the OR, and difficulties in resource accessibility [109]. Distractions in the OR are pervasive, with a reported frequency of one distraction every 30–110 s [110]. A study conducted in a real OR environment investigating distractions in the OR reported that the two most prevalent distractions are those initiated by external personnel, followed by case-irrelevant conversations [111]. Distractions in the OR lead to disruptions, which are classified depending on their impact on patient safety [112]. Minor distractions tend to lead to a major distraction, which compromises care quality [113]. Distractions could have severe consequences on the patient's safety. Distractions in the OR have been correlated with poor team communication [111], while team communication failures are reported as the strongest predictor of surgical errors [109].

Personal Electronic Devices

In an era where technology has infiltrated every key aspect of our social lives, the OR could not be an exception. Distractions from mobile devices have been identified as being among the leading health technology hazards, with even deaths being reported due to personnel being distracted by texting [114, 115]. Answering phone calls or pagers is a frequent distraction in the OR, with an estimated prevalence of 1.9 times per procedure or four times per hour [110, 116]. These distractions are significant enough for the surgeon to cease his/her task and engage entirely with the distracting stimulus [110]. This time interval where the physician is disengaged from the primary mission constitutes an error space, increasing the likelihood of an error.

An interesting randomized crossover study in obstetrics investigated the effect of these distracting stimuli on patient care during virtual salpingectomies conducted by residents [117]. While distracted, 63% of the residents made at least one unsafe clinical decision while operating on the simulator, compromising patient safety [117]. Another study in the field of cardiac surgery investigated the use of cell phones in the OR with independent observers who recorded data from more than 139 h during cardiopulmonary bypass operations [118]. The interaction with personal electronic devices was not limited to patient care, with 5% of the instances regarding non-professional uses, such as taking selfies and browsing social media, with some interactions lasting more than 20 min [118].

Nevertheless, it would be unfair if we did not acknowledge that appropriate use of personal electronic devices could positively impact care quality and patient safety. Personal electronic devices have facilitated rapid communication among peers which allowed rapid responses to emergencies, dramatically increased medical information accessibility, improved data management, and even have various diagnostic and drug reference applications [119, 120].

During periods of criticality, even a few seconds of inattention could have severe consequences to the surgical outcome. Therefore, it is recommended that OR team members create a no-interruption environment where nonessential conversation and activities are prohibited during the operation's critical phases [121]. OR team members should only engage in urgent outside communication, minimize their personal/routine phone calls, keep all phone calls as brief as possible, and ensure that the use of cell phones does not compromise the integrity of the sterile field [107]. Taking and sharing photographs in the OR should follow government and hospital regulations and not compromise the patient's right to privacy and confidentiality [107].

Noise

There are various sources of noise in the OR, which could be either intrinsic or extrinsic. Intrinsic noise sources include music, conversations, functioning equipment, and critical alarms from monitors [107, 121]. On the other hand, extrinsic sources of noise include phone calls, pagers, communication of personnel outside the OR, and OR traffic [107, 121]. The Environmental Protection Agency (EPA) recommends that the level of continuous background noise in the hospital does not exceed 45 decibels a day, while the WHO recommends that the average background environmental noise does not exceed 30 decibels a day [122]. However, in the OR the noise intensity often exceeds the recommended levels [123–125]. Noise exposure could lead to stress responses, tachycardia, irritability, exhaustion, and burnout, contribute to miscommunication, and impair cognitive performance [126–130]. As a result, it could cause medical errors and increase postoperative complication rates [131–133]. A study in general surgery reported that auditory distractions are significantly correlated with higher stress in surgeons and a higher workload in aaesthesiologists [111]. Critical alarms in the OR can be distracting. However, they are necessary because they contribute to patient safety [134]. False alarms are distracting without contributing to the patient safety [135]; therefore, new alarm algorithms that are clinically more useful and less burdensome could be adopted [135].

The power of the OR team to effectively control noise varies, depending on the source. Conversations and traffic could be more effectively monitored. Nonessential conversations and unnecessary traffic should be prohibited during the critical phases of surgery [107, 121]. However, noise transmission from outside sources, such as conversations from corridors, which can be attributed to architecture issues, are more difficult to control and should be addressed when the ORs are designed and maintained [107]. Also, noise from equipment could be challenging to manage and should be considered when surgical instruments are selected [107].

Playing music in the operating room is another debatable topic. Some surgeons prefer to perform their surgical procedures while listening to their favorite tunes while others prefer not to have any music played in the operating room. While music in the operating theater may have a soothing effect on the surgeon and may improve specific task performance, it may also be distracting or may negatively affect proper communication during surgical procedures, especially if the music is high beat and loud. A recent metanalysis of the studies published on this topic revealed that overall, there were more studies supportive of the positive effect of music than its negative effect on surgical task performance with respect to accuracy and speed, especially classical music if played at a low or medium volume. Larger studies will be needed to unequivocally prove the benefit of music and identify what type of music, volume, and timing should be played during the procedure [136].

Disruptive Behavior

Another critical issue to address is disruptive behavior. It is defined as behavior that undermines a culture of safety [137]. Disruptive behavior in the OR includes angry outbursts, yelling, cursing, publicly degrading team members, and being physically abusive [138]. Unfortunately, it has been reported that each surgical procedure includes from one to four instances of high tension [139], with more than 95% of physicians reporting that they regularly encounter disruptive behavior [140]. Such instances distract all OR team members from the task on hand, disorient team communication, and pose a significant compromise to patient safety. A study that investigated tensions in the OR using video-based scenarios reported that while all OR members agreed on the intensity of the conflict, when asked which character was primarily responsible for the conflict, nurses, anesthesiologists, and surgeons believed that their profession had less responsibility for creating tensions [141]. Disrespectful behaviors such as verbal rebuke or berating could intimidate OR members from speaking up, even if they are aware of a situation that could lead to a medical error [142, 143]. It essential to report and condemn any kind of disruptive behavior from any of the OR members [2]. This kind of behavior jeopardizes both the OR team members' and patient's safety [138, 144]. In our opinion, to efficiently address disruptive behavior, healthcare leadership should promote professional behavior as being equally important to surgical skills.

Summary

SSIs are associated with substantial mortality, morbidity, and prolonged hospital stay. Specifically, SSIs are linked with a 2- to 11-fold increased risk of mortality, while 60% of SSIs are estimated to be preventable using evidence-based practices [79, 145]. SSIs are also correlated with a significant financial burden, with their annual cost estimated between $3.5 and $10 billion per year [79]. Evidently, much is still unknown regarding the effect of OR traffic and surgical attire on the risk of SSI development. As we improve our understanding of human–microbial interaction, we will be able to develop targeted interventions to reduce SSIs. We should acknowledge that multiple predisposing factors for SSI development are patient-related, including age, diabetes, obesity, smoking, and alcohol [36, 51, 146].

Nevertheless, our practices could aggravate SSI rates. Increased OR traffic and inappropriate surgical attire are among the modifiable factors that contribute to SSI development. Therefore, following the recommendations could help reduce SSI rates. Personnel should be educated to minimize door openings and keep foot traffic to the essential minimum. Per the recommendations, all OR personnel should wear the appropriate attire when moving among the three designated areas of the OR. Except for attire and traffic, various other practices affect SSI rates, such as preoperative bathing, hair removal, surgical hand scrubbing, antibiotic prophylaxis, anesthesia type, wound classification, and type and duration of the surgical procedure [36, 51, 147, 148]. When SSI rates are properly stratified by operation type and patient-related factors, then the SSI rates could represent the quality of care and be used as a metric for benchmarking and quality control.

Most of our current practices regarding attire reflect a continuation of historic practices rather than evidence-based practices. The underlying reason for this is a complex combination of habit, morals, ignorance, and emotion, particularly fear. Why would anyone not implement a practice that bears no harm to either the provider or the patient, with the risk of potential harm even if the evidence supporting that harm is inadequate? It is essential to understand that developing clinical practice guidelines will always be a trade-off between benefits and potential risks, and when the balance between them is unclear, physicians will naturally adopt a proactive stance. Therefore, guidelines will continue to recommend the enforcement of these practices until high-quality evidence suggests otherwise. Nevertheless, due to this field's nature, large-scale randomized clinical trials on these topics are highly unlikely to occur. As a result, myth and reality will most probably continue to coexist for the imminent future.

Unfortunately, based on the various reports included in this chapter, the idea that the OR is currently a safe, calm, ideal environment to work in is more fiction than reality. OR members continuously face a plethora of potential hazards in the OR. Besides physical harm, OR members encounter multiple psychological challenges, including stress and disruptive behavior. Disruptive behavior should not be tolerated. Professionalism and communication skills are among the core competencies listed by the American Board of Medical Specialties and the Accreditation Council for Graduate Medical Education [149, 150]. We envision a future where professionalism and social skills will be considered as equally important as surgical skills. Healthcare facilities should be proactive regarding disruptive behavior and adopt measures that ameliorate the effects of factors that lead to disruptive behavior, such as emotional stress, before compromising the OR personnel's performance. Prevention is the most critical step toward addressing disruptive behavior [151]. Preventive measures could include team training, standardized communication techniques, and the use of checklists at critical times, which improve team communication, promote respect and familiarity among team members, and empower the OR members to speak up [143, 152, 153]. An unhealthy environment during training could lead to a future disruptive physician; thus, professionalism and communication skills should be a vital part of the training. The performance of a surgeon during training should be evaluated, targeting these particular skills. Finally, monitoring systems and quality control measures that quickly identify and address potential liabilities should be implemented by healthcare facilities to ensure a safe and efficient environment for all the OR inhabitants.

References

1. Salas E, DiazGranados D, Klein C, Burke CS, Stagl KC, Goodwin GF, et al. Does team training improve team performance? A meta-analysis. Hum Factors. 2008;50(6):903–33.
2. Statement on patient safety in the operating room: team care [Internet]. [cited 2020 Sep 28]. https://www.facs.org/about-acs/statements/113-patient-safety
3. de Leval MR, Carthey J, Wright DJ, Farewell VT, Reason JT. Human factors and cardiac surgery: a multicenter study. J Thorac Cardiovasc Surg. 2000;119(4 Pt 1):661–72.
4. Kumar H, Morad R, Sonsati M. Surgical team: improving teamwork, a review. Postgrad Med J. 2019;95(1124):334–9.
5. Spruce L. Back to basics: environmental cleaning hazards. AORN J. 2017;106:424–32.
6. Matern U, Koneczny S. Safety, hazards and ergonomics in the operating room. Surg Endosc. 2007;21(11):1965–9.
7. American Medical Association. Surgical smoke exposure in operating room personnel: a review. 2019;1–8.

8. Link T. Guideline implementation: a safe environment of care. AORN J [Internet]. 2019;110(2):169–179. https://www.nih.jbc.unboundmedicine.com/medline/citation/31355438/Guideline_Implementation:_A_Safe_Environment_of_Care_
9. Hemingway M, Meleis L, Oliver J, Silvestri S. A protocol for the safe use of hazardous drugs in the OR. AORN J. 2020;111:289–300.
10. Hill DS, O'Neill JK, Powell RJ, Oliver DW. Surgical smoke—a health hazard in the operating theatre: a study to quantify exposure and a survey of the use of smoke extractor systems in UK plastic surgery units. J Plast Reconstr Aesthet Surg. 2012;65(7):911–6.
11. Tomita Y, Mihashi S, Nagata K, Ueda S, Fujiki M, Hirano M, et al. Mutagenicity of smoke condensates induced by CO2-laser irradiation and electrocauterization. Mutat Res. 1981;89(2):145–9.
12. Steege AL, Boiano JM, Sweeney MH. Secondhand smoke in the operating room? Precautionary practices lacking for surgical smoke. Am J Ind Med. 2016;59(11):1020–31.
13. Ilce A, Yuzden GE, Yavuz van Giersbergen M. The examination of problems experienced by nurses and doctors associated with exposure to surgical smoke and the necessary precautions. J Clin Nurs. 2017;26(11–12):1555–61.
14. 2017 ACS governors survey: ergonomic injuries and their prevention. The Bulletin [Internet]. [cited 2020 Sep 28]. https://bulletin.facs.org/2018/06/2017-acs-governors-survey-ergonomic-injuries-and-their-prevention/
15. Janki S, Mulder EEAP, Ijzermans JNM, Tran TCK. Ergonomics in the operating room. Surg Endosc. 2017;31(6):2457–66.
16. Hallbeck MS, Law KE, Boughey JC. ASO author reflections: poor ergonomics during surgical procedures may lead to work-related pain and early retirement. Ann Surg Oncol. 2020;27(5):1327–8.
17. Association of Perioperative Registered Nurses. Perioperative standards and recommended practices. Denver: AORN; 2014.
18. Katz JD. Control of the environment in the operating room. Anesth Analg. 2017;125(4):1214–8.
19. Sehulster L, Chinn RYW. Guidelines for environmental infection control in health-care facilities. Recommendations of CDC and the Healthcare Infection Control Practices Advisory Committee (HICPAC). MMWR Recomm Rep. 2003;52(RR-10):1–42.
20. Wagner J, Schreiber K, Cohen R. Improving operating room contamination control. ASHRAE J. 2014;56:18–27.
21. Sprague JG. Development of guidelines for design and construction of hospital and health care facilities. World Hosp Health Serv. 2003;39(3):35–8, 43, 45.
22. Iudicello S, Fadda A. A road map to a comprehensive regulation on ventilation technology for operating rooms. Infect Control Hosp Epidemiol. 2013;34(8):858–60.
23. American Society of Heating, Refrigerating, and Air-Conditioning Engineers, Institute ANS, American Society of Health Care Engineering (ASHE). Ventilation of health care facilities: ASHRAE/ASHE standard. Atlanta: American Society of Heating, Refrigerating, and Air-Conditioning Engineers; 2017.
24. Pokrywka M, Byers K. Traffic in the operating room: a review of factors influencing air flow and surgical wound contamination. Infect Disord Drug Targets. 2013;13(3):156–61.
25. Bédard M, Pelletier-Roy R, Angers-Goulet M, Leblanc P-A, Pelet S. Traffic in the operating room during joint replacement is a multidisciplinary problem. Can J Surg. 2015;58(4):232–6.
26. Elliott S, Parker S, Mills J, Meeusen L, Frana T, Anderson M, et al. STOP: can we minimize OR traffic? AORN J. 2015;102(4):409.e1–7.
27. Lynch RJ, Englesbe MJ, Sturm L, Bitar A, Budhiraj K, Kolla S, et al. Measurement of foot traffic in the operating room: implications for infection control. Am J Med Qual. 2009;24(1):45–52.
28. Whyte W, Shaw BH. The effect of obstructions and thermals in laminar-flow systems. J Hyg (Lond). 1974;72(3):415–23.
29. Beldi G, Bisch-Knaden S, Banz V, Mühlemann K, Candinas D. Impact of intraoperative behavior on surgical site infections. Am J Surg. 2009;198(2):157–62.

30. Belani KG, Albrecht M, McGovern PD, Reed M, Nachtsheim C. Patient warming excess heat: the effects on orthopedic operating room ventilation performance. Anesth Analg. 2013;117(2):406–11.
31. Perez P, Holloway J, Ehrenfeld L, Cohen S, Cunningham L, Miley GB, et al. Door openings in the operating room are associated with increased environmental contamination. Am J Infect Control. 2018;46(8):954–6.
32. Rezapoor M, Alvand A, Jacek E, Paziuk T, Maltenfort MG, Parvizi J. Operating room traffic increases aerosolized particles and compromises the air quality: a simulated study. J Arthroplasty. 2018;33(3):851–5.
33. Alijanipour P, Karam J, Llinás A, Vince KG, Zalavras C, Austin M, et al. Operative environment. J Arthroplasty. 2014;29(2 Suppl):49–64.
34. Brandt C, Hott U, Sohr D, Daschner F, Gastmeier P, Rüden H. Operating room ventilation with laminar airflow shows no protective effect on the surgical site infection rate in orthopedic and abdominal surgery. Ann Surg. 2008;248(5):695–700.
35. Breier A-C, Brandt C, Sohr D, Geffers C, Gastmeier P. Laminar airflow ceiling size: no impact on infection rates following hip and knee prosthesis. Infect Control Hosp Epidemiol. 2011;32(11):1097–102.
36. World Health Organization. Global guidelines for the prevention of surgical site infection [Internet]. 2nd ed. Geneva: World Health Organization. https://apps.who.int/iris/handle/10665/277399
37. Weiser MC, Shemesh S, Chen DD, Bronson MJ, Moucha CS. The effect of door opening on positive pressure and airflow in operating rooms. J Am Acad Orthop Surg. 2018;26(5):e105–13.
38. Mears SC, Blanding R, Belkoff SM. Door opening affects operating room pressure during joint arthroplasty. Orthopedics. 2015;38(11):e991–4.
39. Roth JA, Juchler F, Dangel M, Eckstein FS, Battegay M, Widmer AF. Frequent door openings during cardiac surgery are associated with increased risk for surgical site infection: a prospective observational study. Clin Infect Dis. 2019;69(2):290–4.
40. Minimizing OR traffic may improve patient safety by lowering rates of surgical site infections [Internet]. [cited 2020 Oct 25]. https://www.facs.org/media/press-releases/2016/nsqip-ssi-071816
41. Memarzadeh F. Comparison of operating room ventilation systems in the protection of the surgical site. ASHRAE Trans. 2004;
42. Markel TA, Gormley T, Greeley D, Ostojic J, Wagner J. Wearing long sleeves while prepping a patient in the operating room decreases airborne contaminants. Am J Infect Control. 2018;46(4):369–74.
43. Scaltriti S, Cencetti S, Rovesti S, Marchesi I, Bargellini A, Borella P. Risk factors for particulate and microbial contamination of air in operating theatres. J Hosp Infect. 2007;66(4):320–6.
44. Noguchi C, Koseki H, Horiuchi H, Yonekura A, Tomita M, Higuchi T, et al. Factors contributing to airborne particle dispersal in the operating room. BMC Surg. 2017;17(1):78.
45. Andersson AE, Bergh I, Karlsson J, Eriksson BI, Nilsson K. Traffic flow in the operating room: an explorative and descriptive study on air quality during orthopedic trauma implant surgery. Am J Infect Control. 2012;40(8):750–5.
46. Stauning MT, Bediako-Bowan A, Andersen LP, Opintan JA, Labi A-K, Kurtzhals JAL, et al. Traffic flow and microbial air contamination in operating rooms at a major teaching hospital in Ghana. J Hosp Infect. 2018;99(3):263–70.
47. Alizo G, Onayemi A, Sciarretta JD, Davis JM. Operating room foot traffic: a risk factor for surgical site infections. Surg Infect (Larchmt). 2019;20(2):146–50.
48. Wanta BT, Glasgow AE, Habermann EB, Kor DJ, Cima RR, Berbari EF, et al. Operating room traffic as a modifiable risk factor for surgical site infection. Surg Infect (Larchmt). 2016;17(6):755–60.
49. Parikh SN, Grice SS, Schnell BM, Salisbury SR. Operating room traffic: is there any role of monitoring it? J Pediatr Orthop. 2010;30(6):617–23.

50. Cheng H, Chen BP-H, Soleas IM, Ferko NC, Cameron CG, Hinoul P. Prolonged operative duration increases risk of surgical site infections: a systematic review. Surg Infect (Larchmt). 2017;18(6):722–35.
51. Ban KA, Minei JP, Laronga C, Harbrecht BG, Jensen EH, Fry DE, et al. American College of Surgeons and Surgical Infection Society: surgical site infection guidelines, 2016 update. J Am Coll Surg. 2017;224(1):59–74.
52. Mangram AJ, Horan TC, Pearson ML, Silver LC, Jarvis WR. Guideline for prevention of surgical site infection. Infect Control Hosp Epidemiol. 1999;20(4):247–80. https://www.cambridge.org/core/article/guideline-for-prevention-of-surgical-site-infection-1999/31585A523649826D6497F019D0907A60
53. Chen L, Weg M, Hofmann D, Reisinger H. The Hawthorne effect in infection prevention and epidemiology. Infect Control Hosp Epidemiol. 2015;36:1–7.
54. Patterson P. Curbing OR traffic: finding ways to minimize the flow of personnel. OR Manager. 2012;28(6):1, 9–11.
55. Joyce C. Surgical masks and exposure protection in the perioperative setting. AORN J [Internet]. 2018;107(2):253–256. https://doi.org/10.1002/aorn.12048.
56. AORN guidelines for perioperative practice 2020. [Internet]. 2020. http://online.statref.com/Home/Resolve?id=119756&grpalias=UPHSLPIER
57. Statement on operating room attire. Bull Am Coll Surg. 2016;101(10):47.
58. Belkin NL. The evolution of the surgical mask: filtering efficiency versus effectiveness. Infect Control Hosp Epidemiol. 1997;18(1):49–57.
59. Use of surgical masks in the operating room: a review of the clinical effectiveness and guidelines. Canadian Agency for Drugs & Technologies in Health; 2013.
60. Bahli ZM. Does evidence based medicine support the effectiveness of surgical facemasks in preventing postoperative wound infections in elective surgery? J Ayub Med Coll Abbottabad. 2009;21(2):166–70.
61. Vincent M, Edwards P. Disposable surgical face masks for preventing surgical wound infection in clean surgery. Cochrane Database Syst Rev. 2016;4(4):CD002929.
62. Webster J, Croger S, Lister C, Doidge M, Terry MJ, Jones I. Use of face masks by non-scrubbed operating room staff: a randomized controlled trial. ANZ J Surg. 2010;80(3):169–73.
63. Zhiqing L, Yongyun C, Wenxiang C, Mengning Y, Yuanqing M, Zhenan Z, et al. Surgical masks as source of bacterial contamination during operative procedures. J Orthop Transl. 2018;14:57–62.
64. Bree K, Barnhill S, Rundell W. The dangers of electrosurgical smoke to operating room personnel: a review. Workplace Health Saf. 2017;65(11):517–26.
65. Cowperthwaite L, Holm RL. Guideline implementation: surgical attire. AORN J. 2015;101(2):187–8.
66. Kasuga E, Kawakami Y, Matsumoto T, Hidaka E, Oana K, Ogiwara N, et al. Bactericidal activities of woven cotton and nonwoven polypropylene fabrics coated with hydroxyapatite-binding silver/titanium dioxide ceramic nanocomposite "Earth-plus". Int J Nanomedicine. 2011;6:1937–43.
67. Mariscal A, Lopez-Gigosos RM, Carnero-Varo M, Fernandez-Crehuet J. Antimicrobial effect of medical textiles containing bioactive fibres. Eur J Clin Microbiol Infect Dis. 2011;30(2):227–32.
68. Spruce L, Wood A. Guideline for surgical attire. Surg Infect (Larchmt) [Internet.] 2019;20(6):435–436. https://doi.org/10.1089/sur.2019.161.
69. Slizewski DH, Heberlein E, Meredith JF, Jobe LB, Eichelberger KY. Impact of home versus hospital dressing on bacterial contamination of surgical scrubs in the obstetric setting: a randomized controlled trial. Am J Infect Control. 2018;46(4):379–82.
70. Wright SN, Gerry JS, Busowski MT, Klochko AY, McNulty SG, Brown SA, et al. Gordonia bronchialis sternal wound infection in 3 patients following open heart surgery: intraoperative transmission from a healthcare worker. Infect Control Hosp Epidemiol. 2012;33(12):1238–41.

71. Stapleton EJ, Frane N, Lentz JM, Armellino D, Kohn N, Linton R, et al. Association of disposable perioperative jackets with surgical site infections in a large multicenter health care organization. JAMA Surg. 2019;155(1):15–20.
72. Chow CJ, Hayes LM, Saltzman DA. The impact of perioperative warm-up jackets on surgical site infection: cost without benefit? Am J Surg. 2016;212(5):863–5.
73. Wills BW, Smith WR, Arguello AM, Mcgwin G, Ghanem ES, Ponce BA. Association of surgical jacket and Bouffant use with surgical site infection risk. 2020;35205:1–6.
74. Wills BW, Smith WR, Arguello AM, McGwin G, Ghanem ES, Ponce BA. Association of surgical jacket and Bouffant use with surgical site infection risk. JAMA Surg. 2020;155(4):323–8.
75. Spirling LI, Daniels IR. William Stewart Halsted—surgeon extraordinaire: a story of "drugs, gloves and romance". J R Soc Promot Heal. 2002;122(2):122–4.
76. Idota N, Nakamura M, Akasaka Y, Tsuboi H, Bando R, Ikegaya H. Perforation rates in double latex gloves and protective effects of outer work gloves in a postmortem examination room: a STROBE-compliant study. Medicine (Baltimore). 2019;98(27):e16348.
77. Makama JG, Okeme IM, Makama EJ, Ameh EA. Glove perforation rate in surgery: a randomized, controlled study to evaluate the efficacy of double gloving. Surg Infect (Larchmt). 2016;17(4):436–42.
78. Tanner J, Parkinson H. Double gloving to reduce surgical cross-infection. Cochrane Database Syst Rev. 2006;2006(3):CD003087.
79. Anderson DJ, Podgorny K, Berríos-Torres SI, Bratzler DW, Dellinger EP, Greene L, et al. Strategies to prevent surgical site infections in acute care hospitals: 2014 update. Infect Control Hosp Epidemiol. 2014;35(6):605–27.
80. Kim K, Zhu M, Munro JT, Young SW. Glove change to reduce the risk of surgical site infection or prosthetic joint infection in arthroplasty surgeries: a systematic review. ANZ J Surg. 2019;89(9):1009–15.
81. Hajar Z, Mana TSC, Tomas ME, Alhmidi H, Wilson BM, Donskey CJ. A crossover trial comparing contamination of healthcare personnel during removal of a standard gown versus a modified gown with increased skin coverage at the hands and wrists. Infect Control Hosp Epidemiol. 2019;40(11):1278–80.
82. Mana TSC, Tomas ME, Cadnum JL, Jencson AL, Piedrahita CT, Donskey CJ. A randomized trial of two cover gowns comparing contamination of healthcare personnel during removal of personal protective equipment. Infect Control Hosp Epidemiol. 2018;39(1):97–100.
83. Tomas ME, Cadnum JL, Mana TSC, Jencson AL, Donskey CJ. Seamless suits: reducing personnel contamination through improved personal protective equipment design. Infect Control Hosp Epidemiol. 2016;37:742–4.
84. Kahveci Z, Selcen Kilinc-Balci F, Yorio PL. Critical investigation of glove-gown interface barrier performance in simulated surgical settings. J Occup Environ Hyg. 2019;16(7):498–506.
85. RP first look: new recommended practices for surgical attire. AORN J [Internet]. 2014;100(5):C1–10. https://doi.org/10.1016/S0001-2092(14)01101-6.
86. Elmously A, Gray KD, Michelassi F, Afaneh C, Kluger MD, Salemi A, et al. Operating room attire policy and healthcare cost: favoring evidence over action for prevention of surgical site infections. J Am Coll Surg. 2019;228(1):98–106.
87. Spruce L. Association of Perioperative Registered Nurses clarifies position on surgical attire. J Am Coll Surg. 2019;228:207–8.
88. Elmously A, Pomp A, Michelassi F. Operating room attire policy: the untoward effects of favoring action over evidence: in reply to Spruce. J Am Coll Surg. 2019;228:208–9.
89. Ramos RD, Itani KMF. Emotions, common sense, and evidence in operating room attire. JAMA Surg. 2020;155(4):329.
90. Petro CC, Rosen MJ. What surgeons need to know about the bouffant scandal. JAMA Surg. 2019;154(11):989–90.
91. A statement from the meeting of ACS, AORN, ASA, APIC, AST, and TJC concerning recommendations for operating room attire [Internet]. [cited 2020 Oct 4]. https://www.facs.org/about-acs/consensus-statements/or-attire

92. Kowalski TJ, Kothari SN, Mathiason MA, Borgert AJ. Impact of hair removal on surgical site infection rates: a prospective randomized noninferiority trial. J Am Coll Surg. 2016;223(5):704–11.
93. Kothari SN, Anderson MJ, Borgert AJ, Kallies KJ, Kowalski TJ. Bouffant vs skull cap and impact on surgical site infection: does operating room headwear really matter? J Am Coll Surg. 2018;227(2):198–202.
94. Markel TA, Gormley T, Greeley D, Ostojic J, Wise A, Rajala J, et al. Hats off: a study of different operating room headgear assessed by environmental quality indicators. J Am Coll Surg. 2017;225(5):573–81.
95. Farach SM, Kelly KN, Farkas RL, Ruan DT, Matroniano A, Linehan DC, et al. Have recent modifications of operating room attire policies decreased surgical site infections? An American College of Surgeons NSQIP review of 6,517 patients. J Am Coll Surg. 2018;226(5):804–13.
96. McHugh SM, Corrigan MA, Hill ADK, Humphreys H. Surgical attire, practices and their perception in the prevention of surgical site infection. Surgeon. 2014;12(1):47–52.
97. Salassa TE, Swiontkowski MF. Surgical attire and the operating room: role in infection prevention. J Bone Joint Surg Am. 2014;96(17):1485–92.
98. Friberg B, Friberg S, Ostensson R, Burman LG. Surgical area contamination—comparable bacterial counts using disposable head and mask and helmet aspirator system, but dramatic increase upon omission of head-gear: an experimental study in horizontal laminar air-flow. J Hosp Infect. 2001;47(2):110–5.
99. Spruce L. Back to basics 2.0: surgical attire. AORN J [Internet]. 2020;111(3):349–356. https://doi.org/10.1002/aorn.12978.
100. Link T. Guidelines in practice: surgical attire. AORN J [Internet]. 2020;111(4):425–439. https://doi.org/10.1002/aorn.12991.
101. Owers KL, James E, Bannister GC. Source of bacterial shedding in laminar flow theatres. J Hosp Infect. 2004;58(3):230–2.
102. Shakir IA, Patel NH, Chamberland RR, Kaar SG. Investigation of cell phones as a potential source of bacterial contamination in the operating room. J Bone Joint Surg Am. 2015;97(3):225–31.
103. Chang C-H, Chen S-Y, Lu J-J, Chang C-J, Chang Y, Hsieh P-H. Nasal colonization and bacterial contamination of mobile phones carried by medical staff in the operating room. PLoS One. 2017;12(5):e0175811.
104. Al-Abdalall AHA. Isolation and identification of microbes associated with mobile phones in Dammam in eastern Saudi Arabia. J Family Community Med. 2010;17(1):11–4.
105. Kilic IH, Ozaslan M, Karagoz ID, Zer Y, Davutoglu V. The microbial colonisation of mobile phone used by healthcare staffs. Pak J Biol Sci. 2009;12(11):882–4.
106. Datta P, Rani H, Chander J, Gupta V. Bacterial contamination of mobile phones of health care workers. Indian J Med Microbiol. 2009;27:279–81.
107. Statement on distractions in the operating room. Bull Am Coll Surg 2016;101(10):42–44.
108. Link T. Guideline implementation: team communication. AORN J [Internet]. 2018;108(2):165–177. https://doi.org/10.1002/aorn.12300.
109. Wiegmann DA, ElBardissi AW, Dearani JA, Daly RC, Sundt TM 3rd. Disruptions in surgical flow and their relationship to surgical errors: an exploratory investigation. Surgery. 2007;142(5):658–65.
110. Persoon MC, Broos HJHP, Witjes JA, Hendrikx AJM, Scherpbier AJJM. The effect of distractions in the operating room during endourological procedures. Surg Endosc. 2011;25(2):437–43.
111. Wheelock A, Suliman A, Wharton R, Babu ED, Hull L, Vincent C, et al. The impact of operating room distractions on stress, workload, and teamwork. Ann Surg. 2015;261(6):1079–84.
112. Parker SEH, Laviana AA, Wadhera RK, Wiegmann DA, Sundt TM 3rd. Development and evaluation of an observational tool for assessing surgical flow disruptions and their impact on surgical performance. World J Surg. 2010;34(2):353–61.

113. Joseph A, Khoshkenar A, Taaffe KM, Catchpole K, Machry H, Bayramzadeh S. Minor flow disruptions, traffic-related factors and their effect on major flow disruptions in the operating room. BMJ Qual Saf. 2019;28(4):276–83.
114. Dallas anesthesiologist being sued over deadly surgery admits to texting, reading iPad during procedures [Internet]. [cited 2020 Oct 19]. https://www.dallasobserver.com/news/dallas-anesthesiologist-being-sued-over-deadly-surgery-admits-to-texting-reading-ipad-during-procedures-7134970
115. Top 10 health technology hazards for 2013. Health Devices. 2012;41(11):342–365.
116. Zheng B, Martinec DV, Cassera MA, Swanström LL. A quantitative study of disruption in the operating room during laparoscopic antireflux surgery. Surg Endosc. 2008;22(10):2171–7.
117. Murji A, Luketic L, Sobel ML, Kulasegaram KM, Leyland N, Posner G. Evaluating the effect of distractions in the operating room on clinical decision-making and patient safety. Surg Endosc. 2016;30(10):4499–504.
118. Cohen TN, Shappell SA, Reeves ST, Boquet AJ. Distracted doctoring: the role of personal electronic devices in the operating room. Perioper Care Oper Room Manag [Internet]. 2018;10:10–13. http://www.sciencedirect.com/science/article/pii/S2405603017300365.
119. Prgomet M, Georgiou A, Westbrook JI. The impact of mobile handheld technology on hospital physicians' work practices and patient care: a systematic review. J Am Med Inform Assoc. 2009;16(6):792–801.
120. Attri JP, Khetarpal R, Chatrath V, Kaur J. Concerns about usage of smartphones in operating room and critical care scenario. Saudi J Anaesth. 2016;10(1):87–94.
121. AORN position statement on managing distractions and noise during perioperative patient care. AORN J [Internet]. 2020;111(6):675–680. https://doi.org/10.1002/aorn.13064.
122. Clark C, Paunovic K. WHO environmental noise guidelines for the European region: a systematic review on environmental noise and quality of life, wellbeing and mental health. Int J Environ Res Public Health. 2018;15(11):2400.
123. Keller S, Tschan F, Semmer NK, Holzer E, Candinas D, Brink M, et al. Noise in the operating room distracts members of the surgical team. An observational study. World J Surg. 2018;42(12):3880–7.
124. Shankar N, Malhotra KL, Ahuja S, Tandon OP. Noise pollution: a study of noise levels in the operation theatres of a general hospital during various surgical procedures. J Indian Med Assoc. 2001;99(5):244, 246–7.
125. Wang X, Zeng L, Li G, Xu M, Wei B, Li Y, et al. A cross-sectional study in a tertiary care hospital in China: noise or silence in the operating room. BMJ Open. 2017;7(9):e016316.
126. Basner M, Babisch W, Davis A, Brink M, Clark C, Janssen S, et al. Auditory and non-auditory effects of noise on health. Lancet. 2014;383(9925):1325–32.
127. Witterseh T, Wyon DP, Clausen G. The effects of moderate heat stress and open-plan office noise distraction on SBS symptoms and on the performance of office work. Indoor Air. 2004;14(Suppl 8):30–40.
128. Baker MA, Holding DH. The effects of noise and speech on cognitive task performance. J Gen Psychol. 1993;120(3):339–55.
129. Katz JD. Noise in the operating room. Anesthesiology. 2014;121:894–8.
130. Joseph A, Ulrich R. Sound control for improved outcomes in healthcare settings. Center for Health Design. 2007;4.
131. Dholakia S, Jeans JP, Khalid U, Dholakia S, D'Souza C, Nemeth K. The association of noise and surgical-site infection in day-case hernia repairs. Surgery. 2015;157(6):1153–6.
132. Kurmann A, Peter M, Tschan F, Mühlemann K, Candinas D, Beldi G. Adverse effect of noise in the operating theatre on surgical-site infection. Br J Surg. 2011;98(7):1021–5.
133. Enser M, Moriceau J, Abily J, Damm C, Occhiali E, Besnier E, et al. Background noise lowers the performance of anaesthesiology residents' clinical reasoning when measured by script concordance: a randomised crossover volunteer study. Eur J Anaesthesiol. 2017;34(7):464–70.
134. Communication AE, Competence C. R 3 Report. Int J Qual Heal Care. 2012;(1):3–6.

135. Imhoff M, Kuhls S, Gather U, Fried R. Smart alarms from medical devices in the OR and ICU. Best Pract Res Clin Anaesthesiol. 2009;23(1):39–50.
136. El Boghdady M, Ewalds-Kvist BM. The influence of music on the surgical task performance: a systematic review. Int J Surg. 2020;73:101–12.
137. Preventing violence in the health care setting. Sentinel event alert, Joint Commission 2010;(45):1–3.
138. Leadership skills in the OR, Part II: recognizing disruptive behavior. The Bulletin [Internet]. [cited 2020 Oct 3]. https://bulletin.facs.org/2012/06/leadership-skills-in-the-or-part-ii-recognizing-disruptive-behavior/
139. Lingard L, Reznick R, Espin S, Regehr G, DeVito I. Team communications in the operating room: talk patterns, sites of tension, and implications for novices. Acad Med. 2002;77(3):232–7.
140. Weber DO. Poll results: doctors' disruptive behavior disturbs physician leaders. Physician Exec. 2004;30(5):6–14.
141. Lingard L, Regehr G, Espin S, Devito I, Whyte S, Buller D, et al. Perceptions of operating room tension across professions: building generalizable evidence and educational resources. Acad Med. 2005;80(10 Suppl):S75–9.
142. Gillespie BM, Withers TK, Lavin J, Gardiner T, Marshall AP. Factors that drive team participation in surgical safety checks: a prospective study. Patient Saf Surg. 2016;10:3.
143. Barzallo Salazar MJ, Minkoff H, Bayya J, Gillett B, Onoriode H, Weedon J, et al. Influence of surgeon behavior on trainee willingness to speak up: a randomized controlled trial. J Am Coll Surg. 2014;219(5):1001–7.
144. The disruptive physician: addressing the issues. The Bulletin [Internet]. [cited 2020 Oct 3]. https://bulletin.facs.org/2015/02/the-disruptive-physician-addressing-the-issues/
145. Magill SS, Edwards JR, Bamberg W, Beldavs ZG, Dumyati G, Kainer MA, et al. Multistate point-prevalence survey of health care-associated infections. N Engl J Med. 2014;370(13):1198–208.
146. Korol E, Johnston K, Waser N, Sifakis F, Jafri HS, Lo M, et al. A systematic review of risk factors associated with surgical site infections among surgical patients. PLoS One. 2013;8(12):e83743.
147. Cowperthwaite L, Holm RL. Guideline implementation: preoperative patient skin antisepsis. AORN J. 2015;101(1):71–80.
148. Love KL. Patient care interventions to reduce the risk of surgical site infections. AORN J [Internet]. 2016;104(6):506–515. https://doi.org/10.1016/j.aorn.2016.10.002.
149. ABMS. Standards for initial certification. 2016. https://www.abms.org/media/119927/abms-standards-for-initial-certification.pdf
150. ACGME core competencies—ECHO Resources [Internet]. [cited 2020 Oct 25]. https://www.ecfmg.org/echo/acgme-core-competencies.html
151. John PR, Heitt MC. Disruptive physician behavior: the importance of recognition and intervention and its impact on patient safety. J Hosp Med. 2018;13(3):210–2.
152. Russ S, Rout S, Sevdalis N, Moorthy K, Darzi A, Vincent C. Do safety checklists improve teamwork and communication in the operating room? A systematic review. Ann Surg. 2013;258(6):856–71.
153. Guideline quick view: team communication. AORN J [Internet]. 2018;107(4):531–534. https://doi.org/10.1002/aorn.12125.

10 Handling Surgical Specimens to Decrease Errors in Pathology

Fouad Boulos and Michel Attieh

Introduction

The discipline of pathology is one that largely takes place behind the scenes and is commonly misunderstood by members of the clinical teams. Its role is often reduced to the simple examination of tissue and subsequent issuing of a diagnosis. Although this view represents the essence of what a pathologist is trained to do, it would be a mistake to oversimplify the procedural complexities of diagnostic surgical pathology. The process of obtaining a diagnosis from a surgical specimen is multifaceted and suffers from a myriad of potential sources of error, any one of which can entirely compromise the accuracy of the end result. These errors can occur at any number of junctures, from the admission of the patient to the hospital until the issuing of the final pathology report. In order to better grasp when and how problems may arise, it serves to divide these steps into three distinct stages. The first is the pre-analytical stage, which involves everything that takes place prior to the receipt of the specimen in the pathology department. The second is the analytical stage, which involves the laboratory work including tissue fixation, processing, staining, and interpretation. The third and last is the post-analytical and probably the least complex stage, which involves the drafting and issuing of the final pathology report. Although errors tend to be blamed on the analytical and post-analytical stages of the diagnostic process, many preventable errors occur before the specimen even reaches the pathology lab, contributing either to downright mistakes or to unnecessary delays in the diagnosis and management of patients.

F. Boulos
Department of Pathology and Immunology, Washington University in St. Louis, St. Louis, MO, USA

M. Attieh (✉)
Department of Anatomical Pathology and Laboratory Medicine, American University of Beirut Medical Center, Beirut, Lebanon

J. J. Hoballah et al. (eds.), *Principles of Perioperative Safety and Efficiency*,
https://doi.org/10.1007/978-3-031-41089-5_10

This chapter will focus on the pre-analytical phase of the diagnostic process, listing the potential scenarios where mistakes are likely to occur, and proposing solutions and approaches designed to decrease the frequency and severity of human error.

Although it is quite natural to think of errors in pathology as representing incorrect diagnoses, we believe in expanding the definition of error to encompass actions that result in unnecessary expenses, delays, and confusion, even if they are eventually resolved and an accurate diagnosis is ultimately rendered. Thankfully, the number of instances where a wrong diagnosis is given because of a breakdown of the procedural steps is low. However, the number of instances where a wrong diagnosis could have been given had the pathologists not taken the adequate steps to acquire and verify informational elements that were lacking—or did not fulfill reasonable expectations—is quite high, in our experience. These shortfalls should therefore be regarded as significantly disruptive elements resulting in inefficient or inaccurate outcomes, and all such instances that contribute to the possibility of error should be addressed and remedied individually and systematically.

We shall proceed to divide the pre-analytical phase into its constituent parts, each of which will be analyzed in a separate section. The sections are as follows: patient identification, communication between clinician and pathologist, clinical history, tissue identification and orientation, tissue preservation, and tissue transportation [1, 2].

Patient Identification

Proper patient identification is without a doubt the most fundamental measure to ensure appropriate medical care [3]. A detailed discussion of patient identification procedures is beyond the scope of this chapter, as it will be addressed elsewhere in this textbook. However, patient identification goes beyond doing the correct procedure on the correct patient. It also and very importantly involves the proper identification of the specimens taken from the patients for laboratory testing and pathology examination [4–6]. The greatest number of pre-analytical mistakes related to pathology, based on large studies of thousands of patients, appears to reside in inadequate or inaccurate patient and specimen identification [7, 8]. It has become standard practice by the College of American Pathologists (CAP), Joint Commission International (JCI), and other regulatory agencies' standards to include at least two different identifiers on every patient; this aims to preempt patient mix-up when two different patients have similar identifying information like name, date of birth, or medical record number [9, 10]. The greater the number of identifiers, the lower the likelihood of identifier overlap between two patients. Despite these measures, a common source of specimen mislabeling is batching of specimens and labeling multiple containers in anticipation of a specific procedure, instead of preparing each container for each procedure separately to avoid specimen and container mix-up. Although batching containers across patients is rarely an issue in operating rooms, given the necessary separation and time between procedures, batching the preparation of containers for different specimens on the same patient is common practice.

This frequently results in putting the wrong sample in the wrong container leading, at best, to confusion and inefficiency, and at worst to a mismatch between site and diagnosis. The acquisition of advanced hospital information systems that rely heavily on barcodes and proper identification in order to minimize human error has helped in that respect. It may, however, lead to overreliance on the accuracy of the system, encouraging sloppy practices that will lead to mistakes irrespective of the advances and advantages that medical software provides. For instance, a barcode on the wristband of the patient leading to the opening of the appropriate electronic medical chart and printing of the appropriate labels will not prevent an inattentive healthcare worker from putting the wrong specimen in the wrong container.

Specimen containers should therefore be carefully checked for proper identification and labeling just as carefully as when a phlebotomist draws blood on a patient and puts it in a tube for further testing [11].

Communication Between Clinician and Pathologist

Lack of adequate communication between clinicians and pathologists and between clinicians themselves has affected the healthcare system for decades and continues to play a major role in potential diagnostic and management errors, and in adverse outcomes on multiple medical and non-medical levels [12–14]. We should be cognizant of the fact that patients are acutely aware of—and highly sensitive to—the lack of sufficient communication between members of the medical teams in charge of their care. In the absence of general patient satisfaction, it is doubtful that state-of-the-art medical procedures and knowledge can, by themselves, amount to optimal medical care and outcome. The absence of sufficient communication between the clinician/surgeon and the pathologist is as detrimental as any instance of insufficient communication among medical teams and can manifest in any number of ways. Most frequently, it consists of inadequate sharing of relevant clinical information, or unclear communication of the needed ancillary diagnostic modality [14]. Moreover, in the highly complex and intricate medical ecosystem that has evolved over the recent decades, a surgical procedure may serve the sole purpose of diagnosis, therefore requiring specialized ancillary studies such as molecular testing, flow cytometry, specific predictive immunohistochemical markers, etc. Resections may be therapeutic, or palliative. Resection margins may or may not be relevant, and which margins are especially relevant may not be apparent. A lesion may or may not be grossly visible and may be isolated or one of several. Localization devices may or may not have been inserted to identify the site of the tumor. The information that can be, or needs to be, gleaned from a surgical specimen varies tremendously from one specimen to the other and from one patient to the other. It is the surgeon's solemn responsibility to inform the pathologist of the relevant information and the henceforth-needed diagnostic and clinical tests for the appropriate evaluation and management of the patient.

Another important aspect of proper communication between clinician and pathologist relates to making the pathologist aware of special circumstances associated with a specific tissue sample. These include urgency of the sample, scheduling at odd times when the pathologist and needed ancillary staff may not be readily available, and samples requiring special handling, special media, and unusual diagnostic tests. This frequently not only applies to hematolymphoid and pediatric tumors, but also to a growing number of adult solid neoplasms.

We should remember that most communication occurring between clinician and pathologist takes place on the requisition sheet or within the electronic laboratory information system. Because many hospitals have not yet transitioned to an electronic ordering system and still rely on handwritten requisition sheets, it is important to emphasize the legibility of the information provided on the requisition, be it clinical history, nature of specimen, physician information, among others. An example of poorly written requisition sheets is shown in Fig. 10.1.

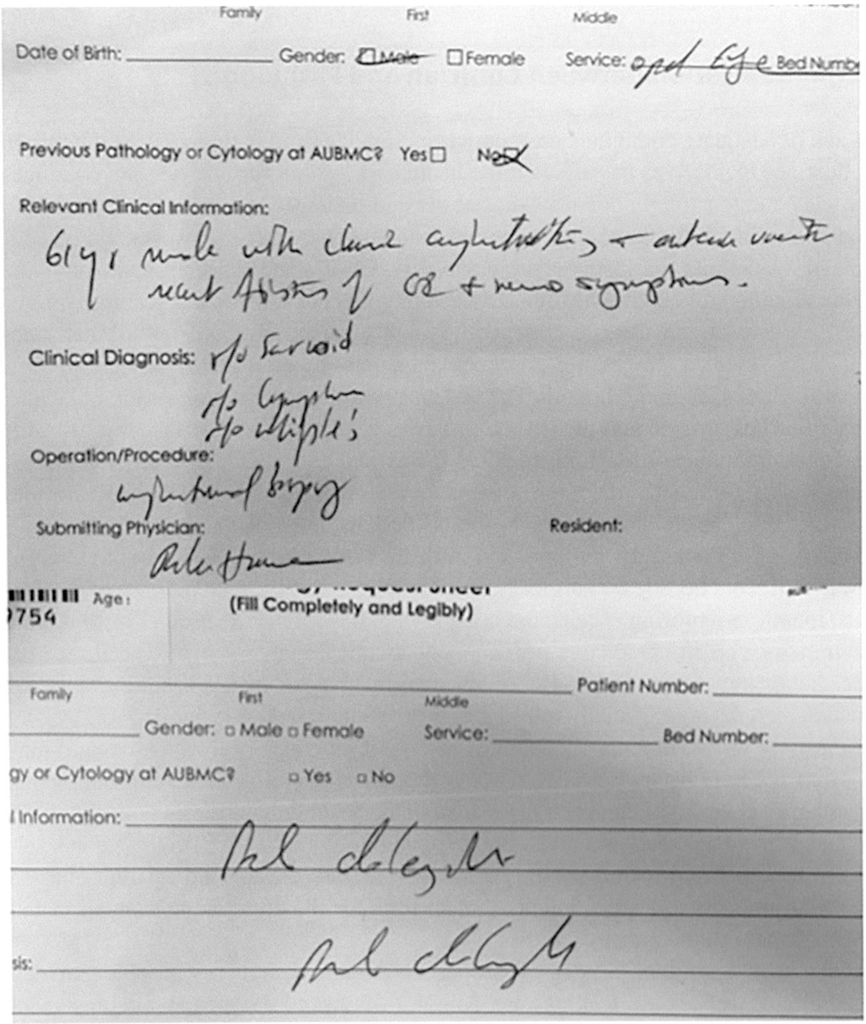

Fig. 10.1 Examples of poorly written notes

Clinical History

This section—pertaining to clinical history—naturally overlaps with the preceding section that discusses communication between pathologist and clinician. But herein we will discuss the importance of including relevant and accurate clinical history, especially if the surgeon/clinician may not be available for immediate inquiry and clarification. The lack of adequate clinical history has affected most practicing pathologists to some extent during their careers. Receiving a specimen with little to no information and no real indication as to the purpose of the surgical procedure can leave a pathologist in a precarious position, vulnerable to unwarranted mistakes. The faith that surgeons often put in a pathologist's ability to make the correct diagnosis or take the appropriate diagnostic measures based on gross and histopathologic features alone is exaggerated, and stems from poor understanding of the intrinsic limitations of the discipline of pathology. Histopathology does not sit in a vacuum, far from the clinical characteristics of the patient in question. It is therefore paramount to reinforce the idea that microscopic changes peculiar to, or characteristic of, a certain condition, may be seen in a number of other conditions as well, and can only be accurately interpreted within the proper clinical context. This is especially relevant when patients undergo surgical resections for recurrent tumors that have not been mentioned as part of the patient's clinical or surgical history. The amount of work, time, and stress that personnel may experience because of a specimen devoid of clinical background is great [15]. The more widespread use of electronic medical records and the accessibility of a patient's clinical information has decreased the amplitude of this problem. However, when patients come in for a surgical procedure after having been managed and treated at other hospitals, and while a clinic note may guide the pathologist toward what the clinician is looking for, the information included in such notes often ends up being rudimentary.

What follows is an actual example from our pathology department. An open biopsy from an abdominal mass was received on a 57-year-old woman. The biopsy harbored an undifferentiated carcinoma. A large panel of immunohistochemical stains was performed with variable nonspecific staining of some markers. A final diagnosis more precise than undifferentiated carcinoma could not be rendered. After many days of working the case up, consulting colleagues, and not being able to contact the surgeon (who was out of the country), examination of the chart revealed, buried within one of the notes, a photocopy of an outside pathology report detailing the findings in a total abdominal hysterectomy procedure that revealed ovarian carcinoma. While this instance did not pose a direct danger of misdiagnosis, and was resolved positively, withholding important information from the pathologist resulted in a waste of time and resources and could have easily ended up with a misinterpretation of the nonspecific findings in the open biopsy, with potential mismanagement of the patient. In another instance, a patient undergoing decortication of diffuse pleural thickening because of metastatic sarcomatoid renal cell carcinoma was misdiagnosed with sarcomatoid mesothelioma because the clinicians omitted the prior history of a malignant renal neoplasm. Understandably, the prognosis in this latter instance may not be significantly altered, but one can easily envision instances where both prognosis and management are significantly compromised by inaccurate or inadequate clinical history.

Another aspect of delivering accurate and complete clinical history includes providing the pathologist with relevant previous material for review. Instances where the patient is undergoing resection of a recurrent tumor, be it locally or at a distant site, are common. Comparing the original to the recurrent/metastatic tumor is very important in order to confidently differentiate a recurrence from a new primary. It is commonly assumed that immunohistochemical staining will provide unequivocal answers as to the type and site of origin of all tumors. This is, however, idealistic, as many tumors share overlapping morphologic and immunohistochemical features, yet carry entirely different management and prognostic characteristics.

In addition, there are many historical elements that may alter the morphology of a resected specimen, or require ancillary testing or more vigilant examination, that may be considered irrelevant by the clinician. These include, but are not limited to, HIV status, EBV infection, administration of steroids in hematolymphoid neoplasms, prior radiation therapy or chemotherapy, exposure to infectious organisms such as tuberculosis or leishmania, travel to possibly endemic areas, etc. Some of these situations may not be intuitive to the clinician, but many are both intuitive and important, yet remain frequently omitted from the clinical information paragraph on the requisition sheet.

Tissue Identification and Orientation

A pathologist cannot overemphasize the importance of stating the exact source of a specimen in order to reach a correct diagnosis. Neighboring organs spawn distinctly different types of neoplastic proliferation. The morphologic overlap between some of these distinct tumors is, however, sufficient to issue a false diagnosis because of incorrect information about the origin of the specimen. It matters if something is renal or suprarenal, rectal or perirectal, gastric or from the gastro-esophageal junction, etc. Naturally, this applies more readily to core biopsies and small surgical specimens lacking the benefit of gross identification, but the principle of accurate designation is not to be taken lightly under any circumstance.

Although laterality will not affect the accuracy of a pathology diagnosis, it remains very important to mention for documentation and medico-legal purposes. In the same vein, a large surgical specimen requiring orientation for adequate evaluation of landmarks and margins should be oriented via three axes, by sutures or special ink applied by the surgeon him/herself. Although sutures are probably the more prevalent method of orienting a specimen, at least in our experience, we believe that a suture marking a single spot does not adequately represent an entire surface as applying ink to it would. The limitation of using sutures is augmented by the distortion an ex vivo specimen may be subjected to following settling, manipulation, and fixation in transportation containers. We do understand, however, that the surgeon may perceive the inking of specimens as cumbersome and may consider the pathologist better suited for such techniques. When knowing exactly which margin is positive and how this positivity will influence further surgical management, an extra effort requiring a rather simple methodology toward a better clinical outcome remains warranted.

Tissue Preservation

The entire discipline of pathology is based on the examination of the architecture and cellular details of tissue excised from the human body. This is only possible if the excised tissue is preserved and prevented from undergoing the otherwise unavoidable degradation process. Formaldehyde is the most commonly used and ubiquitously accepted chemical that accomplishes this function. Once tissue is soaked in formaldehyde, its constituent proteins are cross-linked, and soluble proteins are fixed to structural proteins in a way that maintains tissue integrity, gives mechanical strength, and renders it somewhat resistant to enzymatic digestion and degradation [16, 17]. In other words, it becomes resistant to autolysis. It becomes, therefore, possible to take sections from this tissue and embed them in paraffin. This is then followed by taking thin paraffin tissue sections and putting them on glass slides and staining them with hematoxylin and eosin. If the fixation process is inadequate, then the microscopic detail is lost, and with it, any chance of a reliable or complete diagnosis. This happens most frequently in specimens that sit overnight, either in the surgical suite or in the receiving area, without being transported promptly to surgical pathology. Specimens that are especially sensitive to autolysis are ones that have a mucosal surface, due to the high susceptibility of the mucosa to ischemic damage. Any specimen type can undergo autolytic degeneration to some extent if not properly and promptly handled. Examples of autolysis as seen in hematoxylin and eosin preparations are shown in Fig. 10.2.

Moreover, fixation has become extremely important for adequate pathological assessment, beyond morphologic preservation for histopathologic evaluation. Many tumors, most notably breast cancer, require an array of immunohistochemical stains to adequately predict response to targeted therapies such as hormonal therapy and anti-Her2/neu treatment, among others that will likely be available in the near

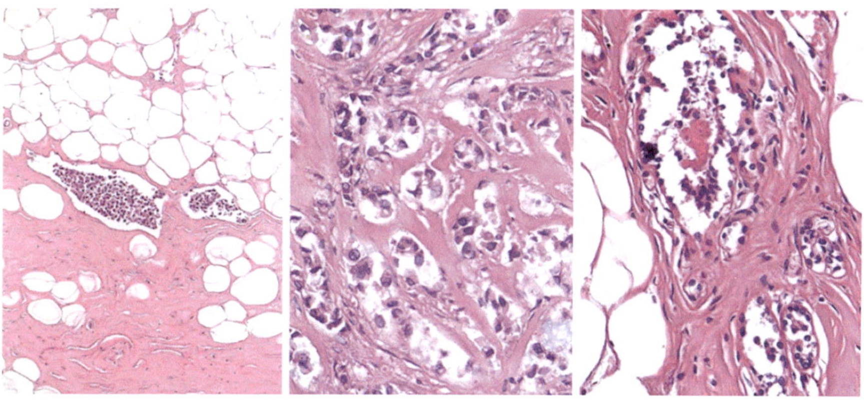

Fig. 10.2 Examples of autolysis as seen on hematoxylin and eosin preparations. The cells appear detached and floating in an empty space. In the sections from breast specimens, the pathologist can hardly determine the grade of the invasive cells or distinguish between in situ carcinoma and lymphatic invasion

future. Such predictive markers are tightly regulated to ensure accuracy and reproducibility of results [18]. As an example, the American Society for Clinical Oncology (ASCO), in conjunction with the College of American Pathologists, have since 2007 issued several reports detailing both testing and scoring requirements based on the available evidence exactly for the purposes of standardization and reproducibility across laboratories, testing facilities, and pathologists. In all of their issued reports, the ASCO/CAP experts have mandated that the tissue be placed in fixative no later than 1 h following surgical resection. This is referred to as cold ischemic time (not to be confused with cold ischemia time, which relates to the disconnection and reconnection of an organ from the systemic vasculature during a surgical procedure) [19, 20]. It may seem like the 1-h threshold of cold ischemic time is quite easy to achieve in the setting of a modern hospital milieu. The real question, however, is how long it takes the fixative to reach the tissue of interest and preserve it for adequate staining and evaluation [21].

As stated above, the fixative that is most widely used and on which all the standard recommendations are based is formaldehyde, in the form of 10% buffered formalin, which is a combination of formaldehyde and a buffer. Formalin infiltrates tissue according to a formula that dictates a decremental rate of penetration reaching approximately 1 mm per hour after the fourth hour. This rate is sufficient for needle biopsies. However, when it comes to larger resection specimens with a tumor in the center of the specimen, several centimeters away from the surgical margin, it is remarkably slow. We bypass this limitation by immediately handling large specimens and sectioning them into multiple 0.5–1 cm slabs in order to expose the maximum surface area possible to formalin and to avoid the all-but-guaranteed ensuing poor fixation and autolysis following delayed exposure to formalin [22].

Another aspect of formalin fixation that is not well known among non-pathologists is the amount of formalin required for the proper fixation of a tissue sample. Appropriate fixation requires an equal volume-to-volume amount of formaldehyde for the fixative to accomplish its function. Given that the formalin used in labs is significantly diluted (10% buffered formalin) the approximate amount of formalin needed for proper fixation is roughly 10 times the volume of the tissue resected. In other words, if an appendix that has a volume of approximately 6 cm^3 is to be properly fixed, it will need approximately 60 mL of formalin. In the case of small specimens and the small containers housing them, this is not a problem. However, when dealing with larger specimens placed within barely large enough containers with hardly any formalin, the issue becomes problematic. The very small amount of formalin barely surrounding the tissue will add to the problem of slow formalin infiltration into the resected surgical specimen.

It is standard practice that specimens removed after-hours will sit overnight in the refrigerator in the operating suite. Refrigeration is an important surrogate for fixation because it delays the degradation of tissue. However, when it comes to the reliability of immunohistochemical markers, refrigeration might not be sufficient to counteract the loss of antigenicity and tissue degradation with ensuing decreased immunoreactivity for the predictive markers, and subsequent high rates of false-negative results [23–25].

The recommendation is to deal with any resected specimen, especially tumor resections, with utmost care and urgency in order to provide the highest quality of service to patients. Appropriately sized containers with a sufficient amount of formalin should be available and should receive the specimen as quickly following excision as possible. This is especially relevant with procedures that take many hours and may result in a specimen sitting on the shelf devoid of proper fixative for longer than necessary. One must, however, note that when it comes to very large specimens, it would be a practical impossibility to surround the resected tissue with formalin 10 times the volume of the tissue itself, which would require a container almost the size of a barrel. However, ensuring that the resected specimen is surrounded by at least the same volume of formalin to allow for proper superficial fixation until the specimen is received in the lab and properly handled, is vital [26, 27].

Tissue Transportation

Serious errors can also occur while the specimen is transported from the surgical suite to the pathology laboratory. These include specimen loss, misplacement of the specimen in a location that exposes it to extremes of temperature leading to tissue deterioration or destruction, and delivering the specimen to sites other than surgical pathology (microbiology, chemistry, or cytogenetics) where it may remain unaccounted for, or subjected to unintended processing procedures that will render the tissue unsuitable for further surgical pathology examination. Such events can be damaging to the medical care and welfare of the patient, especially given that surgical specimens are usually unique and impossible to replace [28].

Notes on Intraoperative Consultation

Although the source of errors related to intraoperative frozen section diagnosis are by far secondary to analytic concerns such as sampling and interpretation, there are rare instances where a frozen section is requested on a small amount of tissue without proper justification of the intraoperative consultation. This may lead to exhaustion of valuable diagnostic material without reaching a final diagnosis, or to subjecting the tissue to freezing artifacts therefore compromising adequate histomorphologic assessment [29]. Such artifacts are magnified by placing the specimen in an aqueous solution, where tissue is likely to absorb significant amounts of fluid, therefore increasing freezing-related changes. Alternatively, putting small pieces of tissue in a completely dry container may cause desiccation of the tissue and may compromise histomorphologic detail. We believe the best practice is to make sure the tissue is in a moderate state of moisture, with a small amount of surrounding saline. A specimen received in formalin, especially if small and quickly affected by the fixative, will be challenging to freeze, as frozen fixed tissue loses the ability to adhere to glass slides. Non-technical issues pertaining to intraoperative consultation include the importance of having a physician or physician-in-training bring the specimen to surgical pathology in order to alert laboratory staff that an intraoperative consultation is requested, and to ensure that the pathologist is aware of the surgeon's specific question, in order to appropriately handle the specimen and provide the needed intraoperative diagnosis.

Interventions and Possible Solutions

Reading through this chapter might leave one with the impression that the process of collecting tissue, processing it, and issuing a diagnosis is nothing short of walking through a minefield. This may be true to some extent, although achieving excellent results with minimal errors is certainly possible if appropriate measures are taken. The traditional approach to problem-solving has often consisted of identifying and incriminating the culprit instead of analyzing the circumstances that lead to the error and responding appropriately to prevent it from recurring. Undoubtedly, many have witnessed a circulation employee drop off a specimen for frozen section, leaving it on the receiving desk without alerting laboratory staff, and being squarely blamed for the incident, while in reality they were covering for a coworker, and were not aware of what a frozen specimen entailed. Rather than attaching blame on an individual, a systems approach emphasizes the process as a whole with respect to the handling and transport of specimens, and policies and procedures formed within a systems approach focus on the precautions that can diminish the risk of errors. The inclusion of a full requisition form accompanying all specimens delivered to the pathology or laboratory department is necessary, especially in the absence of an electronic ordering system. Appropriate training and instructions to fill all the required fields within the requisition sheet is also key. The following information should be completed on the form: patient's name; patient's healthcare facility identification number; patient's unit and/or room number; clinical diagnosis; surgeon's name; source of specimen to include anatomical location where the specimen was removed, side, type of tissue, date and time of collection in the operating room; study requested, for example, frozen section, culture, lymphoma, molecular, etc.; other pertinent clinical information; and the name of circulator who completed documentation and preparation of the specimen for transport to the pathology department. Another very important component of the systems-based approach to decrease errors is chain of custody. Chain of custody tracking needs to be established within the system for handling specimens. The chain of custody process should include the smallest possible number of hand-offs, each of which represents a potential source of error. The pathology, laboratory, and surgery departments should establish a fixed and predictable schedule for transport of surgical specimens for permanent evaluation. Redundancy is an important component of the quality check mechanisms that should be in place. By redundancy we mean repeatedly making sure that all the steps that need to be followed have been followed. We also mean repetitiveness of tasks by the same qualified and adequately trained personnel. Many of the problems discussed in the previous sections can also be circumvented through the use of electronic medical information systems. Relying on software will eliminate the problem of illegibility and will decrease the chances of incompletely filled requisitions by potentially forcing the requesting physician to enter information in the different fields. Unfortunately, forcing a physician to enter a value within the field does not guarantee the accuracy and reliability of the entered value. The single most important intervention toward decreasing the number of errors within pathology is to infuse healthcare workers in charge of every step of the process with a sense of ownership and responsibility, without which all attempts to improve quality and enhance result accuracy stand to fail. As long as automation is partial and human intervention and contribution is an intrinsic part of laboratory and diagnostic processes, focusing on the quality and reliability of the healthcare worker will remain key. Establishing systems to identify weak links and systematic breakdowns in order to effect appropriate modifications is therefore crucial [30].

Conclusion

In the previous paragraphs, we've described many potential sources of error in the handling of specimens prior to receipt within the surgical pathology laboratory. Many of these errors result in inefficiencies and wastage of resources, but the vast majority culminate in a correct final diagnosis. Despite this, procedural inefficiencies and unjustified expenditures on unnecessary tests can easily fall under the scrutiny of a dissatisfied customer and serve as fodder for medico-legal claims. As stated earlier, scientific accuracy is paramount, but its importance is diminished in the wake of patient dissatisfaction. We should therefore consistently strive toward excellence, excellence of both procedure and results, for one cannot materialize without the other. The smallest details will always be where the devil lies, either leading us confidently toward an outstanding product, or throwing us of course into a tempest of finger pointing, impending mediocrity, unsatisfactory patient care, and ultimate breakdown of the standards we have dedicated our careers to uphold.

References

1. Rao S, Masilamani S, Sundaram S, Prathiba D, Rajendiran S. Quality measures in pre-analytical phase of tissue processing: understanding its value in histopathology. J Clin Diagn Res. 2016;10(1):EC7–EC11.
2. Rabinovitch A. The College of American Pathologists laboratory accreditation program. Accred Qual Assur. 2002;7(11):473–6.
3. Valenstein PN, Sirota RL. Identification errors in pathology and laboratory medicine. Clin Lab Med. 2004;24(4):979–96, vii.
4. Francis DL, Prabhakar S, Sanderson SO. A quality initiative to decrease pathology specimen–labeling errors using radiofrequency identification in a high-volume endoscopy center. Am J Gastroenterol. 2009;104(4):972.
5. Marberger M, McConnell JD, Fowler I, Andriole GL, Bostwick DG, Somerville MC, et al. Biopsy misidentification identified by DNA profiling in a large multicenter trial. J Clin Oncol. 2011;29(13):1744.

6. Meyer E, Underwood RS, Padmanabhan V. Patient misidentification in Papanicolaou tests: a systems-based approach to reducing errors. Arch Pathol Lab Med. 2009;133(8):1297–300.
7. Tapper MA, Pethick JC, Dilworth LL, McGrowder DA. Pre-analytical errors at the chemical pathology laboratory of a teaching hospital. J Clin Diagn Res. 2017;11(8):BC16.
8. Nakhleh RE, Zarbo RJ. Surgical pathology specimen identification and accessioning: a College of American Pathologists Q-probes study of 1,004,115 cases from 417 institutions. Arch Pathol Lab Med. 1996;120(3):227.
9. Hawkins R. Managing the pre-and post-analytical phases of the total testing process. Ann Lab Med. 2012;32(1):5–16.
10. Lott R, Tunnicliffe J, Sheppard E, Committee NSfHH. Pre-microscopic examination specimen handling guidelines in the surgical pathology laboratory. College of American Pathologists (CAP) and National Society for Histotechnology Published by HISTOQIP. 2014:1–49.
11. Lott R, Tunnicliffe J, Sheppard E, Santiago J, Hladik C, Nasim M, et al. Practical guide to specimen handling in surgical pathology. Northfield: College of American Pathologists (CAP); 2015. p. 24–52.
12. Nakhleh RE, Gephardt G, Zarbo RJ. Necessity of clinical information in surgical pathology: a College of American Pathologists Q-probes study of 771 475 surgical pathology cases from 341 institutions. Arch Pathol Lab Med. 1999;123(7):615–9.
13. Nakhleh RE, Zarbo RJ. Amended reports in surgical pathology and implications for diagnostic error detection and avoidance: a College of American Pathologists Q-probes study of 1,667,547 accessioned cases in 359 laboratories. Arch Pathol Lab Med. 1998;122(4):303.
14. Troxel DB, Sabella JD. Problem areas in pathology practice. Uncovered by a review of malpractice claims. Am J Surg Pathol. 1994;18(8):821–31.
15. Nakhleh RE. Patient safety and error reduction in surgical pathology. Arch Pathol Lab Med. 2008;132(2):181–5.
16. Fraenkel-Conrat H, Olcott HS. The reaction of formaldehyde with proteins. V. Cross-linking between amino and primary amide or guanidyl groups. J Am Chem Soc. 1948;70(8):2673–84.
17. Fox CH, Johnson FB, Whiting J, Roller PP. Formaldehyde fixation. J Histochem Cytochem. 1985;33(8):845–53.
18. Wolff AC, Hammond MEH, Hicks DG, Dowsett M, McShane LM, Allison KH, et al. Recommendations for human epidermal growth factor receptor 2 testing in breast cancer: American Society of Clinical Oncology/College of American Pathologists clinical practice guideline update. Arch Pathol Lab Med. 2013;138(2):241–56.
19. Wolff AC, Hammond MEH, Schwartz JN, Hagerty KL, Allred DC, Cote RJ, et al. American Society of Clinical Oncology/College of American Pathologists guideline recommendations for human epidermal growth factor receptor 2 testing in breast cancer. Arch Pathol Lab Med. 2007;131(1):18–43.
20. Portier BP, Wang Z, Downs-Kelly E, Rowe JJ, Patil D, Lanigan C, et al. Delay to formalin fixation 'cold ischemia time': effect on ERBB2 detection by in-situ hybridization and immunohistochemistry. Mod Pathol. 2013;26(1):1.
21. Yildiz-Aktas IZ, Dabbs DJ, Bhargava R. The effect of cold ischemic time on the immunohistochemical evaluation of estrogen receptor, progesterone receptor, and HER2 expression in invasive breast carcinoma. Mod Pathol. 2012;25(8):1098.
22. Rolls G. Fixation and fixatives (2)–factors influencing chemical fixation, formaldehyde and glutaraldehyde. Leica Biosystems; 2012. http://www.leicabiosystems.com/pathologyleaders/fixation-and-fixatives-2-factors-influencing-chemical-fixation-formaldehyde-and-glutaraldehyde.
23. Fergenbaum JH, Garcia-Closas M, Hewitt SM, Lissowska J, Sakoda LC, Sherman ME. Loss of antigenicity in stored sections of breast cancer tissue microarrays. Cancer Epidemiol Biomarkers Prev. 2004;13(4):667–72.
24. Khoury T, Sait S, Hwang H, Chandrasekhar R, Wilding G, Tan D, et al. Delay to formalin fixation effect on breast biomarkers. Mod Pathol. 2009;22(11):1457.

25. Hewitt SM, Robinowitz M, Bogen SA, Gown AM, Kalra KL, Otis CN, et al. Quality assurance for design control and implementation of immunohistochemistry assays; approved guideline. 2nd ed. Wayne: Clinical and Laboratory Standards Institute; 2011.
26. Bancroft JD, Gamble M. Theory and practice of histological techniques. Philadelphia: Elsevier Health Sciences; 2008.
27. Lott R. HQIP: H&E staining. HQIP—a final critique. Chicago: College of American Pathologists; 2010.
28. Krishnan RP, Ramani P, Sherlin HJ, Sukumaran G, Ramasubramanian A, Jayaraj G, et al. Surgical specimen handover from operation theater to laboratory: a survey. Ann Maxillofac Surg. 2018;8(2):234.
29. Thomson AM, Wallace WA. Fixation artefact in an intra-operative frozen section: a potential cause of misinterpretation. J Cardiothorac Surg. 2007;2(1):45.
30. Association of Surgical Technologists. AST standards of practice for handling and care of surgical specimens. http://www.ast.org/uploadedFiles/Main_Site/Content/About_Us/Standard_Handling_Care_Surgical_Specimens.pdf. Accessed 19 Aug 2019.

Blood Transfusion Safety in the Operating Room

11

Nathan D. Neilsen, Roman Dudaryk, and Daniel Dante Yeh

Introduction

The aphorism "Blood Is Life" is likely truer nowhere than within the confines of the operating room. While blood transfusion finally became a life-saving reality in the twentieth century, thereby vastly expanding the range of survivable operations and injuries, it still remains an imperfect science, with both overt and non-overt risks and consequences. Potential safety issues regarding blood transfusion in the operating room range from risks posed by blood products directly and physiological alterations resulting from transfusion to the uncertainties that surround transfusion strategies and blood product selection. In this chapter, we will describe the most common safety concerns and measures of mitigation that pertain to blood transfusion in the surgical patient. However, it must be noted that this is a very broad topic, and one to which a significant portion of the field of transfusion medicine is dedicated. Thus, what we present here should be considered an introduction, rather than a comprehensive discussion.

N. D. Neilsen
Section of Transfusion Medicine and Therapeutic Pathology,
Division of Pulmonary, Critical Care, and Sleep Medicine,
University of New Mexico School of Medicine,
Albuquerque, NM, USA

R. Dudaryk
Department of Anesthesiology, University of Miami, Miami, FL, USA

Ryder Trauma Center, Jackson Memorial Hospital, Miami, FL, USA

D. D. Yeh (✉)
Denver Health Medical Center, Denver, CO, USA
e-mail: Daniel.yeh@dhha.org

J. J. Hoballah et al. (eds.), *Principles of Perioperative Safety and Efficiency*,
https://doi.org/10.1007/978-3-031-41089-5_11

Following a general review of blood transfusion safety practices and risks common to all transfusions, the remainder of the first portion of this chapter will focus on safety considerations that apply to special scenarios, in particular emergency blood transfusions and massive transfusion events. The second portion of the chapter will address safety considerations regarding blood product selection and transfusion strategies, with a particular emphasis on the management of major hemorrhage. Finally, we will conclude with a brief discussion on transfusion reduction strategies, now widely referred to as patient blood management.

Blood Products: Risks and Precautions

Risks of Transfusion

There are two general categories of risk with all blood transfusions—risks posed directly from the transfused products and risks due to the interaction between the blood products and the recipient. Significant direct risks include transfusion-transmitted infections (TTIs), hemolytic transfusion reactions, and anaphylactic reactions. Donor-recipient interaction risks include nosocomial infection, transfusion-related immunomodulation (TRIM), transfusion-associated circulatory overload (TACO), and transfusion-related acute lung injury (TRALI).

Transfusion Transmitted Infections (TTI)

All blood intended for transfusion is tested for transfusion-transmitted pathogens such as hepatitis B and C viruses (HBV, HCV) and human immunodeficiency virus (HIV). The tests used to screen donated blood are listed in Table 11.1. Yet despite these precautions, the risk of TTI cannot be entirely eliminated, varying from a one in two million chance for HIV infection from a single transfusion to 1 in 5000 for the transfusion of a bacterially contaminated platelet unit (Table 11.2) [1].

Historically, bacterial contamination of blood components leading to a septic transfusion reaction accounted for 11–17% of Food and Drug Administration (FDA)-reported transfusion fatalities [2]. Fortunately, the incidence has declined since the mid-2000s due to more intensive screening of platelet units and, more recently, the advent of pathogen inactivation systems. Despite such advances, platelets are by far the most commonly implicated blood product for such complications, accounting for ~70% of all septic transfusion reactions, while comprising less than 15% of total blood products transfused [3, 4].

Table 11.1 Pathogen screening tests for donated blood

Infectious disease pathogen	Laboratory tests used	Frequency of tests
Hepatitis B virus (HBV)	Hepatitis B surface antigen (HBsAg) detection	Every donation
	Hepatitis B core antibody (anti-HBc) detection	
	Nucleic acid amplification testing (NAT) for HBV	
Hepatitis C virus (HCV)	Hepatitis C virus antibody (anti-HCV) detection	Every donation
	Nucleic acid amplification testing (NAT) for HCV	
Human immunodeficiency virus types 1 and 2 (HIV)	HIV-1 and HIV-2 antibody (anti-HIV-1 and anti-HIV-2) detection	
	Nucleic acid amplification testing (NAT) for HIV-1	Every donation
Human T-lymphotropic virus types I and II (HTLV)	HTLV-I and HTLV-II antibody (anti-HTLV-I and anti-HTLV-II) detection	Every donation
Treponema pallidum (syphilis)	Anti-treponemal antibody detection	Every donation
West Nile virus (WNV)	Nucleic acid amplification testing (NAT) for WNV	Every donation
Zika virus (ZIKV)	Nucleic acid amplification testing (NAT) for ZikV	Every donation
Bacterial contamination	Bacterial culture	Every platelet donation
Babesia	Nucleic acid amplification test (NAT) and antibody for *B. microti*	Performed on donations in Babesia-endemic regions
Trypanosoma cruzi (Chagas disease)	*T. cruzi* antibody detection	All first-time donors tested
Cytomegalovirus (CMV)	CMV antibody detection	Performed on some donations for special needs recipients

Source: Centers for Disease Control and Prevention. https://www.cdc.gov/bloodsafety/basics.html

Table 11.2 Risks of transfusion transmitted infection per unit transfused

Pathogen	Risk per unit
HIV	1:2,000,000
HBV	1:300,000
HCV	1:1,500,000
West Nile virus	1:350,000
HTLV-II	1:~3,000,000
Bacterial contamination (RBC)	1:38,500
Bacterial contamination (Platelets)	1:5000

Adapted from: Petrides M, AuBuchon J. To Transfuse or Not to Transfuse: An Assessment of Risks and Benefits. In: Mintz PD, ed. *Transfusion Therapy: Clinical Principles and Practice, 3rd Edition.* Bethesda, Maryland, USA: AABB Press; 2011: 855-899

Hemolytic Transfusion Reactions

ABO-incompatible transfusions are more common than expected (~1:38,000). While less than 50% of these cases will have any clinical symptoms, 2% will directly lead to death (historical fatality risk of 1 per 1,800,000 transfusions) [5]. The National Healthcare Safety Network of the Centers for Disease Control and Prevention (CDC) reported only one to four deaths per year attributed to ABO incompatibility from 2012 to 2016 [6]. Given that approximately 21 million blood products are transfused annually in the USA, this provides an updated estimate of ABO-incompatible fatality rates of 1:5,000,000–1:20,000,000.

Mortality due to non-ABO incompatibility hemolytic transfusion reactions appear to be as common, if not more so, than ABO-incompatibility-mediated reactions, accounting for 2–13% of transfusion attributable deaths from 2012 to 2016 (Table 11.3). The etiology of these non-ABO compatibility reactions is complex, ranging from frank mistransfusion ("wrong product and/or wrong patient") to evanescent antibody levels (resulting in anamnestic immune responses) to unpreventable donor-recipient antigen-antibody mismatch in uncrossmatched transfusions. Physiologically, non-ABO hemolytic transfusion reactions typically result from the interaction of recipient antibodies and non-ABO antigens on transfused red blood cells (RBCs), most commonly those in the Rh system (D, C, c, E, e antigens), Duffy system (Fy^a, Fy^b), MNS system (M, N, S, s) and most notably, the Kell (K, k) and Kidd systems (Jk^a, Jk^b). Less frequently, these reactions can result from the interaction of antibodies in donor plasma (in transfused plasma or platelet products) and the recipient's RBC antigens [7, 8].

The majority of the fatalities from non-ABO incompatibility events are due to extravascular hemolysis, resulting in the delayed destruction of the incompatible transfused RBCs (typically 3–10 days post-transfusion). Less commonly, non-ABO transfusion reactions (typically due to Kell and Kidd antigens) can result in acute hemolytic transfusion reactions that mimic ABO-incompatible transfusion reactions, presenting with vasodilatory shock, disseminated intravascular coagulation, and renal failure [7, 9].

Clinically, non-ABO mediated hemolytic reactions are most likely to occur with "emergency" transfusions (where blood products are provided before full compatibility testing can be completed) and transfusions where the recipient's transfusion history is unknown or unavailable. Some RBC alloantibodies can drop below the level of detection of standard testing, resulting in false compatibility results, and later results in an anamnestic immune response and delayed hemolysis [10–12]. The classic example of alloantibodies that can evanesce below the level of detection but still cause severe, even fatal, transfusion reactions are those of the Kidd system (Jk^a, Jk^b). This phenomenon has led to the transfusion medicine aphorism "Kidd Kills!"

Table 11.3 Transfusion-associated fatalities by complication, FY 2012–2016

Complication	FY12 (no.)	FY12 (%)	FY13 (no.)	FY13 (%)	FY14 (no.)	FY14 (%)	FY15 (no.)	FY15 (%)	FY 16 (no.)	FY16 (%)	Total (no.)	Total (%)
Anaphylaxis	2	5	–	0	2	7	2	5	5	12	**11**	**6**
Contamination	3	8	5	13	1	3	5	14	5	12	**19**	**10**
HTR (ABO)	3	8	1	3	4	13	2	5	4	9	**14**	**8**
HTR (non-ABO)	5	13	5	13	4	13	4	11	1	2	**19**	**10**
Hypotensive reaction	–		–	0	1	3	1	3	1	2	**3**	**2**
TACO	8	21	13	34	5	17	11	30	19	44	**56**	**30**
TRALI*	17	45	14	37	13	43	12	32	8	19	**64**	**34**

Source: Federal Drug Administration Center for Biologics Evaluation and Research (CBER). Fatalities Reported to FDA Following Blood Collection and Transfusion Annual Summary for FY2016. https://www.fda.gov/media/111226/download

TRIM and Nosocomial Infection

The precise nature and mechanisms of TRIM have yet to be fully elucidated or understood though it is thought to be at the root of increased rates of perioperative infections, nosocomial pneumonia, sepsis, and cancer recurrence [13–16]. A comprehensive systematic review of 20 studies reported an odds ratio of 3.45 for postoperative bacterial infection in transfused trauma patients compared to the non-transfused [17]. Additionally, the number of blood products transfused is also associated with increased infection rates, with a clear dose-dependent correlation between number of RBC units transfused and the risk of development of infection [18, 19]. Unfortunately, various initiatives to mitigate the potential for TRIM, chief among them leukocyte reduction, have generally not been successful [20, 21].

TACO and TRALI

In recent years, the two leading causes of transfusion-associated fatalities have been TACO and TRALI. According to recent CDC data (Table 11.3), TACO surpassed TRALI in 2016 as the most common cause of transfusion-associated mortality, reaching 44%. However, the numbers reported for each complication are likely to be a gross underrepresentation due to a lack of recognition, complex confounding factors, and underreporting from clinical facilities. At least one source has suggested that TRALI alone accounts for over 150 patient deaths per year [1], and deaths due to TACO likely far outstrip this number.

Nevertheless, TRALI incidence in the USA has markedly decreased as the result of mitigation strategies aimed to reduce or eliminate plasma-containing components (plasma, platelets, whole blood) from female donors containing anti-leukocyte antibodies that are responsible for the majority of TRALI fatalities. Although not mandated by the FDA, since 2007, individual blood product manufacturers have been gradually shifting to the use of all-male donor plasma, though exceptions still exist for AB plasma, given its relative scarcity. The Association for the Advancement of Blood & Biotherapies (AABB), formerly known as the American Association of Blood Banks, now requires that all plasma-containing components and whole blood for transfusion must be collected from men, nulliparous women, or women who have tested negative for human leukocyte antigen antibodies [22].

As the risk of TRALI has decreased, the contribution of TACO to morbidity and mortality has become more pronounced, and is likely to rise further in coming years as surveillance and reporting efforts become more established and clinical awareness rises.

Type and Screen/Type and Crossmatch Process in Perioperative Environment

Aside from the peri-processing and storage safety precautions detailed above, one of the earliest safety steps in the clinical transfusion process is the "type and screen/crossmatch" (n.b.: the nomenclature of this test can vary). This test is performed in order to avoid major, potentially life-threatening, transfusion reactions due to donor–recipient incompatibility of ABO and Rh-D antigens. The test has three parts: first, the recipient's blood type and Rh D status are determined ("type"); second, the recipient's serum is tested for common and clinically significant antibodies ("screen"); third, a small amount of the recipient's serum is mixed with a small amount of the potential donor RBC unit(s)—the mixture can then be visually examined under a microscope or analyzed via automated platform. If the potential transfusion is incompatible, antibodies in the recipient serum will cause agglutination in the donor RBCs.

In theory, once the recipient's blood type is known, a transfusion of ABO-compatible blood could be given. However, simply because a potential RBC unit is ABO-compatible, the possibility of an incompatible transfusion remains—the transfusion recipient may have alloantibodies against uncommon non-ABO RBC antigens which are not identified during standard screening, or the recipient has antibodies that are of low enough titer not to be detected during screening (a false negative screen) but can result in a delayed anamnestic immune response. Both scenarios can lead to transfusion reactions (varying from trivial to fatal) if the transfused RBCs carry these antigens. The crossmatch portion of the "type and cross" is performed in order to prevent these types of reactions.

"Computer crossmatch," also known as "electronic crossmatch," is a relatively new, more efficient alternative to the serological crossmatch detailed above. This process allows for a rapid and efficient donor–recipient crossmatching process without the need for contact between donor RBCs and recipient sera. As sensitivity of commercially available antibody screens have improved with time, the necessity for traditional serologic crossmatching has declined. The electronic crossmatch has the following steps: first, the ABO/Rh typing from both donor and recipient are verified twice (two concordant blood samples). Next, recipient serum is screened for the absence of antibodies. Finally, the blood bank computer system compares and verifies ABO and Rh D types of the donor and recipient for compatibility. This process is as safe as serological crossmatch and is FDA approved as an alternative to the traditional "type and cross," provided that the recipient has had their ABO/Rh status tested *at least twice* and is not known to possess clinically significant RBC alloantibodies. The major advantage of electronic crossmatch is the rapid availability of RBCs for emergency transfusion (under 1 min) vs. conventional serologic testing (45 min). It is important to note that if the recipient has a positive antibody screen or has a history of alloantibodies, then the traditional serologic crossmatch *must* be performed.

Safety Considerations Specific to Emergency Blood Product Utilization

Emergency Red Blood Cell Transfusions

In patients who require emergent RBC transfusion, it is sometimes necessary to transfuse RBC units prior to the completion of routine blood bank compatibility testing, which may take 45 min or longer to complete. Such units are referred to as "emergency release" units and are exclusively group O in order to avoid potential ABO incompatibility reactions. However, because standard donor–recipient compatibility testing is not performed for these transfusions, nor is a recipient antibody screen available prior to transfusion, the risk of transfusion reactions mediated by non-ABO alloantibodies cannot be discounted.

A 2003 study reported a 2% prevalence of clinically significant RBC alloantibodies in a population of patients at risk for requiring urgent, uncrossmatched transfusions [23]. The same study estimated a rate of RBC alloimmunization of up to 4% among patients admitted to the emergency department. While the transfusion of uncrossmatched blood has been well documented in the military setting for decades [24], these results cannot be reliably applied to a non-combat population. More recently, studies from the civilian trauma literature have reported no acute hemolytic transfusion reactions (AHTRs), leading to the claim that uncrossmatched transfusions are safe in this setting. A longitudinal single-center study of over 1,000 emergency department RBC transfusions discovered clinically significant alloantibodies in 6% of transfused individuals, resulting in 3% of cases receiving antigen incompatible RBC units, and one case of non-ABO alloantibody-mediated HTR (0.1% of emergency release transfused units) [25]. Several studies have corroborated this finding, demonstrating a 0.02–0.5% rate of detectable hemolysis (acute *and* delayed) following uncrossmatched RBC transfusions [26, 27].

Overall, the transfusion of uncrossmatched RBC units is a relatively safe intervention with a very low risk of significant adverse reactions although close monitoring of recipients with (subsequently identified) clinically significant antibodies for evidence of hemolysis is recommended.

Emergency Plasma Transfusions

Recent years have seen a large increase in the amount of plasma used in emergency situations before the recipient's ABO/Rh type can be confirmed. This is especially true in cases of trauma, where RBC:plasma transfusion ratios now routinely approach 1:1. Since group AB plasma lacks ABO antibodies (anti-A, anti-B, anti-AB), it has historically been the standard choice for plasma transfusion when the recipient's blood type is unknown, the so-called universal plasma. This steady rise in emergent, uncrossmatched plasma use has put an untenable strain on blood suppliers as hospital blood banks attempt to keep AB plasma at 10–20% of the plasma stores, despite AB donors representing only 4% of the donor pool.

As a result of this unsustainable demand for AB plasma, some academic hospitals have trialed the use of group A plasma as an alternative. In the initial studies, no significant hemolysis was reported amongst B or AB patients who received "incompatible" group A plasma. This lack of harm has been further confirmed with wider clinical adoption [28]. There are several potential reasons for the observed lack of harm arising from group A plasma transfusions to the ~15% of the population who are non-A. First, as part of TRALI mitigation strategies, almost all group A plasma units now come from male donors, and group A male plasma typically have low titers of anti-B antibodies. Second, many centers are pre-screening the anti-B titers in A plasma units and selecting only those with low titers of anti-B for emergency use. Third, transfused anti-B antibodies are diluted into much larger recipient total blood volumes, likely reaching clinically irrelevant levels. Fourth, in the setting of emergent transfusion support, the recipients would be receiving group O RBC units, and consequently, the proportion of B or AB RBC units available for the anti-B to bind to will be progressively reduced. Finally, 80% of B or AB patients are "secretors," with soluble group B antigen in their plasma. As anti-B antibodies preferentially bind to free plasma B antigens over RBC membrane-bound ones, in these cases much of the anti-B antibodies will be "neutralized" before they can cause any clinically relevant effects. Consequently, it is a reasonable *a priori* assumption that group A plasma use is safe for emergency transfusion. This assumption has been borne out in ever more frequent clinical practice [28, 29].

It should be noted, however, that the safety of this practice has only been established in emergency situations and should *not* be applied to non-emergent ones. Routine plasma transfusions should still follow conventional ABO compatibility rules. Furthermore, even in emergency situations, it is still essential to obtain a blood sample from the recipient as soon as possible so that the transfusions service can switch to ABO-specific products as soon as possible, for both inventory and safety purposes.

Specific Safety Considerations for Massive Blood Transfusion

Massive transfusion was originally (arbitrarily) defined as the transfusion of ≥10 units RBC units in a 24-h period, though newer, evidence-based definitions have been proposed (see the "Massive Transfusion Protocols" section below). Aside from the standard risks associated with conventional blood transfusion detailed above, massive blood transfusion carries with it additional risks (see Table 11.4 for a comprehensive list of complications) [30]. Specific complications more likely to occur with massive transfusion than with standard intraoperative transfusion practice include hypothermia, coagulopathy, electrolyte abnormalities, and acid-base disturbances. Additionally, higher rates of multiorgan failure and potentially TRALI and TACO have also been reported in massive transfusion recipients [31].

Hypothermia is a common occurrence in massive transfusion scenarios for several reasons, but the use of large quantities of blood products can be a major contributor. As RBCs and plasma units are typically stored at between 1 and 6 °C, they can precipitate a rapid drop in core body temperature if they are not warmed prior to transfusion. This risk of hypothermia has been mitigated by various rapid infusion systems currently available on the market (e.g., Belmont® Rapid Infuser).

Coagulopathy is also a common occurrence among individuals receiving massive transfusion for numerous reasons, the constitution of the transfused blood products themselves contributing significantly. Simply, the standard process for producing blood components results in products that are diluted with crystalloid-based preservative solutions—a combination of 1 unit of RBC, 1 unit of plasma, and 1 unit of platelets results in a markedly diluted mixture (hematocrit of ~29%, platelet count 85,000/mcL, coagulation factor activity ~62% of normal) as compared to whole blood [30]. Nearly one-third of the volume of a unit of RBC is comprised of preservative solutions, and crystalloids may be infused as "carrier" fluids as well. Therefore, the clinician must maintain vigilance, as a dilutional coagulopathy is still possible even when transfusing equal amounts of RBC, plasma, and platelets [30, 32].

Table 11.4 Complications associated with massive blood transfusion

Acute	
	Acute hemolytic transfusion reactions
	Febrile nonhemolytic transfusion reactions
	TRALI
	TACO
	Allergic reactions
	Bacterial sepsis
	Hypocalcemia
	Hypokalemia, hyperkalemia
	Acidosis
	Hypothermia
	Dilutional coagulopathy
	Dilutional thrombocytopenia
Delayed	
	Delayed hemolytic transfusion reactions
	TRIM
	Microchimerism
	Transfusion-transmitted diseases
	Posttransfusion graft-vs-host disease
	Posttransfusion purpura

Source: Sihler KC, Napolitano LM. Complications of massive transfusion. Chest 2010;137(1):209–20.

Both hypo- and hyperkalemia are seen in massive transfusion events. Hyperkalemia occurs due to an accumulation of potassium in the extracellular fluid component of RBC units and increases with duration of storage. In fact, potassium concentrations in RBC units can range from 7 to 77 mEq/L. Patients with underlying renal injury or severe tissue injury (e.g., rhabdomyolysis or myonecrosis) are most at risk, and cases of hyperkalemic cardiac arrest have been reported with rapid transfusion through central venous catheters [33]. Hypokalemia is likely an even more common phenomenon, with incidence rates in excess of 50% in two studies of massively transfused surgical patients [34]. Multiple mechanisms account for the development of hypokalemia, first among them the restoration of RBC membrane ATPase pumps that become dormant during cold storage of RBC units—this results in potassium influx into RBCs as they "warm up" post-transfusion. Consequently, plasma potassium levels should be carefully monitored in any patient who requires massive transfusion.

Hypocalcemia, and to a lesser degree, hypomagnesemia, occurs in massive transfusion because stored blood products are anticoagulated with citrate, which binds both calcium and magnesium. In massive transfusion scenarios, citrate concentrations can reach 40–140 times normal levels, and life-threatening hypocalcemia can result [35]. Arterial blood *ionized* calcium levels should be monitored closely, as serum (total) calcium measures are not reliable in the settings and can be falsely normal or even elevated.

Metabolic alkalosis is a frequent finding in patients who required massive transfusion due to the metabolism of the citrate preservative in blood products into bicarbonate by the liver. As such, the development of a metabolic acidosis in this setting indicates tissue hypoperfusion and/or hepatic impairment.

Transfusion Strategies: Risks, Benefits, and Precautions

Blood transfusion therapy began as whole blood transfusion [36]. In the middle of the twentieth century, blood banks began to separate whole blood into its components: "packed" red blood cells, fresh frozen plasma (FFP), cryoprecipitate, and platelets. The practice of transfusing only individual components gained widespread adoption as an efficacious and cost-effective method of treating clinically stable anemia or correcting coagulopathy. This practice also led to wide acceptance of crystalloid-based resuscitation and delayed administration of plasma and platelets, eventually leading to a situation when dilutional coagulopathy became a very common sequela of this approach. Gradually, whole blood became unavailable for transfusion in the civilian sector. However, due to logistical obstacles related to blood bank processing and storage, the military continued to utilize whole blood by necessity. Studies emerging from military conflicts over the past two decades have demonstrated the survival benefits of transfusing whole fresh, warm blood to injured warriors [37]. The next logical evolution was to "reconstruct" whole blood by transfusing fractionated blood components in the same ratios from which they were deconstructed.

In 2007, Borgman et al. reported that for combat-injured soldiers receiving massive transfusion (defined as ≥10 units RBC in 24 h), those receiving higher amounts of FFP ("high ratio") had higher survival rates compared to those receiving lower amounts of FFP ("low ratio") [38]. This seminal publication triggered a cascade of interest. Recognizing that military studies have unique demographics and injury mechanism, studies in civilian trauma centers were subsequently performed using similar methodology and also reported that higher ratios of plasma and platelets were associated with improved survival [39, 40].

The term "damage control resuscitation" or "hemostatic resuscitation" has thus come to refer to a strategy of transfusing FFP and platelets at ratios approximating the ratios found in whole blood [41–44]. Animal studies have demonstrated that "1:1" FFP: RBC transfusion ratios result in decreased systemic inflammation, improved platelet function, and attenuated organ injury when compared to "1:2" FFP:RBC transfusion ratio [45, 46]. Interestingly, damage control resuscitation has been associated with higher rates of successful non-operative management of severe blunt liver injuries [47].

Military studies have reported that transfusion of fresh whole blood to combat-injured soldiers resulted in improved outcomes when compared to those receiving individual blood components [48]. Indeed, using a prescreened donor pool and a "walking blood bank," [49], military surgeons are able to receive fresh whole blood within 27 min of request [50]. At present, whole blood is unavailable for routine use in civilian practice, though there is significant interest in making it a therapeutic option [51]. A single-center trial randomized trauma patients to receive either whole blood or component therapy. After excluding those with severe traumatic brain injury, the whole blood group received significantly fewer blood products overall [52]. However, additional research is required before whole blood can be expanded out of the research setting in civilian trauma.

The PROMMTT (prospective, observational, multicenter, major trauma transfusion) study was conducted at 10 U.S. Level 1 trauma centers and demonstrated decreased 6-h mortality in patients receiving FFP:RBC ratios of 1:1 or greater compared to those receiving less than 1:2 [53]. Subsequent to the PROMMTT study, the PROPPR (pragmatic, randomized optimal platelet and plasma ratios) trial randomized massively bleeding patients to receive FFP:platelets:RBC in 1:1:1 ratio or 1:1:2. This trial did not show improvement in 24-h or 30-day all-cause mortality associated with the higher ratio transfusion strategy, but demonstrated better clinical hemostasis (a secondary outcome) in the high ratio group. Importantly, patients receiving higher volumes of FFP and platelets did not experience higher rates of 23 pre-specified complications, including ARDS, multiorgan failure, and infectious complications [54]. At present, the PROPPR trial represents the highest quality evidence on the topic of transfusion ratios in severely injured patients requiring massive transfusion. Yet many questions remain, for example, it is not known whether the same purported benefits of "balanced" blood component transfusion extend to non-trauma populations. Similarly, while much attention has been focused on the risk/benefits of plasma ratios, much remains unknown regarding platelet transfusion [40, 55, 56]. Recent evidence suggests that platelet transfusions are associated with lung injury, even in the setting of "hemostatic resuscitation" [57]. Finally, it must be acknowledged that the PROPPR trial was a *negative* trial that failed to prove superiority of 1:1:1 transfusion over 1:1:2 for its primary endpoint. An optimal transfusion ratio for all patients may not exist, and within a single patient, the optimal transfusion ratio may vary over time as the disease course evolves.

Acute Traumatic Coagulopathy

"Dilutional" coagulopathy occurs when hemorrhage is followed by volume replacement with crystalloid or low FFP:platelets:RBC ratios, leading to prolonged conventional coagulation tests—international normalized ratio (INR) and activated partial thromboplastin time (aPTT). However, it is recognized that coagulopathy can occur before any resuscitation fluids have been given, often present at the scene before arrival of rescue agents [58]. This phenomenon was initially termed "acute traumatic coagulopathy" (ATC) [59], which occurs in 24–31% of severely injured patients [59–63], and is associated with significantly higher mortality rates [59, 60, 62, 63]. ATC, also known as "systemic acquired coagulopathy," "endogenous acute coagulopathy," "traumatic coagulopathy," "trauma associated coagulopathy," and "early trauma-induced coagulopathy," has been shown to develop in the presence of tissue hypoperfusion and severe traumatic injury [58, 64]. It appears to be related to activation of protein C and is associated with depletion of multiple coagulation factors, including I, II, V, VII, VIII, IX, and X [59, 65–68]. Interestingly, ATC was found to be significantly aggravated by crystalloid resuscitation and mitigated by whole blood transfusion [69].

Viscoelastic Testing (VET)

Traditional laboratory coagulation studies require up to 80 min to receive results, whereas actionable results from thromboelastography (TEG) and rotational thromboelastometry (ROTEM)—two forms of viscoelastic testing—can be obtained within 5 min [70, 71]. VET tracings provide insight into the dynamic nature of anticoagulation, demonstrating objective measurements for clot initiation, strengthening, stabilization, and lysis (Fig. 11.1). Reproducible patterns are discernable in abnormal conditions such as coagulopathy, platelet deficiency, fibrinolysis, and hypercoagulopathy (Fig. 11.2). TEG and ROTEM have been used for decades in cardiac surgery, and strategies of factor replacement therapy guided by viscoelastic testing have been shown to result in decreased exposure to allogeneic blood products, lower incidence of postoperative acute kidney injury, fewer thromboembolic events, and lower rates of re-exploration for bleeding [73]. In trauma patients, TEG results obtained within 5 min can rapidly diagnose ATC (decreased maximal amplitude) and accurately predict the need for massive transfusion [70, 71, 74]. Goal-directed, VET-guided trauma resuscitation resulted in higher survival despite lower utilization of plasma and platelets when compared to standard conventional coagulation test-driven resuscitation [75–77].

Interestingly, TEG investigations have identified two subtypes of fibrinolytic dysfunction occurring immediately after trauma: (1) hyperfibrinolysis, a state of enhanced fibrinolytic activity; and (2) fibrinolysis shutdown, a state of impaired fibrinolysis. Both derangements, representing opposite ends of the spectrum, are associated with higher mortality rates than normal physiologic fibrinolysis [78–84]. In animal models, plasma infusion was superior to saline to attenuate hyperfibrinolysis and led to superior survival [85].

Although still a relatively new and rare practice in trauma, VET-guided resuscitation strategies are being developed and tested at several trauma centers in the USA. In theory, a VET-guided algorithm would quickly identify the need for

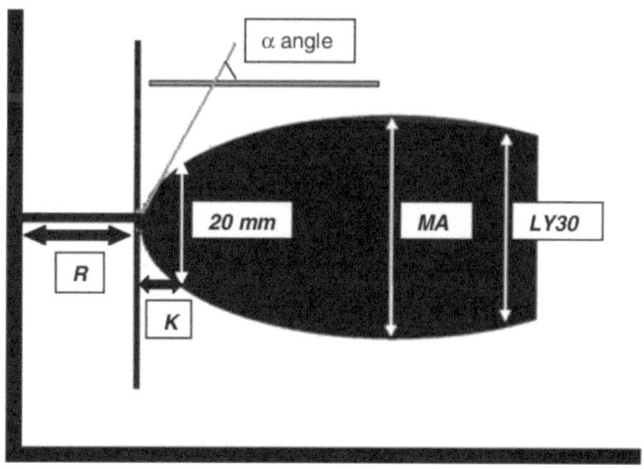

Fig. 11.1 VET tracings provide insight into the dynamic nature of anticoagulation, demonstrating objective measurements for clot initiation, strengthening, stabilization, and lysis [72]

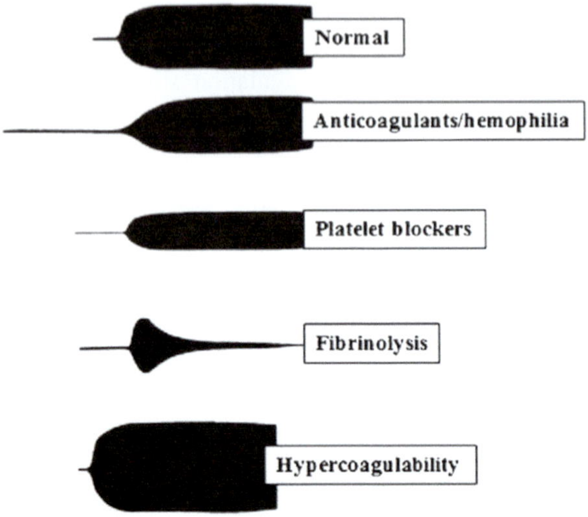

Fig. 11.2 Reproducible patterns are discernable in abnormal conditions such as coagulopathy, platelet deficiency, fibrinolysis, and hypercoagulopathy [72]

VET parameter	Interpretation	Treatment
ACT R-time Clot Time (CT)	Prolonged with factor deficiency, severe hemodilution	Plasma
K-time Clot Formation Time (CFT)	Increased with hypofibrinogenemia ± platelet dysfunction	Cryoprecipitate OR Fibrinogen concentrate ± Plasma
α-angle	Decreased with hypofibrinogenemia or platelet dysfunction	Cryoprecipitate (or fibrinogen concentrate)
Maximal Amplitude Maximum Clot Firmness	Decreased with platelet dysfunction ± hypofibrinogenemia	Platelets, ± cryoprecipitate
LY-30 CL30	Increased with accelerated fibrinolysis	Tranexamic acid OR aminocaproic acid

Reprinted with permission from Bryan Cotton

Fig. 11.3 Example of a possible VET-guided transfusion response strategy. *ACT* activated clotting time, *LY-30 %* clot lysed after 30 min, *MA* maximal amplitude, *R-time* reaction time, *VET* viscoelastic testing

massive transfusion, determine which phase of coagulation is deranged, prescribe which specific component should be transfused in response, and provide rapid feedback on the efficacy of such treatment. An example of a possible VET-guided transfusion response strategy is illustrated in Fig. 11.3.

Massive Transfusion Protocols

Massive transfusion (presently most often defined as the receipt of ≥10 units RBCs in 24 h) [86] occurs in up to 5% of all trauma patients [87–89]. Massive transfusion protocols (MTP) are hospital-level sets of rules and regulations guiding logistics of rapid delivery of blood products in pre-specified ratios for patients with massive transfusion requirements. Beyond "activation," however, additional challenges include ongoing delivery and termination of the MTP. Over-transfusion should be avoided; transfusion or RBCs to a supraphysiologic hematocrit >40% does not confer additional survival benefit and may be harmful [90]. Similarly, transfusion of FFP in ratios greater than 1:1 does not confer additional benefit and may similarly cause harm [91]. One major challenge for nearly all MTPs is plasma availability, as it takes up to 40 min to thaw frozen plasma. Without immediately available pre-thawed or liquid ("never frozen") plasma, it is difficult to accomplish a true 1:1:1 transfusion ratio in the early period after patient arrival [92].

Before-and-after studies have reported that institution of a formal MTP is associated with improved outcomes in multiorgan failure, infectious complications, ventilator-free days, and mortality [93–95]. One study reported that incorporation of a predictive score (assessment of blood consumption score) in the pre-hospital setting to shorten the time to receive thawed plasma after hospital arrival resulted in higher FFP:RBC transfusion ratio and was associated with improved overall and penetrating trauma mortality [96]. Although increased volumes of transfusion are associated with lower survival rates [97], at this time, there is no upper limit of transfusion volume which has been shown to be futile [98, 99]. One case report described a trauma patient who received 173 units of RBC and 176 units of FFP in the first 30 h, with the patient ultimately recovering and returning to work [100].

As stated above, the "traditional" definition of massive transfusion (MT) was the transfusion of 10 units or more of RBCs in a 24-h period. However, this definition has been criticized as arbitrary and inaccurate [86], as observational evidence has demonstrated that in survivors the majority of transfusions occur in the first 6 h [101, 102]. Recently, two newer definitions for massive transfusion have been proposed: *critical administration threshold (CAT)* [103] and *resuscitation intensity (RI)* [104]. A patient is defined as "CAT+" if he/she received three or more RBC units within any single hour. Resuscitation intensity (RI) attempts to quantify all forms of resuscitation fluid; the following quantities are thus redefined as "1 unit of resuscitation fluid": 1000 mL crystalloid, 500 mL colloid, 1 RBC unit, 1 FFP unit, 1 apheresis platelet unit [104]. Thus, a patient receiving 1 L of saline, 2 units of RBC, and 1 unit of FFP would be defined as RI 4. These data-driven definitions address some of the limitations (namely survivorship bias) inherent in the original definition. For example, Savage et al. examined patients receiving blood transfusion within the first 24 h and reported that CAT identified 75% of all deaths, compared to only 33% identified by the traditional MT definition [103]. Another advantage of using the CAT+ definition is the ability to analyze the effects of FFP transfusion *concurrent* with RBC transfusions per hour. The traditional MT definition cannot distinguish between alternating transfusions of RBC and FFP from 10 units of RBC transfused followed by 10 units of FFP transfused. Savage et al. demonstrated that concurrent

FFP transfusions were associated with improved survival compared to non-concurrent FFP transfusions [105]. Secondary analysis of the PROMMT study revealed higher mortality rates in patients receiving >4 units of RBC per hour at any point in the first 6 h [106]. Both CAT and an RI of >4 U have been validated as more accurate than the traditional definition in predicting early mortality [103, 107].

Interestingly, the practice of "hemostatic resuscitation" has shifted the epidemiology of massive transfusions, with at least one study reporting that a practice change to early and aggressive FFP transfusion was associated with decreased requirements for massive transfusion and overall blood component utilization [108].

Prediction

The accumulated evidence may be summarized as: for patients requiring massive transfusion, balanced ratio blood product resuscitation should be initiated as early as possible. For transfusions not meeting the threshold definitions for "massive," however, the transfusion of plasma is wasteful at best and harmful at worst. The conundrum facing the clinician at the outset is the accurate prediction of volume of transfusion that will be required in the bleeding patient [86]. Clinical gestalt has been demonstrated to be insufficiently accurate [109] and therefore, multiple predictive scoring systems have been developed (Table 11.5), including TASH (trauma-associated severe hemorrhage) score [110], PWH (Prince of Wales Hospital/Rainer) score [111], Vandromme score [112], ABC (assessment of blood consumption)

Table 11.5 Commonly used variables in massive transfusion scores [86]

	ABC [33]	TASH [22]	Schreiber et al. (2007) [24]	McLaughlin et al. (2008) [21]	ETS[a] [23]	PWH [36]
Hypotension	X	X	–	X	X	X
Hemoglobin/hematocrit	–	X	X	X	–	X
Intra-abdominal fluid	X	X	–	–	X	X
Pelvic or long bone fracture	–	X	–	–	X	X
Tachycardia	X	X	–	X	–	X
Base deficit	–	X	–	–	–	X
Gender	–	X	–	–	–	–
Admission from scene	–	–	–	–	X	–
Traffic accident	–	–	–	–	X	–
Fall (>3 m)	–	–	–	–	X	–
Penetrating mechanism	X	–	X	–	–	–
INR	–	–	X	–	–	–
PH	–	–	–	X	–	–
Age	–	–	–	–	X	–
GCS	–	–	–	–	–	X

[a] Score designed to predict the need for any transfusion not only the need for a MT

score [113], Schreiber score [114], MTS (massive transfusion score) [115, 116], traumatic bleeding severity score (TBSS) [117], and Larsen score [118], among others [119, 120]. Some scores have been independently externally validated while others have not. As with all clinical prediction/decision rules, the more accurate the score, the more input variables it requires and the less likely the bedside clinician will use it; contrarily, the simpler the score, the less accurate are its predictions. Some scores require specialized imaging (e.g., to visualize intra-abdominal fluid) while others require laboratory testing (e.g., INR). At this time, no single score has been universally adopted for clinical use.

Other Populations

It should be emphasized that the bulk of the literature supporting damage control resuscitation in MT scenarios is for adult patients. For pediatric patients, the existing evidence is conflicting. Two studies have been conducted in children injured in the theater of war and have not proven a survival benefit with transfusion of higher ratios of FFP and platelets [121, 122]. However, these studies have limited applicability to civilian trauma practice, as >95% of the subjects in those studies were injured by penetrating injury mechanism. Single-institution civilian studies with small sample sizes have reported no survival benefit with higher FFP:RBC transfusion ratios [123–125]. A more recent civilian study examining the pediatric Trauma Quality Improvement Program (TQIP) database reported improved survival at 24 h for high (>1:1) and medium (>= 1:2 and <1:1) FFP:RBC ratio compared to low (<1:2) ratio transfusion [126]. However, platelet transfusion ratios were not associated with mortality rates.

Non-massive Transfusion

It is unclear if "damage control resuscitation" is similarly beneficial in patients receiving non-massive transfusions. Inaba et al. reported that patients receiving plasma for non-massive transfusion did not have improved survival rates, and experienced an increased rate of complications (particularly respiratory complications) in a dose-dependent manner [127]. Others have also reported increased complications in critically ill non-trauma surgical patients receiving FFP compared to patients who did not receive FFP [128].

Non-trauma Patients

Implementation of a formal massive transfusion protocol is associated with reduced crystalloid and blood product utilization, lower rates of complications, and improved survival rates [93, 129–132] and the majority of trauma hospitals now have a formal institutionalized MTP for trauma patients [133, 134], as recommended by practice management guidelines [135]. However, in clinical practice, the majority of massive transfusions occur in *non*-trauma patients [97, 136–139] and MTPs have now been extended beyond the population to other patient populations [140–144]. Notably, several studies have *not* reported survival benefits of high FFP:RBC ration transfusion strategies in bleeding non-trauma patients [139, 144–147]. Indeed, for some massive transfusion patients (e.g., non-surgical), high FFP:RBC ratios are associated with *increased* mortality [139].

Tranexamic Acid

Tranexamic acid (TXA) is a synthetic drug (lysine derivative) that is used as an antifibrinolytic. Conceptually, it helps stabilize the clot and prevents premature dissolution. Pre-clinical studies have demonstrated that TXA reverses hyperfibrinolysis and traumatic coagulopathy, even in the setting of severe acidemia [148, 149]. Additionally, TXA has been shown to provide a protective effect to the intestinal barrier function in hemorrhagic shock [150].

Studies in humans have been conflicting, and the role of TXA is a topic of ongoing investigation. TXA has been studied in a variety of hemorrhage conditions including upper gastrointestinal bleeding, orthotopic liver transplantation, orthopedic surgery, transurethral prostatic surgery, and oral surgery in patients with hemophilia or therapeutic anticoagulation [151, 152]. The vast majority of scientific evidence favors its use, as it appears to decrease the need for blood transfusion in surgery [153] and decrease mortality without any increased risk of adverse events, including thrombosis, in non-traumatic bleeding [151]. The WOMAN trial randomized 20,060 women with post-partum hemorrhage to receive either TXA or placebo and demonstrated significantly lower rates of death due to bleeding in the subjects receiving TXA without any increase in adverse events [154]. The CRASH-2 study was another massive randomized trial which enrolled 20,211 adult trauma patients from 274 hospitals across 40 countries, randomizing injured subjects to either TXA or placebo [155]. Subjects receiving TXA had significantly reduced rates of all-cause mortality (14.5% vs. 16.0%) and risk of death due to bleeding (4.9% vs. 5.7%). Interestingly, there seems to be a significant time-dependent effect of TXA; receipt of TXA within 3 h of injury conferred the most benefit, whereas TXA receipt beyond 3 h of injury seemed to *increase* the risk of death due to bleeding [156].

However, there have been two major criticisms of the CRASH-2 trial: (1) the majority of subjects were enrolled from developing or middle-income countries without mature massive transfusion protocols; and (2) only half of the enrolled subjects (50.4 and 51.3%) actually received blood transfusion. To address the former criticism, the military application of tranexamic acid in trauma emergency resuscitation (MATTERs) study was performed, which confirmed the benefit of TXA administration (with or without cryoprecipitate) in terms of coagulopathy measures and survival [157, 158].

After the publication of the CRASH-2 trial in 2010, many hospitals began to incorporate TXA into their massive transfusion protocols (MTPs). A recent survey revealed that approximately 50% of hospitals participating in the ACS-TQIP (American College of Surgeons Trauma Quality Improvement Project) program include TXA in their MTP [133]. Some researchers have reported a beneficial impact on multiple organ failure and all-cause mortality [159], while one study reported increased mortality with TXA use [160], and another reported significantly higher odds of thromboembolic complications in those receiving TXA without any increase in survival [161].

In terms of clot durability, hyperfibrinolysis and fibrinolytic shutdown represent two opposite ends of the spectrum, with the former representing a fragile clot and the latter representing pathologic clot durability. Given the mechanism of action of TXA, those with hyperfibrinolysis would theoretically gain the most benefit from TXA [162]. However, clinical evidence demonstrating this benefit is lacking. One study failed to find any mortality benefit associated with TXA administration in patients with hyperfibrinolysis (defined as LY-30 ≥ 3%) on rapid TEG [163]. Khan et al. performed a post-hoc analysis of the PROPPR trial, focusing only on those patients with admission hyperfibrinolysis. In a propensity score-matched analysis, receipt of TXA was not associated with improved long-term survival [164]. Emerging evidence suggests that even those with physiologic fibrinolysis may be harmed by TXA administration [165].

Of more concern, however, is that TXA has been implicated in the development of later fibrinolytic shutdown (LY30 ≤ 0.8%) and worse outcomes [166].

At this time, TXA is conditionally recommended [135] with two caveats: (1) if TXA is to be given, it should be given only within 3 h of injury; (2) in centers with access to viscoelastic testing, TXA administration should be given only to patients with evidence of hyperfibrinolysis and should be avoided in those with evidence of fibrinolytic shutdown or physiologic fibrinolysis [167]. Additional research is clearly needed to better define optimal patient selection.

"The Safest Transfusion of All": Strategies to Avoid Operative Transfusion

Patient Blood Management

Despite the many processes in place to ensure the safety of blood products in the USA, including pre-donation donor screening, extensive post-donation pathogen testing, pre-transfusion crossmatch and compatibility protocols, and post-transfusion surveillance programs, blood transfusion is not a risk-free procedure, and will likely never be one. While the directly attributable mortality rate from transfusion is extremely low (43 FDA-reported fatalities/21,000,000 transfused blood products in 2016) [6], the only 100% safe transfusion is the one that never happens. This fact, coupled with the observation that many transfused patients fail to benefit clinically from the procedure as well as the rising healthcare costs associated with blood transfusion, has led to the development of patient blood management (PBM) programs worldwide.

Principles of PBM can be applied at all three phases of surgery: preoperative, intraoperative, and postoperative [168]. Preoperatively, the major element of PBM is the identification and treatment of anemia prior to surgery. Preoperative anemia, if identified sufficiently in advance (i.e., more than 30 days prior to anticipated surgery), can often be addressed with the combination of erythropoietin and oral or parenteral iron supplementation. The mitigation of preoperative anemia has been shown to markedly reduce the incidence of perioperative transfusion [169, 170].

Intraoperatively, PBM programs focus on the minimization of intraoperative blood loss—this not only incorporates surgical techniques designed to reduce hemorrhage, but also incorporates pharmacological interventions such as the perioperative use of TXA and fibrin sealants. For example, a meta-analysis of over 120 trials demonstrated that the use of TXA reduced the probability of blood transfusion by 38% [153]. For surgical procedures with significant expected blood loss, the incorporation of techniques such as intraoperative blood salvage and acute normovolemic hemodilution can markedly reduce the need for allogenic blood transfusion [168].

Postoperatively, PBM emphasizes efforts to reduce blood losses whenever possible. Simple interventions such as reducing the frequency and volume of phlebotomy can have a major impact on overall transfusion frequency [171]. The reduction in postoperative surgical drain use can also reduce transfusion requirements [172]. Iron supplementation postoperatively has been shown to reduce postoperative transfusion requirements in some settings though overall data are limited at this time [173].

PBM initiatives are becoming rapidly incorporated into the inpatient and, particularly, surgical landscape, and should be considered a major element of surgical safety programs for the foreseeable future.

Conclusion

Blood product transfusion remains an essential aspect of high-quality, modern perioperative care, though not without risk. Complications directly related to the transfused products and those related to the blood-recipient interaction are rare, but may be serious or deadly, and are more commonly associated with emergency transfusions. Emergency transfusion of uncrossmatched RBC and plasma shows promise in initial investigations, but more research is required before widespread implementation can be recommended.

Massive transfusion (MT) is a special case of emergency blood product transfusion that has received considerable recent attention, mainly in trauma patients. Updated definitions of MT have been developed to replace the original arbitrary definition and to better reflect the clinical reality of rapid bleeding. Massive transfusion protocols have been implemented in nearly all mature trauma centers in the USA and are also being extended to patients with non-traumatic causes of hemorrhage. The ideal transfusion ratios of plasma and platelets to RBC remain a topic of active investigation. Viscoelastic testing provides more granular and real-time information about coagulation dynamics than traditional coagulation tests, and VET-guided transfusion practice may result in more efficient use of blood bank resources and, ultimately, better patient care.

References

1. Petrides MAJ. To transfuse or not to transfuse: an assessment of risks and benefits. In: Mintz P, editor. Transfusion therapy: clinical principles and practice. 3rd ed. Bethesda: AABB Press; 2011. p. 855–99.
2. Brecher ME, Hay SN. Bacterial contamination of blood components. Clin Microbiol Rev. 2005;18(1):195–204.

3. Rao PL, Strausbaugh LJ, Liedtke LA, Srinivasan A, Kuehnert MJ. Bacterial infections associated with blood transfusion: experience and perspective of infectious diseases consultants. Transfusion. 2007;47(7):1206–11.
4. CDC. Morbidity and mortality weekly report. Fatal bacterial infections associated with platelet transfusions—United States, 2004. CDC. 2005. https://www.cdc.gov/mmWR/preview/mmwrhtml/mm5407a2.htm.
5. Linden JV, Wagner K, Voytovich AE, Sheehan J. Transfusion errors in New York State: an analysis of 10 years' experience. Transfusion. 2000;40(10):1207–13.
6. FDA's Center for Biologics Evaluation and Research (CBER). Fatalities reported to FDA following blood collection and transfusion annual summary for fiscal year 2016. FDA. https://www.fda.gov/media/111226/download.
7. Strobel E. Hemolytic transfusion reactions. Transfus Med Hemother. 2008;35(5):346–53.
8. Tormey CA, Hendrickson JE. Transfusion-related red blood cell alloantibodies: induction and consequences. Blood. 2019;133(17):1821–30.
9. Davenport RD. Pathophysiology of hemolytic transfusion reactions. Semin Hematol. 2005;42(3):165–8.
10. Vamvakas EC, Pineda AA, Reisner R, Santrach PJ, Moore SB. The differentiation of delayed hemolytic and delayed serologic transfusion reactions: incidence and predictors of hemolysis. Transfusion. 1995;35(1):26–32.
11. Hendrickson JE, Hillyer CD. Noninfectious serious hazards of transfusion. Anesth Analg. 2009;108(3):759–69.
12. Delaney M, Wendel S, Bercovitz RS, Cid J, Cohn C, Dunbar NM, et al. Transfusion reactions: prevention, diagnosis, and treatment. Lancet. 2016;388(10061):2825–36.
13. Ploeg A, Bateman RM, Sharpe MD, Jagger JE, Ellis CG, Solé-Violán J, et al. Nosocomial infections after peripheral arterial bypass surgery. World J Surg. 2007;31(8):1687–92.
14. Gunst MA, Minei JP. Transfusion of blood products and nosocomial infection in surgical patients. Curr Opin Crit Care. 2007;13(4):428–32.
15. Izuel Rami M, García Erce JA, Gómez-Barrera M, Cuenca Espiérrez J, Abad Sazatornil R, Rabanaque Hernández MJ. [Relationship between allogeneic blood transfusion, iron deficiency and nosocomial infection in patients with hip fracture]. Med Clin (Barc). 2008;131(17):647–652. [In Spanish].
16. Rosmarakis ES, Prapas SN, Rellos K, Michalopoulos A, Samonis G, Falagas ME. Nosocomial infections after off-pump coronary artery bypass surgery: frequency, characteristics, and risk factors. Interact Cardiovasc Thorac Surg. 2007;6(6):759–67.
17. Hill GE, Frawley WH, Griffith KE, Forestner JE, Minei JP. Allogeneic blood transfusion increases the risk of postoperative bacterial infection: a meta-analysis. J Trauma. 2003;54(5):908–14.
18. Taylor RW, Manganaro L, O'Brien J, Trottier SJ, Parkar N, Veremakis C. Impact of allogenic packed red blood cell transfusion on nosocomial infection rates in the critically ill patient. Crit Care Med. 2002;30(10):2249–54.
19. Chelemer SB, Prato BS, Cox PM Jr, O'Connor GT, Morton JR. Association of bacterial infection and red blood cell transfusion after coronary artery bypass surgery. Ann Thorac Surg. 2002;73(1):138–42.
20. Vamvakas EC. The abandoned controversy surrounding universal white blood cell reduction. Blood Transfus. 2014;12(2):143–5.
21. Simancas-Racines D, Osorio D, Martí-Carvajal AJ, Arevalo-Rodriguez I. Leukoreduction for the prevention of adverse reactions from allogeneic blood transfusion. Cochrane Database Syst Rev. 2015;(12):CD009745.
22. Otrock ZK, Liu C, Grossman BJ. Transfusion-related acute lung injury risk mitigation: an update. Vox Sang. 2017;112(8):694–703.
23. Saverimuttu J, Greenfield T, Rotenko I, Crozier J, Jalaludin B, Harvey M. Implications for urgent transfusion of uncrossmatched blood in the emergency department: the prevalence of clinically significant red cell antibodies within different patient groups. Emerg Med (Fremantle). 2003;15(3):239–43.

24. Barnes A Jr, Allen TE. Transfusions subsequent to administration of universal donor blood in Vietnam. JAMA. 1968;204(8):695–7.
25. Goodell PP, Uhl L, Mohammed M, Powers AA. Risk of hemolytic transfusion reactions following emergency-release RBC transfusion. Am J Clin Pathol. 2010;134(2):202–6.
26. Radkay L, Triulzi DJ, Yazer MH. Low risk of hemolysis after transfusion of uncrossmatched red blood cells. Immunohematology. 2012;28(2):39–44.
27. Mulay SB, Jaben EA, Johnson P, Badjie K, Stubbs JR. Risks and adverse outcomes associated with emergency-release red blood cell transfusion. Transfusion. 2013;53(7):1416–20.
28. Zielinski MD, Johnson PM, Jenkins D, Goussous N, Stubbs JR. Emergency use of prethawed Group A plasma in trauma patients. J Trauma Acute Care Surg. 2013;74(1):69–74; discussion 74–5.
29. Stubbs JR, Zielinski MD, Berns KS, Badjie KS, Tauscher CD, Hammel SA, et al. How we provide thawed plasma for trauma patients. Transfusion. 2015;55(8):1830–7.
30. Sihler KC, Napolitano LM. Complications of massive transfusion. Chest. 2010;137(1):209–20.
31. Moore FA, Moore EE, Sauaia A, Blood transfusion. An independent risk factor for postinjury multiple organ failure. Arch Surg. 1997;132(6):620–4; discussion 624–5.
32. Levy JH. Massive transfusion coagulopathy. Semin Hematol. 2006;43(1 Suppl 1):S59–63.
33. Smith HM, Farrow SJ, Ackerman JD, Stubbs JR, Sprung J. Cardiac arrests associated with hyperkalemia during red blood cell transfusion: a case series. Anesth Analg. 2008;106(4):1062–9, table of contents.
34. Lee TL, Lun KC. Review of problems of massive blood transfusion in a surgical intensive care unit. Ann Acad Med Singapore. 1985;14(1):175–84.
35. Ludbrook J, Wynn V. Citrate intoxication; a clinical and experimental study. Br Med J. 1958;2(5095):523–8.
36. Spinella PC, Cap AP. Whole blood: back to the future. Curr Opin Hematol. 2016;23(6):536–42.
37. Spinella PC, Perkins JG, Grathwohl KW, Beekley AC, Holcomb JB. Warm fresh whole blood is independently associated with improved survival for patients with combat-related traumatic injuries. J Trauma. 2009;66(4 Suppl):S69–76.
38. Borgman MA, Spinella PC, Perkins JG, Grathwohl KW, Repine T, Beekley AC, et al. The ratio of blood products transfused affects mortality in patients receiving massive transfusions at a combat support hospital. J Trauma. 2007;63(4):805–13.
39. Holcomb JB, Wade CE, Michalek JE, Chisholm GB, Zarzabal LA, Schreiber MA, et al. Increased plasma and platelet to red blood cell ratios improves outcome in 466 massively transfused civilian trauma patients. Ann Surg. 2008;248(3):447–58.
40. Holcomb JB, Zarzabal LA, Michalek JE, Kozar RA, Spinella PC, Perkins JG, et al. Increased platelet: RBC ratios are associated with improved survival after massive transfusion. J Trauma. 2011;71(2 Suppl 3):S318–28.
41. Beekley AC. Damage control resuscitation: a sensible approach to the exsanguinating surgical patient. Crit Care Med. 2008;36(7 Suppl):S267–74.
42. Duchesne JC, Barbeau JM, Islam TM, Wahl G, Greiffenstein P, McSwain NE Jr. Damage control resuscitation: from emergency department to the operating room. Am Surg. 2011;77(2):201–6.
43. Duchesne JC, McSwain NE Jr, Cotton BA, Hunt JP, Dellavolpe J, Lafaro K, et al. Damage control resuscitation: the new face of damage control. J Trauma. 2010;69(4):976–90.
44. Holcomb JB, Jenkins D, Rhee P, Johannigman J, Mahoney P, Mehta S, et al. Damage control resuscitation: directly addressing the early coagulopathy of trauma. J Trauma. 2007;62(2):307–10.
45. Makley AT, Goodman MD, Belizaire RM, Friend LA, Johannigman JA, Dorlac WC, et al. Damage control resuscitation decreases systemic inflammation after hemorrhage. J Surg Res. 2012;175(2):e75–82.
46. Sillesen M, Johansson PI, Rasmussen LS, Jin G, Jepsen CH, Imam A, et al. Fresh frozen plasma resuscitation attenuates platelet dysfunction compared with normal saline in a large animal model of multisystem trauma. J Trauma Acute Care Surg. 2014;76(4):998–1007.

47. Shrestha B, Holcomb JB, Camp EA, Del Junco DJ, Cotton BA, Albarado R, et al. Damage-control resuscitation increases successful nonoperative management rates and survival after severe blunt liver injury. J Trauma Acute Care Surg. 2015;78(2):336–41.
48. Auten JD, Lunceford NL, Horton JL, Galarneau MR, Galindo RM, Shepps CD, et al. The safety of early fresh, whole blood transfusion among severely battle injured at US Marine Corps forward surgical care facilities in Afghanistan. J Trauma Acute Care Surg. 2015;79(5):790–6.
49. Garcia Hejl C, Martinaud C, Macarez R, Sill J, Le Golvan A, Dulou R, et al. The implementation of a multinational "walking blood bank" in a combat zone: the experience of a health service team deployed to a medical treatment facility in Afghanistan. J Trauma Acute Care Surg. 2015;78(5):949–54.
50. Cahill BP, Stinar TR. Improving the emergency whole blood program. Mil Med. 2011;176(11):1287–91.
51. Pivalizza EG, Stephens CT, Sridhar S, Gumbert SD, Rossmann S, Bertholf MF, et al. Whole blood for resuscitation in adult civilian trauma in 2017: a narrative review. Anesth Analg. 2018;127(1):157–62.
52. Cotton BA, Podbielski J, Camp E, Welch T, del Junco D, Bai Y, et al. A randomized controlled pilot trial of modified whole blood versus component therapy in severely injured patients requiring large volume transfusions. Ann Surg. 2013;258(4):527–32; discussion 532–3.
53. Holcomb JB, del Junco DJ, Fox EE, Wade CE, Cohen MJ, Schreiber MA, et al. The prospective, observational, multicenter, major trauma transfusion (PROMMTT) study: comparative effectiveness of a time-varying treatment with competing risks. JAMA Surg. 2013;148(2):127–36.
54. Holcomb JB, Tilley BC, Baraniuk S, Fox EE, Wade CE, Podbielski JM, et al. Transfusion of plasma, platelets, and red blood cells in a 1:1:1 vs a 1:1:2 ratio and mortality in patients with severe trauma: the PROPPR randomized clinical trial. JAMA. 2015;313(5):471–82.
55. Hallet J, Lauzier F, Mailloux O, Trottier V, Archambault P, Zarychanski R, et al. The use of higher platelet: RBC transfusion ratio in the acute phase of trauma resuscitation: a systematic review. Crit Care Med. 2013;41(12):2800–11.
56. Lustenberger T, Frischknecht A, Brüesch M, Keel MJ. Blood component ratios in massively transfused, blunt trauma patients—a time-dependent covariate analysis. J Trauma. 2011;71(5):1144–50; discussion 1150–1.
57. Kornblith LZ, Robles AJ, Conroy AS, Redick BJ, Howard BM, Hendrickson CM, et al. Predictors of postinjury acute respiratory distress syndrome: lung injury persists in the era of hemostatic resuscitation. J Trauma Acute Care Surg. 2019;87(2):371–8.
58. Floccard B, Rugeri L, Faure A, Saint Denis M, Boyle EM, Peguet O, et al. Early coagulopathy in trauma patients: an on-scene and hospital admission study. Injury. 2012;43(1):26 32.
59. Brohi K, Singh J, Heron M, Coats T. Acute traumatic coagulopathy. J Trauma. 2003;54(6):1127–30.
60. Duchesne JC, Islam TM, Stuke L, Timmer JR, Barbeau JM, Marr AB, et al. Hemostatic resuscitation during surgery improves survival in patients with traumatic-induced coagulopathy. J Trauma. 2009;67(1):33–7; discussion 37–9.
61. Engels PT, Rezende-Neto JB, Al Mahroos M, Scarpelini S, Rizoli SB, Tien HC. The natural history of trauma-related coagulopathy: implications for treatment. J Trauma. 2011;71(5 Suppl 1):S448–55.
62. MacLeod JB, Lynn M, McKenney MG, Cohn SM, Murtha M. Early coagulopathy predicts mortality in trauma. J Trauma. 2003;55(1):39–44.
63. Niles SE, McLaughlin DF, Perkins JG, Wade CE, Li Y, Spinella PC, et al. Increased mortality associated with the early coagulopathy of trauma in combat casualties. J Trauma. 2008;64(6):1459–63; discussion 1463–5.
64. Brohi K, Cohen MJ, Ganter MT, Schultz MJ, Levi M, Mackersie RC, et al. Acute coagulopathy of trauma: hypoperfusion induces systemic anticoagulation and hyperfibrinolysis. J Trauma. 2008;64(5):1211–7; discussion 1217.

65. Cohen MJ, Call M, Nelson M, Calfee CS, Esmon CT, Brohi K, et al. Critical role of activated protein C in early coagulopathy and later organ failure, infection and death in trauma patients. Ann Surg. 2012;255(2):379–85.
66. Cohen MJ, Kutcher M, Redick B, Nelson M, Call M, Knudson MM, et al. Clinical and mechanistic drivers of acute traumatic coagulopathy. J Trauma Acute Care Surg. 2013;75(1 Suppl 1):S40–7.
67. Rizoli SB, Scarpelini S, Callum J, Nascimento B, Mann KG, Pinto R, et al. Clotting factor deficiency in early trauma-associated coagulopathy. J Trauma. 2011;71(5 Suppl 1):S427–34.
68. Shaz BH, Winkler AM, James AB, Hillyer CD, MacLeod JB. Pathophysiology of early trauma-induced coagulopathy: emerging evidence for hemodilution and coagulation factor depletion. J Trauma. 2011;70(6):1401–7.
69. Sheppard FR, Schaub LJ, Cap AP, Macko AR, Moore HB, Moore EE, et al. Whole blood mitigates the acute coagulopathy of trauma and avoids the coagulopathy of crystalloid resuscitation. J Trauma Acute Care Surg. 2018;85(6):1055–62.
70. Davenport R, Manson J, De'Ath H, Platton S, Coates A, Allard S, et al. Functional definition and characterization of acute traumatic coagulopathy. Crit Care Med. 2011;39(12):2652–8.
71. Cotton BA, Faz G, Hatch QM, Radwan ZA, Podbielski J, Wade C, et al. Rapid thrombelastography delivers real-time results that predict transfusion within 1 hour of admission. J Trauma. 2011;71(2):407–14; discussion 414–7.
72. da Luz LT, Nascimento B, Rizoli S. Thrombelastography (TEG(R)): practical considerations on its clinical use in trauma resuscitation. Scand J Trauma Resusc Emerg Med. 2013;21:29.
73. Deppe AC, Weber C, Zimmermann J, Kuhn EW, Slottosch I, Liakopoulos OJ, et al. Point-of-care thromboelastography/thromboelastometry-based coagulation management in cardiac surgery: a meta-analysis of 8332 patients. J Surg Res. 2016;203(2):424–33.
74. Holcomb JB, Minei KM, Scerbo ML, Radwan ZA, Wade CE, Kozar RA, et al. Admission rapid thrombelastography can replace conventional coagulation tests in the emergency department: experience with 1974 consecutive trauma patients. Ann Surg. 2012;256(3):476–86.
75. Gonzalez E, Moore EE, Moore HB, Chapman MP, Chin TL, Ghasabyan A, et al. Goal-directed hemostatic resuscitation of trauma-induced coagulopathy: a pragmatic randomized clinical trial comparing a viscoelastic assay to conventional coagulation assays. Ann Surg. 2016;263(6):1051–9.
76. Schöchl H, Nienaber U, Maegele M, Hochleitner G, Primavesi F, Steitz B, et al. Transfusion in trauma: thromboelastometry-guided coagulation factor concentrate-based therapy versus standard fresh frozen plasma-based therapy. Crit Care. 2011;15(2):R83.
77. Tapia NM, Chang A, Norman M, Welsh F, Scott B, Wall MJ Jr, et al. TEG-guided resuscitation is superior to standardized MTP resuscitation in massively transfused penetrating trauma patients. J Trauma Acute Care Surg. 2013;74(2):378–85; discussion 385–6.
78. Moore HB, Moore EE, Liras IN, Gonzalez E, Harvin JA, Holcomb JB, et al. Acute fibrinolysis shutdown after injury occurs frequently and increases mortality: a multicenter evaluation of 2540 severely injured patients. J Am Coll Surg. 2016;222(4):347–55.
79. Chapman MP, Moore EE, Moore HB, Gonzalez E, Morton AP, Chandler J, et al. The "Death Diamond": rapid thrombelastography identifies lethal hyperfibrinolysis. J Trauma Acute Care Surg. 2015;79(6):925–9.
80. Roberts DJ, Kalkwarf KJ, Moore HB, Cohen MJ, Fox EE, Wade CE, et al. Time course and outcomes associated with transient versus persistent fibrinolytic phenotypes after injury: a nested, prospective, multicenter cohort study. J Trauma Acute Care Surg. 2019;86(2):206–13.
81. Taylor JR 3rd, Fox EE, Holcomb JB, Rizoli S, Inaba K, Schreiber MA, et al. The hyperfibrinolytic phenotype is the most lethal and resource intense presentation of fibrinolysis in massive transfusion patients. J Trauma Acute Care Surg. 2018;84(1):25–30.
82. Moore HB, Moore EE, Gonzalez E, Chapman MP, Chin TL, Silliman CC, et al. Hyperfibrinolysis, physiologic fibrinolysis, and fibrinolysis shutdown: the spectrum of postinjury fibrinolysis and relevance to antifibrinolytic therapy. J Trauma Acute Care Surg. 2014;77(6):811–7; discussion 817.

83. Moore EE, Moore HB, Gonzalez E, Chapman MP, Hansen KC, Sauaia A, et al. Postinjury fibrinolysis shutdown: rationale for selective tranexamic acid. J Trauma Acute Care Surg. 2015;78(6 Suppl 1):S65–9.
84. Kutcher ME, Cripps MW, McCreery RC, Crane IM, Greenberg MD, Cachola LM, et al. Criteria for empiric treatment of hyperfibrinolysis after trauma. J Trauma Acute Care Surg. 2012;73(1):87–93.
85. Moore HB, et al. Shock-induced systemic hyperfibrinolysis is attenuated by plasma-first resuscitation. J Trauma Acute Care Surg. 2015;79(6):897–904.
86. Cantle PM, Cotton BA. Prediction of massive transfusion in trauma. Crit Care Clin. 2017;33(1):71–84.
87. Brockamp T, Nienaber U, Mutschler M, Wafaisade A, Peiniger S, Lefering R, et al. Predicting on-going hemorrhage and transfusion requirement after severe trauma: a validation of six scoring systems and algorithms on the TraumaRegister DGU. Crit Care. 2012;16(4):R129.
88. Rose AH, Kotzé A, Doolan D, Norfolk DR, Bellamy MC. Massive transfusion—evaluation of current clinical practice and outcome in two large teaching hospital trusts in Northern England. Vox Sang. 2009;97(3):247–53.
89. Como JJ, Dutton RP, Scalea TM, Edelman BB, Hess JR. Blood transfusion rates in the care of acute trauma. Transfusion. 2004;44(6):809–13.
90. Long K, Heaney JB, Simms ER, McSwain NE, Duchesne JC. When enough is enough: impact of packed red blood cells in massive transfusion outcomes. Am Surg. 2013;79(8):810–4.
91. Davenport R, Curry N, Manson J, De'Ath H, Coates A, Rourke C, et al. Hemostatic effects of fresh frozen plasma may be maximal at red cell ratios of 1:2. J Trauma. 2011;70(1):90–5; discussion 95–6.
92. Ho AM, Holcomb JB, Ng CS, Zamora JE, Karmakar MK, Dion PW. The traditional vs "1:1:1" approach debate on massive transfusion in trauma should not be treated as a dichotomy. Am J Emerg Med. 2015;33(10):1501–4.
93. Cotton BA, Au BK, Nunez TC, Gunter OL, Robertson AM, Young PP. Predefined massive transfusion protocols are associated with a reduction in organ failure and postinjury complications. J Trauma. 2009;66(1):41–8; discussion 48–9.
94. Riskin DJ, Tsai TC, Riskin L, Hernandez-Boussard T, Purtill M, Maggio PM, et al. Massive transfusion protocols: the role of aggressive resuscitation versus product ratio in mortality reduction. J Am Coll Surg. 2009;209(2):198–205.
95. Johansson PI, Stensballe J. Effect of haemostatic control resuscitation on mortality in massively bleeding patients: a before and after study. Vox Sang. 2009;96(2):111–8.
96. Heelan Gladden AA, et al. Effect of pre-hospital use of the assessment of blood consumption score and pre-thawed fresh frozen plasma on resuscitation and trauma mortality. J Am Coll Surg. 2019;228(2):141–7.
97. Dzik WS, Ziman A, Cohn C, Pai M, Lozano M, Kaufman RM, et al. Survival after ultramassive transfusion: a review of 1360 cases. Transfusion. 2016;56(3):558–63.
98. Vaslef SN, Knudsen NW, Neligan PJ, Sebastian MW. Massive transfusion exceeding 50 units of blood products in trauma patients. J Trauma. 2002;53(2):291–5; discussion 295–6.
99. Velmahos GC, Chan L, Chan M, Tatevossian R, Cornwell EE 3rd, Asensio JA, et al. Is there a limit to massive blood transfusion after severe trauma? Arch Surg. 1998;133(9):947–52.
100. Brotman S, Lamonica C, Cowley RA. Massive transfusion without major complications after trauma. Am J Emerg Med. 1986;4(6):514–5.
101. de Biasi AR, Stansbury LG, Dutton RP, Stein DM, Scalea TM, Hess JR. Blood product use in trauma resuscitation: plasma deficit versus plasma ratio as predictors of mortality in trauma (CME). Transfusion. 2011;51(9):1925–32.
102. Kashuk JL, Moore EE, Johnson JL, Haenel J, Wilson M, Moore JB, et al. Postinjury life threatening coagulopathy: is 1:1 fresh frozen plasma:packed red blood cells the answer? J Trauma. 2008;65(2):261–70; discussion 270–1.
103. Savage SA, Zarzaur BL, Croce MA, Fabian TC. Redefining massive transfusion when every second counts. J Trauma Acute Care Surg. 2013;74(2):396–400; discussion 400–2.

104. Rahbar E, Fox EE, del Junco DJ, Harvin JA, Holcomb JB, Wade CE, et al. Early resuscitation intensity as a surrogate for bleeding severity and early mortality in the PROMMTT study. J Trauma Acute Care Surg. 2013;75(1 Suppl 1):S16–23.
105. Savage SA, Zarzaur BL, Croce MA, Fabian TC. Time matters in 1:1 resuscitations: concurrent administration of blood: plasma and risk of death. J Trauma Acute Care Surg. 2014;77(6):833–8.
106. Moren AM, Hamptom D, Diggs B, Kiraly L, Fox EE, Holcomb JB, et al. Recursive partitioning identifies greater than 4 U of packed red blood cells per hour as an improved massive transfusion definition. J Trauma Acute Care Surg. 2015;79(6):920–4.
107. Meyer DE, Cotton BA, Fox EE, Stein D, Holcomb JB, Cohen M, et al. A comparison of resuscitation intensity and critical administration threshold in predicting early mortality among bleeding patients: a multicenter validation in 680 major transfusion patients. J Trauma Acute Care Surg. 2018;85(4):691–6.
108. Kautza BC, Cohen MJ, Cuschieri J, Minei JP, Brackenridge SC, Maier RV, et al. Changes in massive transfusion over time: an early shift in the right direction? J Trauma. 2012;72(1):106–11.
109. Pommerening MJ, Goodman MD, Holcomb JB, Wade CE, Fox EE, Del Junco DJ, et al. Clinical gestalt and the prediction of massive transfusion after trauma. Injury. 2015;46(5):807–13.
110. Yucel N, Lefering R, Maegele M, Vorweg M, Tjardes T, Ruchholtz S, et al. Trauma associated severe hemorrhage (TASH)-score: probability of mass transfusion as surrogate for life threatening hemorrhage after multiple trauma. J Trauma. 2006;60(6):1228–36; discussion 1236–7.
111. Rainer TH, Ho AM, Yeung JH, Cheung NK, Wong RS, Tang N, et al. Early risk stratification of patients with major trauma requiring massive blood transfusion. Resuscitation. 2011;82(6):724–9.
112. Vandromme MJ, Griffin RL, McGwin G Jr, Weinberg JA, Rue LW 3rd, Kerby JD. Prospective identification of patients at risk for massive transfusion: an imprecise endeavor. Am Surg. 2011;77(2):155–61.
113. Nunez TC, Voskresensky IV, Dossett LA, Shinall R, Dutton WD, Cotton BA. Early prediction of massive transfusion in trauma: simple as ABC (assessment of blood consumption)? J Trauma. 2009;66(2):346–52.
114. Schreiber MA, Perkins J, Kiraly L, Underwood S, Wade C, Holcomb JB. Early predictors of massive transfusion in combat casualties. J Am Coll Surg. 2007;205(4):541–5.
115. Callcut RA, Cripps MW, Nelson MF, Conroy AS, Robinson BB, Cohen MJ. The Massive Transfusion Score as a decision aid for resuscitation: learning when to turn the massive transfusion protocol on and off. J Trauma Acute Care Surg. 2016;80(3):450–6.
116. Callcut RA, Cotton BA, Muskat P, Fox EE, Wade CE, Holcomb JB, et al. Defining when to initiate massive transfusion: a validation study of individual massive transfusion triggers in PROMMTT patients. J Trauma Acute Care Surg. 2013;74(1):59–65, 67–8; discussion 66–7.
117. Ogura T, Nakamura Y, Nakano M, Izawa Y, Nakamura M, Fujizuka K, et al. Predicting the need for massive transfusion in trauma patients: the Traumatic Bleeding Severity Score. J Trauma Acute Care Surg. 2014;76(5):1243–50.
118. Larson CR, et al. Association of shock, coagulopathy, and initial vital signs with massive transfusion in combat casualties. J Trauma. 2010;69(Suppl 1):S26–32.
119. Hsu JM, Hitos K, Fletcher JP. Identifying the bleeding trauma patient: predictive factors for massive transfusion in an Australasian trauma population. J Trauma Acute Care Surg. 2013;75(3):359–64.
120. McLaughlin DF, Niles SE, Salinas J, Perkins JG, Cox ED, Wade CE, et al. A predictive model for massive transfusion in combat casualty patients. J Trauma. 2008;64(2 Suppl):S57–63; discussion S63.
121. Cannon JW, Johnson MA, Caskey RC, Borgman MA, Neff LP. High ratio plasma resuscitation does not improve survival in pediatric trauma patients. J Trauma Acute Care Surg. 2017;83(2):211–7.
122. Edwards MJ, Lustik MB, Clark ME, Creamer KM, Tuggle D. The effects of balanced blood component resuscitation and crystalloid administration in pediatric trauma patients

requiring transfusion in Afghanistan and Iraq 2002 to 2012. J Trauma Acute Care Surg. 2015;78(2):330–5.
123. Hendrickson JE, Shaz BH, Pereira G, Parker PM, Jessup P, Atwell F, et al. Implementation of a pediatric trauma massive transfusion protocol: one institution's experience. Transfusion. 2012;52(6):1228–36.
124. Nosanov L, Inaba K, Okoye O, Resnick S, Upperman J, Shulman I, et al. The impact of blood product ratios in massively transfused pediatric trauma patients. Am J Surg. 2013;206(5):655–60.
125. Hwu RS, Spinella PC, Keller MS, Baker D, Wallendorf M, Leonard JC. The effect of massive transfusion protocol implementation on pediatric trauma care. Transfusion. 2016;56(11):2712–9.
126. Butler EK, Mills BM, Arbabi S, Bulger EM, Vavilala MS, Groner JI, et al. Association of blood component ratios with 24-hour mortality in injured children receiving massive transfusion. Crit Care Med. 2019;47(7):975–83.
127. Inaba K, Branco BC, Rhee P, Blackbourne LH, Holcomb JB, Teixeira PG, et al. Impact of plasma transfusion in trauma patients who do not require massive transfusion. J Am Coll Surg. 2010;210(6):957–65.
128. Sarani B, Dunkman WJ, Dean L, Sonnad S, Rohrbach JI, Gracias VH. Transfusion of fresh frozen plasma in critically ill surgical patients is associated with an increased risk of infection. Crit Care Med. 2008;36(4):1114–8.
129. Cotton BA, Gunter OL, Isbell J, Au BK, Robertson AM, Morris JA Jr, et al. Damage control hematology: the impact of a trauma exsanguination protocol on survival and blood product utilization. J Trauma. 2008;64(5):1177–82; discussion 1182–3.
130. Cotton BA, et al. Damage control resuscitation is associated with a reduction in resuscitation volumes and improvement in survival in 390 damage control laparotomy patients. Ann Surg. 2011;254(4):598–605.
131. Duchesne JC, Kimonis K, Marr AB, Rennie KV, Wahl G, Wells JE, et al. Damage control resuscitation in combination with damage control laparotomy: a survival advantage. J Trauma. 2010;69(1):46–52.
132. O'Keeffe T, Refaai M, Tchorz K, Forestner JE, Sarode R. A massive transfusion protocol to decrease blood component use and costs. Arch Surg. 2008;143(7):686–90; discussion 690–1.
133. Camazine MN, Hemmila MR, Leonard JC, Jacobs RA, Horst JA, Kozar RA, et al. Massive transfusion policies at trauma centers participating in the American College of Surgeons Trauma Quality Improvement Program. J Trauma Acute Care Surg. 2015;78(6 Suppl 1):S48–53.
134. Schuster KM, Davis KA, Lui FY, Maerz LL, Kaplan LJ. The status of massive transfusion protocols in United States trauma centers: massive transfusion or massive confusion? Transfusion. 2010;50(7):1545–51.
135. Cannon JW, Khan MA, Raja AS, Cohen MJ, Como JJ, Cotton BA, et al. Damage control resuscitation in patients with severe traumatic hemorrhage: a practice management guideline from the Eastern Association for the Surgery of Trauma. J Trauma Acute Care Surg. 2017;82(3):605–17.
136. Campos A, Muñoz M, García-Erce JA, Ramírez G. [Incidence and mortality of massive transfusion in a university hospital: study of the period 2001-2005]. Med Clin (Barc). 2007;129(10):366–371. [In Spanish].
137. Halmin M, Chiesa F, Vasan SK, Wikman A, Norda R, Rostgaard K, et al. Epidemiology of massive transfusion: a binational study from Sweden and Denmark. Crit Care Med. 2016;44(3):468–77.
138. Johansson PI, Hansen MB, Sorensen H. Transfusion practice in massively bleeding patients: time for a change? Vox Sang. 2005;89(2):92–6.
139. Mesar T, Larentzakis A, Dzik W, Chang Y, Velmahos G, Yeh DD. Association between ratio of fresh frozen plasma to red blood cells during massive transfusion and survival among patients without traumatic injury. JAMA Surg. 2017;152(6):574–80.

140. Baumann Kreuziger LM, Morton CT, Subramanian AT, Anderson CP, Dries DJ. Not only in trauma patients: hospital-wide implementation of a massive transfusion protocol. Transfus Med. 2014;24(3):162–8.
141. McDaniel LM, Neal MD, Sperry JL, Alarcon LH, Forsythe RM, Triulzi D, et al. Use of a massive transfusion protocol in nontrauma patients: activate away. J Am Coll Surg. 2013;216(6):1103–9.
142. Pacheco LD, Saade GR, Costantine MM, Clark SL, Hankins GD. The role of massive transfusion protocols in obstetrics. Am J Perinatol. 2013;30(1):1–4.
143. Saule I, Hawkins N. Transfusion practice in major obstetric haemorrhage: lessons from trauma. Int J Obstet Anesth. 2012;21(1):79–83.
144. Sommer N, Schnüriger B, Candinas D, Haltmeier T. Massive transfusion protocols in nontrauma patients: a systematic review and meta-analysis. J Trauma Acute Care Surg. 2019;86(3):493–504.
145. Kauvar DS, Sarfati MR, Kraiss LW. Intraoperative blood product resuscitation and mortality in ruptured abdominal aortic aneurysm. J Vasc Surg. 2012;55(3):688–92.
146. Khan H, Belsher J, Yilmaz M, Afessa B, Winters JL, Moore SB, et al. Fresh-frozen plasma and platelet transfusions are associated with development of acute lung injury in critically ill medical patients. Chest. 2007;131(5):1308–14.
147. Sambasivan CN, Kunio NR, Nair PV, Zink KA, Michalek JE, Holcomb JB, et al. High ratios of plasma and platelets to packed red blood cells do not affect mortality in nonmassively transfused patients. J Trauma. 2011;71(2 Suppl 3):S329–36.
148. Debarros M, Hatch Q, Porta CR, Salgar S, Izenberg S, DuBose J, et al. Tranexamic acid corrects fibrinolysis in the presence of acidemia in a swine model of severe ischemic reperfusion. J Trauma Acute Care Surg. 2014;76(3):625–33.
149. Porta CR, Nelson D, McVay D, Salgar S, Eckert M, Izenberg S, et al. The effects of tranexamic acid and prothrombin complex concentrate on the coagulopathy of trauma: an in vitro analysis of the impact of severe acidosis. J Trauma Acute Care Surg. 2013;75(6):954–60.
150. Diebel ME, Diebel LN, Manke CW, Liberati DM, Whittaker JR. Early tranexamic acid administration: a protective effect on gut barrier function following ischemia/reperfusion injury. J Trauma Acute Care Surg. 2015;79(6):1015–22.
151. Dunn CJ, Goa KL. Tranexamic acid: a review of its use in surgery and other indications. Drugs. 1999;57(6):1005–32.
152. Huang F, Wu D, Ma G, Yin Z, Wang Q. The use of tranexamic acid to reduce blood loss and transfusion in major orthopedic surgery: a meta-analysis. J Surg Res. 2014;186(1):318–27.
153. Ker K, Edwards P, Perel P, Shakur H, Roberts I. Effect of tranexamic acid on surgical bleeding: systematic review and cumulative meta-analysis. BMJ. 2012;344:e3054.
154. WOMAN Trial Collaborators. Effect of early tranexamic acid administration on mortality, hysterectomy, and other morbidities in women with post-partum haemorrhage (WOMAN): an international, randomised, double-blind, placebo-controlled trial. Lancet. 2017;389(10084):2105–16.
155. Shakur H, Roberts I, Bautista R, Caballero J, Coats T, et al. Effects of tranexamic acid on death, vascular occlusive events, and blood transfusion in trauma patients with significant haemorrhage (CRASH-2): a randomised, placebo-controlled trial. Lancet. 2010;376(9734):23–32.
156. Roberts I, Shakur H, Afolabi A, Brohi K, Coats T, Dewan Y, et al. The importance of early treatment with tranexamic acid in bleeding trauma patients: an exploratory analysis of the CRASH-2 randomised controlled trial. Lancet. 2011;377(9771):1096–101; 1101.e1–2.
157. Morrison JJ, Dubose JJ, Rasmussen TE, Midwinter MJ. Military application of tranexamic acid in trauma emergency resuscitation (MATTERs) study. Arch Surg. 2012;147(2):113–9.
158. Morrison JJ, Ross JD, Dubose JJ, Jansen JO, Midwinter MJ, Rasmussen TE. Association of cryoprecipitate and tranexamic acid with improved survival following wartime injury: findings from the MATTERs II study. JAMA Surg. 2013;148(3):218–25.

159. Cole E, Davenport R, Willett K, Brohi K. Tranexamic acid use in severely injured civilian patients and the effects on outcomes: a prospective cohort study. Ann Surg. 2015;261(2):390–4.
160. Valle EJ, Allen CJ, Van Haren RM, Jouria JM, Li H, Livingstone AS, et al. Do all trauma patients benefit from tranexamic acid? J Trauma Acute Care Surg. 2014;76(6):1373–8.
161. Myers SP, Kutcher ME, Rosengart MR, Sperry JL, Peitzman AB, Brown JB, et al. Tranexamic acid administration is associated with an increased risk of posttraumatic venous thromboembolism. J Trauma Acute Care Surg. 2019;86(1):20–7.
162. Chapman MP, Moore EE, Ramos CR, Ghasabyan A, Harr JN, Chin TL, et al. Fibrinolysis greater than 3% is the critical value for initiation of antifibrinolytic therapy. J Trauma Acute Care Surg. 2013;75(6):961–7.
163. Harvin JA, Peirce CA, Mims MM, Hudson JA, Podbielski JM, Wade CE, et al. The impact of tranexamic acid on mortality in injured patients with hyperfibrinolysis. J Trauma Acute Care Surg. 2015;78(5):905–9; discussion 909–11.
164. Khan M, Jehan F, Bulger EM, O'Keeffe T, Holcomb JB, Wade CE, et al. Severely injured trauma patients with admission hyperfibrinolysis: is there a role of tranexamic acid? Findings from the PROPPR trial. J Trauma Acute Care Surg. 2018;85(5):851–7.
165. Moore HB, Moore EE, Huebner BR, Stettler GR, Nunns GR, Einersen PM, et al. Tranexamic acid is associated with increased mortality in patients with physiological fibrinolysis. J Surg Res. 2017;220:438–43.
166. Meizoso JP, Dudaryk R, Mulder MB, Ray JJ, Karcutskie CA, Eidelson SA, et al. Increased risk of fibrinolysis shutdown among severely injured trauma patients receiving tranexamic acid. J Trauma Acute Care Surg. 2018;84(3):426–32.
167. Moore HB, Moore EE, Chapman MP, Hansen KC, Cohen MJ, Pieracci FM, et al. Does tranexamic acid improve clot strength in severely injured patients who have elevated fibrin degradation products and low fibrinolytic activity, measured by thrombelastography? J Am Coll Surg. 2019;229(1):92–101.
168. Butcher A, Richards T. Cornerstones of patient blood management in surgery. Transfus Med. 2018;28(2):150–7.
169. Quinn EM, Meland E, McGinn S, Anderson JH. Correction of iron-deficiency anaemia in colorectal surgery reduces perioperative transfusion rates: a before and after study. Int J Surg. 2017;38:1–8.
170. Froessler B, Palm P, Weber I, Hodyl NA, Singh R, Murphy EM. The important role for intravenous iron in perioperative patient blood management in major abdominal surgery: a randomized controlled trial. Ann Surg. 2016;264(1):41–6.
171. Yeh DD. A clinician's perspective on laboratory utilization management. Clin Chim Acta. 2014;427:145–50.
172. Parker MJ, Roberts CP, Hay D. Closed suction drainage for hip and knee arthroplasty. A meta-analysis. J Bone Joint Surg Am. 2004;86(6):1146–52.
173. Khalafallah AA, Yan C, Al-Badri R, Robinson E, Kirkby BE, Ingram E, et al. Intravenous ferric carboxymaltose versus standard care in the management of postoperative anaemia: a prospective, open-label, randomised controlled trial. Lancet Haematol. 2016;3(9):e415–25.

Part II

System Design and Improvement

Detecting and Reporting Errors, Complications, and Adverse Events

12

Majed El Hechi and Haytham M. A. Kaafarani

Introduction

Much of modern thinking about safety systems evolved out of military aviation [1]. Until World War II, aviation accidents were blamed primarily on individuals, and "safety culture" simplistically translated to motivating people to "be safe." Throughout the war, United States generals lost aircraft and pilots in domestic operations because of system errors and came to realize that planning for safety was as important as planning for combat. For this reason, several military aviation safety centers were created in the early 1950s. Gradually, the field evolved and eventually disseminated into the commercial sector. Around the 1970s, the risk of dying on a commercial flight was 1 in two million. By the 1990s, the risk had decreased to 1 in eight million [2].

In healthcare, the importance of patient safety and quality of care came decades later. The two landmark reports, "To Err Is Human" and "Crossing the Quality Chasm," released by the Institute of Medicine in the early 2000s, estimated that between 44,000 and 98,000 patients died every year in the United States because of medical errors. The same reports highlighted that efforts aimed at measuring the quality of care were insufficient, and that medical errors were often caused by flawed systems from a patient safety perspective [2, 3]. Applying

M. El Hechi
Department of Surgery, Massachusetts General Hospital, Boston, MA, USA

H. M. A. Kaafarani (✉)
Division of Trauma, Emergency Surgery and Surgical Critical Care, Department of Surgery, Massachusetts General Hospital, Boston, MA, USA
e-mail: hkaafarani@mgh.harvard.edu

J. J. Hoballah et al. (eds.), *Principles of Perioperative Safety and Efficiency*,
https://doi.org/10.1007/978-3-031-41089-5_12

these healthcare statistics to modern professional aviation equates to nearly 200 jumbo jets crashing every year, or one Boeing 747 airplane crashing every other day [4]. This staggering insight led to the rapid rise in patient safety as a field in healthcare and the launch of many initiatives worldwide to improve patient safety, such as the "100,000 lives campaign" by the Institute for Healthcare Improvement (IHI) in 2004 [5].

Nearly all the success stories of the patient safety movement in the last two decades included robust methodologies to detect and report adverse events and errors, as one cannot improve what one cannot or does not measure. This chapter will describe the evolution of adverse event and error detection-and-reporting systems in surgery, as well as classification tools that allow for risk adjustment.

Detection and Reporting Systems

Institutional Detection and Reporting: Mortality and Morbidity Conferences

In the early 1900s, after discovering the poor quality of documentation in hospital records and the corresponding problems with patient safety and care, Ernest A. Codman, a surgeon at the Massachusetts General Hospital, developed a system where patient outcomes were documented, and adverse events were systematically reviewed and their causative errors categorized [6]. This initiative led to the creation of the "Minimum Standard" system, which was adopted by the American College of Surgeons in 1919 [7]. The aforementioned standard required that hospital staff meet, review, and analyze their clinical experience in various departments at regular intervals, with the intent to inquire whether the "end result" achieved was optimal. The "minimum standard system" still occurs in all surgical departments across the United States in the form of a morbidity and mortality (M&M) conference. The M&M conferences are the primary mechanism by which surgical departments monitor, report, analyze, and learn from surgical complications [8]. In 1983, it was mandated that all departments with surgical training programs hold "a weekly review of all current complications and deaths, including radiologic and pathologic correlation of surgical specimens and autopsies." [9] However, despite its educational value, it has been repeatedly suggested that these conferences alone are an insufficient quality-assurance mechanism for the modern and continuously evolving surgical practice [2, 3, 10]. Multiple studies have specifically shown that the error detection sensitivity of M&M conferences is 25% at best [8]. Consequently, it became evident that additional systems for quality measurement, error reporting, and provider feedback are needed to improve the safety and quality of surgical care [11, 12]. Specifically, prospective data collection that incorporates risk-adjusted performance feedback were deemed essential for reducing errors, changing physician behavior, and improving surgical outcomes [13–15].

Administratively Derived National Detection and Reporting Systems

Patient Safety Indicators

In the 1990s, to improve detection and reporting of medical errors, the Agency for Healthcare Research and Quality (AHRQ) developed quality indicators based from the Healthcare Cost and Utilization Project (HCUP) database of inpatient data. Thirty-three quality indicators were developed from administrative data that measured inpatient mortality as well as the rates of specific procedures being performed in the healthcare system. As information on the performance of quality indicators was gathered, they were refined and developed further.

The joint effort between Stanford University and University of California, San Francisco, yielded a set of 20 provider-level Patient Safety Indicators (PSIs) that use International Classification of Diseases, Ninth Revision, Clinical Modification (ICD-9-CM) diagnoses, procedures, and diagnosis-related groups (DRGs). After extensive evaluation and revision by clinical panels and expert reviewers, the PSIs were made readily available to providers in 2003 at no cost. Subsequently, seven area-level quality indicators were added to the list (Table 12.1) [16]. Select PSIs were later endorsed for hospital profiling and pay-for-performance purposes [17]. Notably, The National Quality Forum adopted 10 PSIs, [18] and the Centers for

Table 12.1 Provider and area-level patient safety indicators

Patient Safety Indicators

Provider-Level Indicators

- PSI 02 - Death rate in low-mortality diagnosis related groups (DRGs)
- PSI 03 - Pressure ulcer rate
- PSI 04 - Death rate among surgical inpatients with serious treatable conditions
- PSI 05 - Retained surgical item or unretrieved device fragment count
- PSI 06 - Iatrogenic pneumothorax rate
- PSI 07 - Central venous catheter-related blood stream infection rate
- PSI 08 - Postoperative hip fracture rate
- PSI 09 - Perioperative hemorrhage or hematoma rate
- PSI 10 - Postoperative physiologic and metabolic derangement rate
- PSI 11 - Postoperative respiratory failure rate
- PSI 12 - Perioperative pulmonary embolism or deep vein thrombosis rate
- PSI 13 - Postoperative sepsis rate
- PSI 14 - Postoperative wound dehiscence rate
- PSI 15 - Accidental puncture or laceration rate
- PSI 16 - Transfusion reaction count
- PSI 17 - Birth trauma rate – injury to neonate
- PSI 18 - Obstetric trauma rate – vaginal delivery with instrument
- PSI 19 - Obstetric trauma rate-vaginal delivery without instrument
- PSI 90 - Patient Safety for Selected Indicators

Area-Level Indicators

- PSI 21 - Retained surgical item or unretrieved device fragment rate
- PSI 22 - Iatrogenic pneumothorax rate
- PSI 23 - Central venous catheter-related blood stream infection rate
- PSI 24 - Postoperative wound dehiscence rate
- PSI 25 - Accidental puncture or laceration rate
- PSI 26 - Transfusion reaction rate
- PSI 27 - Postoperative hemorrhage or hematoma rate

Source: AHRQ Quality Indicators. https://www.qualityindicators.ahrq.gov/Downloads/Modules/PSI/V50/PSI_Brochure.pdf

Medicare and Medicaid Services (CMS) publicly reported on six individual PSIs as well as a PSI composite measure [19].

With the use of PSIs in public reporting, concerns emerged about the ability of these indicators to identify true events and reflect hospital performance. Administrative data is known for its coding variability and inconsistency regarding diagnoses and procedures, and as a result of PSIs being derived from it, they were intended to serve as "indicators" for potentially preventable inpatient complications and for use in quality improvement initiatives and monitoring trends, rather than definitive measures [16]. Nonetheless, given these concerns, the AHRQ conducted the PSI Validation Pilot Project to assess the criterion validity of several of the PSIs in a volunteer sample of nonfederal hospitals, [20–24] with validation of additional PSIs undertaken by an alliance of 113 academic medical centers and their affiliated hospitals, the United Health Care (UHC). Positive predictive value, the proportion of flagged cases confirmed by chart review to have the PSI event, ranged from 32% for decubitus ulcer to 91% for accidental puncture or laceration [20–24]. These studies led to recommendations for coding changes to enhance the specificity and PPV of certain indicators and provided guidelines for the use of individual PSIs. Moreover, the individual PSIs were validated in Veterans Affairs hospitals, which demonstrated that some PSIs perform better than others and that overall, the PSIs have moderate to high sensitivities and specificities [22–24].

Despite being cost efficient, the PSIs present several disadvantages and challenges. Being administratively derived rendered PSIs unable to determine the root causes of events. Namely, they do not cover important areas of patient safety events because of the absence of relevant information from administrative data, such as adverse drug events. Moreover, they rely heavily on ICD-9-CM codes. This is an issue, since a wide range of clinical diagnoses can be represented by a single ICD-9-CM code. Lastly, it has been repeatedly questioned whether the clinical accuracy of administrative coding can be completely trusted.

Global Trigger Tools

Another response to the need for a practical, less labor-intensive approach to assessing patient safety came in the form of the Global Trigger Tool (GTT), developed by the Institute for Healthcare Improvement (IHI) in 2003 [25]. The GTT utilizes two to three nurses or pharmacists to review and analyze patient charts for a "trigger" [26]. Triggers may include a medication stop order, abnormal lab result, or the use of an antidote medication. For instance, the administration of naloxone to a patient already hospitalized would act as a trigger that a patient received a harmful dose of opioid medication. Fifty-three different triggers were created, some of which apply to all patients and others that apply only to specific populations or specific settings of care. The trigger tools are significant due to their efficiency. Whereas a complete chart review of all medical records would be expensive and labor-intensive, triggers alert the safety personnel to possible adverse events that warrant a medical chart review [27]. The detection of a trigger initiates an investigation into whether an adverse event actually occurred or not, and additionally evaluates the severity of the event [28]. This feature has the possibility of being integrated into the electronic medical record to allow for automation and increased efficiency of this process.

Nonetheless, several drawbacks with trigger tools immediately surfaced. The IHI emphasizes that the GTT will not identify all sources of patient harm, notably, events with low severity [26]. Moreover, the reliability of trigger tools is significantly influenced by the level of training and the experience of reviewers, as well as their familiarity with the clinical setting being evaluated. A study found that the Global Trigger Tool had poor inter-rater reliability for the detection and grading of adverse events between reviewers experienced in the use of the tool [29]. Finally, most existing trigger tools have been used to identify adverse events in the inpatient setting. Although some studies have thought to develop trigger tools for ambulatory care, there is relatively little data on the accuracy and reliability of these tools [30].

Clinically Derived National Detection and Reporting Systems

In 1994, the National Surgical Quality Improvement Program (NSQIP) was conceived in the Veterans Affairs (VA) healthcare system. [31–36] This outcome-based program records the performance of all VA hospitals performing major surgery and, adjusting for patient preoperative risk, compares these hospitals by the ratio of observed to expected (O/E) adverse events. The results are then provided to each hospital and used to identify areas of substandard performance and potential excess adverse events (Fig. 12.1) [15]. The NSQIP was widely accepted

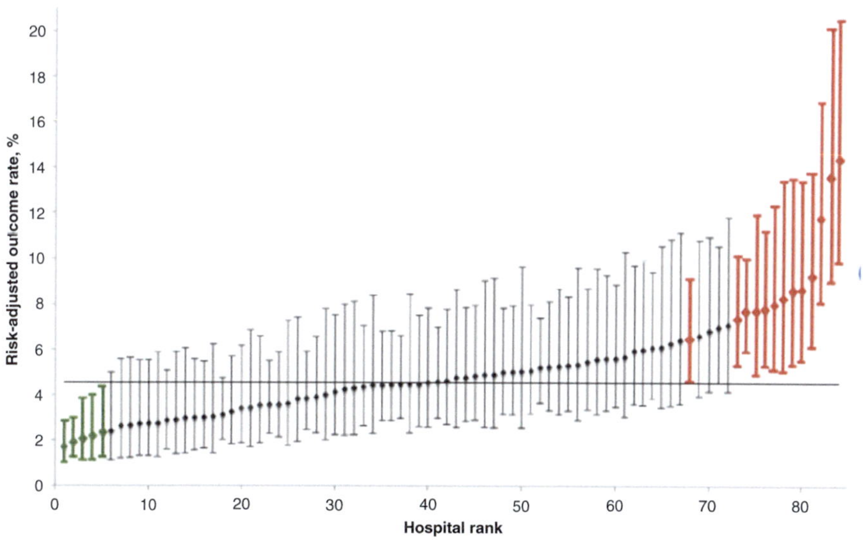

Fig. 12.1 Example performance report (any complication, hospitals with at least 125 cases/year, laparoscopic gastric bypass procedures). Diamonds: hospital risk-adjusted outcomes rates with 95% CIs. Green: low outliers, have 95% CIs less than the average outcomes rate. Red: high outliers, have 95% CIs greater than the average outcomes rate. Solid horizontal line, overall mean outcomes rate. (Source: https://www.researchgate.net/figure/Example-performance-report-any-complication-hospitals-with-at-least-125-cases-year_fig1_263283398. *May be subject to copyright*)

by VA surgeons and managers and has provided annual outcome reports that have resulted in significant improvements to the standard of surgical care. Between 1991 and 2002, unadjusted 30-day morbidity and mortality rates for major non-cardiac surgery in the VA system decreased from 17.4% to 9.9% and 3.2% to 2.3%, respectively [14].

With the solid success in the VA system, the NSQIP was subsequently adapted for use in the private sector [14, 15, 37] with trained, audited nurse reviewers collecting 30-day complication and mortality rates based on standardized definitions. Eventually, the American College of Surgeons (ACS) made this program available to private sector hospitals with the ACS-NSQIP and is using it as its platform for promoting quality and safety [8]. ACS-NSQIP derives its data from the patient's medical charts, as opposed to other quality programs that rely on claims or administrative data that are easy to obtain [38]. While this process is labor- and time-intensive, the accuracy and clinical utility of the data gathered is of superior quality. Similarly, clinically derived, field-specific quality improvement programs have since been created, such as the Trauma Quality Improvement Program (TQIP) and the Metabolic and Bariatric Surgery Accreditation and Quality Improvement Program (MBSAQIP).

Vizient

Vizient, formerly known as University HealthSystem Consortium (UHC), is the largest member-driven, healthcare performance improvement company in the United States. It empowers healthcare professionals and scientists to deliver exceptional, cost-effective care to every patient, and helps develop new approaches to patient care. It contains data representing over 97% of United States academic medical centers and 160 community hospitals. The database contains demographic, financial, and clinical information including hospital length of stay, complication rate, readmission rate, mortality rate, medication use, hospital-acquired conditions, and direct cost [39]. Additionally, the Vizient database allows for some degree of risk adjustment based on well-established risk models for certain outcomes [40]. However, the Vizient database lacks specific patient characteristics, and users are unable to determine the timing of complications with regard to the date of surgery [39].

Surgical Care Improvement Project (SCIP)

In 2002, the Surgical Care Improvement Project (SCIP) was introduced by the Centers for Medicare and Medicaid Services (CMS) in partnership with national organizations, such as the American Hospital Association, Centers for Disease Control and Prevention (CDC), the Institute for Healthcare Improvement, and The Joint Commission [41]. It targets complications that account for a significant portion of preventable morbidity and aims to improve cost effectiveness [42]. The specific SCIP initiatives are published in the Specifications Manual for National Inpatient Quality Measures (Specifications Manual), which is a constantly evolving manual [42]. For instance, a goal of this program is to reduce the rates of postoperative surgical infections. The three core preventative measures that specifically relate to healthcare-associated infections (HAIs) include: [41]

1. The initiation of prophylactic antibiotics within 1 h before surgical incisions (or within 2 h if the patient is receiving vancomycin or fluoroquinolones)
2. The use of prophylactic antibiotics appropriate for the specific procedures of the patient
3. The discontinuation of prophylactic antibiotics within 24 h of surgery completion, but within 48 h for cardiothoracic surgery.

While SCIP reporting is mandatory, reporting measures are not universally enforced, and it is postulated that tighter enforcement of SCIP measures in hospitals that are not complying consistently can lead to a substantial improvement in surgical site infection (SSI) rates. This can significantly reduce the current societal burden of the estimated 750,000–1,000,000 annual SSIs, which includes an economic annual excess cost of $1.6 billion [41]. Other SCIP projects include the prevention of venous thromboembolism and adverse cardiac events.

Anesthesia-Related Intraoperative Adverse Events: Anesthesia Information Management Systems (AIMS)

The adoption of anesthesia information management systems (AIMS), the primary function of which is to collect intraoperative data that enables anesthesia care providers to create a more reliable and accurate anesthesia record, has been shown to improve patient care and quality assurance and has enabled the development of mandatory quality assurance (QA) reporting systems for adverse events (AEs) [43].

AIMS includes an "outcomes" section, in which the presence or absence of all intraoperative anesthesia AEs can be entered. Examples of anesthesia AE include, but are not limited to, airway, pulmonary, cardiovascular, neurologic, and physical injury events, as well as adverse drug reactions, transfusion reactions, emergence, and case cancelations. However, the completion of this documentation was not required for the finalization of documentation. Consequently, entries were sparse and the capture rate of AEs was inconsistent [44].

When AIMS is implemented, a decrease in the rate of anesthesia-related AEs can be observed. In one academic center that required in a non-punitive manner entry of AEs in the AIMS, compliance with the reporting process increased from <10% in the pre-intervention period to 97% post-intervention and was sustained over the first 2 years of the program. Over that period, the documented AE rate significantly decreased from 1.23 to 0.64%. The decrease occurred mainly in the group of preventable AEs, whereas the rate of unpreventable AEs was unchanged. At another institution, once AIMS was implemented, the AE rate decreased from 4.20 to 1.36% over a 7-year period. It is reasonable to assume that, because providers were expected to report QA data for every surgical case, a focus on reporting complications improved the culture of safety over time [44].

Classification Systems

Access to reliable and consistent risk-adjusted outcome data is necessary to improve and benchmark surgical performance. In the absence of reliable markers of outcome, reporting raw, unadjusted performance data to patients to identify "top" physicians or hospitals can be misleading. The challenge is always to create and use scale systems, which, while maintaining simplicity, are still accurate and generalizable [45]. Severity classification systems of AEs can help.

Postoperative Adverse Events

Clavien-Dindo Classification

In 1992, Clavien et al. published a classification system intended to standardize the recording of postoperative complications [46]. In this classification, the extent of treatment required to prevent or treat the adverse effects of a certain complication defined its severity on a four-level grading system (Table 12.2) [45]. The

Table 12.2 Clavien-Dindo classification of postoperative complications

Grade	Definition
Grade I	Any deviation from the normal postoperative course without the need for pharmacological treatment or surgical, endoscopic, and radiological interventions
	Allowed therapeutic regimens are: drugs as antiemetics, antipyretics, analgetics, diuretics, electrolytes, and physiotherapy. This grade also includes wound infections opened at the bedside
Grade II	Requiring pharmacological treatment with drugs other than such allowed for grade I complications
	Blood transfusions and total parenteral nutrition are also included
Grade III	Requiring surgical, endoscopic or radiological intervention
Grade IIIa	Intervention not under general anesthesia
Grade IIIb	Intervention under general anesthesia
Grade IV	Life-threatening complication (including CNS complications)[a] requiring IC/ICU management
Grade IVa	Single organ dysfunction (including dialysis)
Grade IVb	Multiorgan dysfunction
Grade V	Death of a patient
Suffix "d"	If the patient suffers from a complication at the time of discharge (see examples in Table 12.2). The suffix "d" (for "disability") is added to the respective grade of complication. This label indicates the need for a follow-up to fully evaluate the complication

CNS central nervous system, *IC* intermediate care, *ICU* intensive care unit

Source: Dindo D, Demartines N, Clavien P-A. Classification of surgical complications: a new proposal with evaluation in a cohort of 6336 patients and results of a survey. Annals of surgery. 2004;240(2):205

[a] Brain hemorrhage, ischemic stroke, subarachnoidal bleeding, but excluding transient ischemic attacks

classification has since been used in many studies and large-scale database research [46–48]. The system was revised internationally, incorporating more objective criteria and some flexibility by allowing a contraction of grades to adjust to the patient population studied. This revised system [49] rapidly gained acceptance and became increasingly used in large-scale trials.

Accordion Classification

A newer modified classification (the Accordion Classification) for surgical complications was introduced by Strasberg and colleagues in 2009 [50]. The Accordion Severity Grading System is named after its ability to expand to accommodate the range of complications found in large complex studies, while contracting for smaller studies. The expansion or contraction exclusively happens within the "severe" complications section. In the contracted state, the classification has only four levels, headed by self-evident terms rather than grades. For large and complex studies, such as those involving complex procedures such as esophageal or pancreatic resection, where many severe complications may be expected, there is good reason to subdivide and expand the severe category to fully describe the range of complications.

The Clavien-Dindo and Accordion classifications have played a crucial research and quality-improvement role as a common language to report and compare postoperative complications within and across surgical departments, institutions, and researchers [45, 50–53].

Intraoperative Adverse Events

Up until nearly a decade ago, most surgical patient safety efforts had exclusively focused on postoperative adverse events, and successfully established a common language to nationally and internationally discuss postoperative complications [46, 49, 54–57]. Intraoperatively, however, surgeons relied principally on their surgical instinct and clinical assessment of the operative course to determine postoperative course and guide clinical care [58]. While most physicians believed that intraoperative management contributes importantly to overall outcomes, quantitative metrics of the quality of intraoperative care were not available [59]. Thus, attention was shifted toward what happens in the "black box" of the operating room. Subsequently, it was shown that patients who suffer intraoperative adverse events (iAEs) have a 41% increase in hospital costs on average, directly attributable to the occurrence of the iAE. The increase in cost is not confined to the immediate cost of addressing the iAE, but also extends to all categories of postoperative care, such as laboratory, radiology, medication, and nutritional charges. Beyond their financial implications for all stakeholders, the true significance of iAEs lies in the quality and safety of care delivered to patients. Thus, by tracking, measuring the effects, and developing systems to reduce the occurrence and/or severity of iAEs, we can achieve higher value healthcare delivery by simultaneously controlling costs and improving patient outcomes [60]. In 2006, a review of malpractice claims at four liability insurers revealed that more than 75% of closed claims related to surgical care resulted from iAEs [61].

Surgical Apgar Score

In 2007, Gawande et al. derived and validated a 10-point Surgical Apgar Score which was developed using three intraoperative parameters that were independent predictors of 30-day major complications: estimated blood loss (EBL), lowest heart rate (HR), and the lowest mean arterial pressure (MAP) during the operation. The beta coefficients of the variables were used to weigh the points allocated to each variable in a 10-point score. The score effectively predicted major postoperative complications within 30 days of both general and vascular surgery [62]. The Surgical Apgar Score successfully integrated components of patient susceptibility, procedure complexity, and operative performance to provide a measure of immediate postoperative condition and prognostication [63]. While the Surgical Apgar Score was potentially useful as a reporting mechanism for iAE, it was not capable of detecting and properly classifying iAEs.

A major challenge that existed in detecting and reporting of iAEs included considerable variability in reporting iAEs in operative notes. Even when reported in mortality and morbidity conferences, the rate of capture of their occurrences was very low [64, 65]. This was mainly due to the absence of a clear definition for what constitutes an iAE or the surgeon's personal interpretation of the clinical significance of the incident [60]. A compelling need to generate not only risk-adjusted but also severity-adjusted rates of iAEs was present, as from a patient transparency perspective, severity-adjusted rates of iAEs are more relevant than the crude incidence of such events.

Surgical Intraoperative Adverse Event Classification Scheme

In 2013, using a methodology that combined clinically and administratively generated data and the 15th Patient Safety Indicator (accidental puncture or laceration) algorithms created by the AHRQ, the Massachusetts General Hospital and Harvard Medical School developed a six-point severity classification scale for iAE (Table 12.3) [66]. The classification tool was created to be a quality assessment and improvement tool at the hospital, regional, and national levels, as opposed to being a tool to screen for iAEs. To maintain objectivity and ease of identification and reproducibility, the scale severity classification was based on the extent of therapeutic intervention needed to mitigate its effect [66]. On validation, the scale had excellent inter-rater reliability. It also had external validity: high-grade iAEs were correlated with higher risks of surgical site infections, systemic sepsis, failure to wean off the ventilator, and a prolonged postoperative length of stay, compared to lower grade iAEs. A subsequent study by Bohnen et al. [67] quantified the impact of iAEs on postoperative outcome, suggesting that the risk of 30-day mortality is more than tripled and the risk of 30-day complications is more than doubled after the occurrence of an iAE, even when that iAE is addressed intraoperatively. Furthermore, an anonymous survey of Boston surgeons in 2017 reported that most surgeons encountered one to six iAEs in the past 12 months of practice. In that same study, approximately half the surgeons pointed out the lack of a standardized iAE reporting system, the absence of a clear iAE definition, and fear of litigation as the three most important barriers to iAE reporting [68]. Thus, the true incidence of iAEs

Table 12.3 Intraoperative adverse event severity classification scheme

Class	Description
I	Injury requiring no repair within the same procedure (e.g., cauterization, use of prothrombotic material, small vessel ligation)
II	Injury requiring surgical repair, without organ removal or a change in the originally planned procedure (e.g., any suture repair, patch repair)
III	Injury requiring tissue or organ removal with completion of the originally planned procedure
IV	Injury requiring a significant change[a] and/or incompletion of the originally planned procedure
V	Missed intraoperative injury requiring re-operation within 7 days
VI	Intraoperative death
Suffix T	Add if injury required transfusion of ≥2 U blood

Source: Kaafarani HM, Mavros MN, Hwabejire J, Fagenholz P, Yeh DD, Demoya M, et al. Derivation and validation of a novel severity classification for intraoperative adverse events. Journal of the American College of Surgeons. 2014;218(6):1120–8

[a] Excludes minimally invasive to open conversions

remained difficult to assess due to the lack of a standardized method for surgeons to systematically report iAEs.

Subsequently, a prospective study assessed the incidence of iAEs through surgeon self-reporting (surgeons' willingness to provide this information). The findings suggested that surgeons are willing to admit and report their iAEs, evidenced by a high response rate to the inquiries, and having a similar response rate in cases with and without iAEs. These findings were pleasantly surprising, given the potential medicolegal, professional, and emotional impact of reporting intraoperative mishaps. However, there was systematic underreporting of all iAEs, especially iAEs of low severity, with only 1 in 10 of class I iAEs being self-reported. This may be because of both the lack of a clear iAE definition and their subjective interpretation of what is clinically insignificant, expected, or inconsequential [69].

The "black box" nature of the operating room and medicolegal and professional impact of iAEs pose a serious challenge to accurately detecting iAEs. The aforementioned study suggested that operative report review is, in fact, more reliable than self-reporting, but occasionally misses potentially relevant iAEs that were self-reported by surgeons, yet not documented in the chart. That being said, the true incidence of iAEs is undoubtedly higher than either method, and the search continues for the optimal method to detect and report iAEs that is independent from the surgeon's willingness to self-report or the variation in operative report documentation among different surgeons [69]. Thus, the authors strongly advocate for a consistent and reliable system for iAE detection, reporting, and simultaneous robust risk adjustment. Risk adjustment will be crucial to avoid penalizing the surgeon willing to operate on higher risk patients. For a system to be established and ultimately improve the quality of patient care, a culture change in the world of surgery will be necessary, and such a system will need to be conceived under the protective umbrella of peer review to avoid medicolegal repercussions.

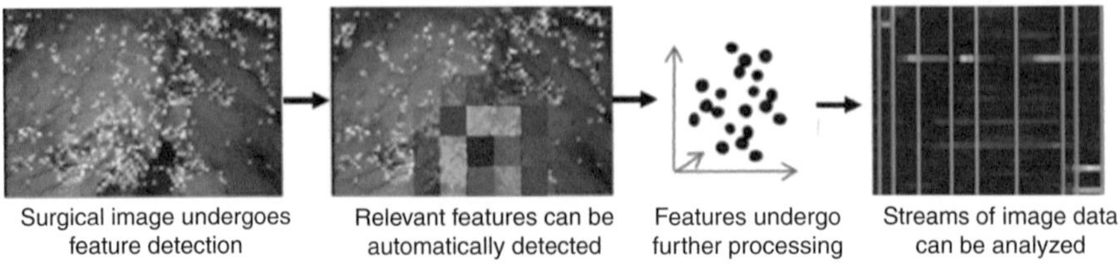

Fig. 12.2 Computer vision utilizes mathematical techniques to analyze visual images or video streams as quantifiable features such as color, texture, and position that can then be used within a dataset to identify statistically meaningful events such as bleeding. (Source: Hashimoto DA, Rosman G, Rus D, Meireles OR. Artificial intelligence in surgery: promises and perils. Annals of surgery. 2018;268(1):70–6. *May be subject to copyright*)

Theoretical solutions to this matter include having a peer surgeon review video recordings of procedures to identify iAEs. However, this is costly from both an equipment perspective and the time needed for trained personnel [69]. Alternatively, this could prove cost-effective and accurate in the near future with the promise of artificial intelligence (AI) and the advent of one of its core subfields, image recognition, and computer vision [70]. Computer vision describes machine understanding of images and videos, where advances have resulted in machines achieving human-level capabilities in object and scene recognition [71]. One important healthcare-related application of computer vision includes image acquisition and interpretation in image-guided surgery [72]. For instance, real-time analysis of laparoscopic video yielded 92.8% accuracy in automated identification of the steps of a sleeve gastrectomy, and even made notice of missing or unexpected steps [73]. Videos contain a wealth of actionable data, where it is estimated that 1 minute of high-definition surgical video contains 25 times the amount of data found in a high-resolution computed tomography image [74–76].

Thus, although predictive video analysis is in its infancy, such work provides proof-of-concept that AI can be leveraged to process massive amounts of surgical data to identify or even predict the occurrence of iAEs in real time (Fig. 12.2). Until this technology becomes readily available and implementable, the authors believe that a simple measure, such as adding a "Did an iAE occur?" question to the "time out" phase at the end of a surgical procedure is a good start if a standardized iAE definition is used [69].

Conclusion

In the interest of our patients, transparency of surgical errors, including iAEs, is important in a culture that embodies patient safety and aims at understating and improving the shortcomings and limitations of the care we deliver today. Seeking systems of adverse events reporting that are accurate, risk-adjusted, severity-adjusted, and reasonably automated carries the premise of revolutionizing the quality of care we provide as surgeons.

References

1. Miller CO. In: Wiener EL, editor. Human factors in aviation. San Diego: Academic Press; 1988.
2. Havens DH, Boroughs L. "To err is human": a report from the Institute of Medicine. J Pediatr Health Care. 2000;14(2):77–80.
3. Institute of Medicine (US) Committee on Quality of Health Care in America. Crossing the quality chasm: a new health system for the 21st century. Washington: National Academies Press (US); 2001.
4. Stahel PF. Learning from aviation safety: a call for formal "readbacks" in surgery. Patient Saf Surg. 2008;2:21.
5. Wachter RM, Pronovost PJ. The 100,000 lives campaign: a scientific and policy review. Jt Comm J Qual Patient Saf. 2006;32(11):621–7.
6. Codman EA. The classic: a study in hospital efficiency: as demonstrated by the case report of first five years of private hospital. Clin Orthop Relat Res. 2013;471(6):1778–83.
7. Codman EA. The "minimum standard" document: American College of Surgeons. https://www.facs.org/about-acs/archives/pasthighlights/minimumhighlight.
8. Hutter MM, Rowell KS, Devaney LA, Sokal SM, Warshaw AL, Abbott WM, et al. Identification of surgical complications and deaths: an assessment of the traditional surgical morbidity and mortality conference compared with the American College of Surgeons-National Surgical Quality Improvement Program. J Am Coll Surg. 2006;203(5):618–24.
9. American Congress of Obstetricians and Gynecologists Education. Program requirements for residency education in surgery. 2004.
10. Gordon LA. Gordon's guide to the surgical morbidity and mortality conference. Philadelphia: Hanley & Belfus; 1994.
11. Longo DR, Hewett JE, Ge B, Schubert S. The long road to patient safety: a status report on patient safety systems. JAMA. 2005;294(22):2858–65.
12. Wachter RM. The end of the beginning: patient safety five years after 'to err is human' Health Aff. 2004;23(Suppl 1):W4–534–45.
13. Birkmeyer NJ, Birkmeyer JD. Strategies for improving surgical quality—should payers reward excellence or effort? vol. 354. Waltham: Massachusetts Medical Society; 2006. p. 864.
14. Khuri SF, Daley J, Henderson W, Hur K, Demakis J, Aust JB, et al. The Department of Veterans Affairs' NSQIP: the first national, validated, outcome-based, risk-adjusted, and peer-controlled program for the measurement and enhancement of the quality of surgical care. Ann Surg. 1998;228(4):491.
15. Fink AS, Campbell DA Jr, Mentzer RM Jr, Henderson WG, Daley J, Bannister J, et al. The National Surgical Quality Improvement Program in non-veterans administration hospitals: initial demonstration of feasibility. Ann Surg. 2002;236(3):344.
16. Kaafarani HM, Rosen AK. Using administrative data to identify surgical adverse events: an introduction to the Patient Safety Indicators. Am J Surg. 2009;198(5):S63–8.
17. Fraser I. AHRQ quality indicators: guide to patient safety indicators version 3.1. Department of Health and Human Services/Agency for Healthcare Research and Quality. 2007.
18. AHRQ Quality Indicators. Guide to patient safety indicators. Rockville: Agency for Healthcare Research and Quality; 2003.
19. Miller DC, Filson CP, Wallner LP, Montie JE, Campbell DA, Wei JT. Comparing performance of morbidity and mortality conference and National Surgical Quality Improvement Program for detection of complications after urologic surgery. Urology. 2006;68(5):931–7.
20. Zrelak PA, Sadeghi B, Utter GH, Baron R, Tancredi DJ, Geppert JJ, et al. Positive predictive value of the Agency for Healthcare Research and Quality Patient Safety Indicator for central line-related bloodstream infection ("selected infections due to medical care"). J Healthc Qual. 2011;33(2):29–36.
21. White RH, Sadeghi B, Tancredi DJ, Zrelak P, Cuny J, Sama P, et al. How valid is the ICD-9-CM based AHRQ patient safety indicator for postoperative venous thromboembolism? Med Care. 2009;47:1237–43.

22. Utter GH, Cuny J, Sama P, Silver MR, Zrelak PA, Baron R, et al. Detection of postoperative respiratory failure: how predictive is the Agency for Healthcare Research and Quality's Patient Safety Indicator? J Am Coll Surg. 2010;211(3):347–54.e29.
23. Utter GH, Zrelak PA, Baron R, Tancredi DJ, Sadeghi B, Geppert JJ, et al. Positive predictive value of the AHRQ accidental puncture or laceration patient safety indicator. Ann Surg. 2009;250(6):1041–5.
24. Sadeghi B, Baron R, Zrelak P, Utter GH, Geppert JJ, Tancredi DJ, et al. Cases of iatrogenic pneumothorax can be identified from ICD-9-CM coded data. Am J Med Qual. 2010;25(3):218–24.
25. Allison JJ, Wall TC, Spettell CM, Calhoun J, Fargason CA Jr, Kobylinski RW, et al. The art and science of chart review. Jt Comm J Qual Improv. 2000;26(3):115–36.
26. Agency for Healthcare Research and Quality. Triggers and trigger tools. 2019. https://psnet.ahrq.gov/primers/primer/33/Triggers-and-Trigger-Tools.
27. Classen DC, Resar R, Griffin F, Federico F, Frankel T, Kimmel N, et al. 'Global trigger tool' shows that adverse events in hospitals may be ten times greater than previously measured. Health Aff. 2011;30(4):581–9.
28. Weingart SN, Davis RB, Palmer RH, Cahalane M, Beth Hamel M, Mukamal K, et al. Discrepancies between explicit and implicit review: physician and nurse assessments of complications and quality. Health Serv Res. 2002;37(2):483–98.
29. Schildmeijer K, Nilsson L, Årestedt K, Perk J. Assessment of adverse events in medical care: lack of consistency between experienced teams using the global trigger tool. BMJ Qual Saf. 2012;21(4):307–14.
30. Rosen AK, Mull HJ, Kaafarani H, Nebeker J, Shimada S, Helwig A, et al. Applying trigger tools to detect adverse events associated with outpatient surgery. J Patient Saf. 2011;7(1):45–59.
31. Young G, Charns M, Desai K, Daley J, Henderson W, Khuri S, editors. Patterns of coordination and clinical outcomes: a study of surgical services. Health Serv Res. 1998;33(5 Pt 1):1211–1236.
32. Khuri SF, Daley J, Henderson W, Hur K, Gibbs JO, Barbour G, et al. Risk adjustment of the postoperative mortality rate for the comparative assessment of the quality of surgical care: results of the National Veterans Affairs Surgical Risk Study. J Am Coll Surg. 1997;185(4):315–27.
33. Khuri SF, Daley J, Henderson W, Barbour G, Lowry P, Irvin G, et al. The National Veterans Administration Surgical Risk Study: risk adjustment for the comparative assessment of the quality of surgical care. J Am Coll Surg. 1995;180(5):519–31.
34. Gibbs J, Clark K, Khuri S, Henderson W, Hur K, Daley J. Validating risk-adjusted surgical outcomes: chart review of process of care. Int J Qual Health Care. 2001;13(3):187–96.
35. Gibbs J, Cull W, Henderson W, Daley J, Hur K, Khuri SF. Preoperative serum albumin level as a predictor of operative mortality and morbidity: results from the National VA Surgical Risk Study. Arch Surg. 1999;134(1):36–42.
36. Daley J, Forbes MG, Young GJ, Charns MP, Gibbs JO, Hur K, et al. Validating risk-adjusted surgical outcomes: site visit assessment of process and structure. J Am Coll Surg. 1997;185(4):341–51.
37. Khuri SF, Daley J, Henderson WG. The comparative assessment and improvement of quality of surgical care in the Department of Veterans Affairs. Arch Surg. 2002;137(1):20–7.
38. Iezzoni LI. Assessing quality using administrative data. Ann Intern Med. 1997;127:666–74.
39. Karhade AV, Larsen AM, Cote DJ, Dubois HM, Smith TR. National databases for neurosurgical outcomes research: options, strengths, and limitations. Neurosurgery. 2017;83(3):333–44.
40. Birdas TJ, Rozycki GF, Dunnington GL, Stevens L, Liali V, Schmidt CM. "Show me the data": a recipe for quality improvement success in an academic surgical department. J Am Coll Surg. 2019;228(4):368–73.
41. Cataife G, Weinberg DA, Wong H-H, Kahn KL. The effect of surgical care improvement project (SCIP) compliance on surgical site infections (SSI). Med Care. 2014;52:S66–73.
42. Rosenberger LH, Politano AD, Sawyer RG. The surgical care improvement project and prevention of post-operative infection, including surgical site infection. Surg Infect. 2011;12(3):163–8.

43. Stol IS, Ehrenfeld JM, Epstein RH. Technology diffusion of anesthesia information management systems into academic anesthesia departments in the United States. Anesth Analg. 2014;118(3):644–50.
44. Wanderer JP, Gratch DM, Jacques PS, Rodriquez LI, Epstein RH. Trends in the prevalence of intraoperative adverse events at two academic hospitals after implementation of a mandatory reporting system. Anesth Analg. 2018;126(1):134–40.
45. Clavien PA, Barkun J, De Oliveira ML, Vauthey JN, Dindo D, Schulick RD, et al. The Clavien-Dindo classification of surgical complications: five-year experience. Ann Surg. 2009;250(2):187–96.
46. Clavien PA, Sanabria JR, Strasberg SM. Proposed classification of complications of surgery with examples of utility in cholecystectomy. Surgery. 1992;111(5):518–26.
47. Clavien PA, Camargo CA Jr, Croxford R, Langer B, Levy GA, Greig PD. Definition and classification of negative outcomes in solid organ transplantation. Application in liver transplantation. Ann Surg. 1994;220(2):109.
48. Ghobrial RM, Freise CE, Trotter JF, Tong L, Ojo AO, Fair JH, et al. Donor morbidity after living donation for liver transplantation. Gastroenterology. 2008;135(2):468–76.
49. Dindo D, Demartines N, Clavien P-A. Classification of surgical complications: a new proposal with evaluation in a cohort of 6336 patients and results of a survey. Ann Surg. 2004;240(2):205.
50. Muysoms F, Deerenberg E, Peeters E, Agresta F, Berrevoet F, Campanelli G, et al. Recommendations for reporting outcome results in abdominal wall repair. Hernia. 2013;17(4):423–33.
51. Yui R, Satoi S, Toyokawa H, Yanagimoto H, Yamamoto T, Hirooka S, et al. Less morbidity after introduction of a new departmental policy for patients who undergo open distal pancreatectomy. J Hepatobiliary Pancreat Sci. 2014;21(1):72–7.
52. Tefekli A, Karadag MA, Tepeler K, Sari E, Berberoglu Y, Baykal M, et al. Classification of percutaneous nephrolithotomy complications using the modified Clavien grading system: looking for a standard. Eur Urol. 2008;53(1):184–90.
53. Yoon PD, Chalasani V, Woo HH. Use of Clavien-Dindo classification in reporting and grading complications after urological surgical procedures: analysis of 2010 to 2012. J Urol. 2013;190(4):1271–4.
54. Strasberg SM, Linehan DC, Hawkins WG. The Accordion severity grading system of surgical complications. Ann Surg. 2009;250(2):177–86.
55. Griffin F, Classen D. Detection of adverse events in surgical patients using the trigger tool approach. BMJ Qual Saf. 2008;17(4):253–8.
56. Khuri SF, Henderson WG, Daley J, Jonasson O, Jones RS, Campbell DA Jr, et al. Successful implementation of the Department of Veterans Affairs' National Surgical Quality Improvement Program in the private sector: the patient safety in surgery study. Ann Surv. 2008;248(2):329–36.
57. Hall BL, Richards K, Ingraham A, Ko CY. New approaches to the National Surgical Quality Improvement Program: the American College of Surgeons experience. Am J Surg. 2009;198(5):S56–62.
58. Hartley M, Sagar P. The surgeon's 'gut feeling' as a predictor of post-operative outcome. Ann R Coll Surg Engl. 1994;76(6 Suppl):277–8.
59. Vincent C, Moorthy K, Sarker SK, Chang A, Darzi AW. Systems approaches to surgical quality and safety: from concept to measurement. Ann Surg. 2004;239(4):475.
60. Ramly EP, Larentzakis A, Bohnen JD, Mavros M, Chang Y, Lee J, et al. The financial impact of intraoperative adverse events in abdominal surgery. Surgery. 2015;158(5):1382–8.
61. Rogers SO Jr, Gawande AA, Kwaan M, Puopolo AL, Yoon C, Brennan TA, et al. Analysis of surgical errors in closed malpractice claims at 4 liability insurers. Surgery. 2006;140(1):25–33.
62. Gawande AA, Kwaan MR, Regenbogen SE, Lipsitz SA, Zinner MJ. An Apgar score for surgery. J Am Coll Surg. 2007;204(2):201–8.
63. Regenbogen SE, Lancaster RT, Lipsitz SR, Greenberg CC, Hutter MM, Gawande AA. Does the Surgical Apgar Score measure intraoperative performance? Ann Surg. 2008;248(2):320.

64. Dimick JB, Pronovost PJ, Cowan JA, Lipsett PA. Complications and costs after high-risk surgery: where should we focus quality improvement initiatives? J Am Coll Surg. 2003;196(5):671–8.
65. Kalish RL, Daley J, Duncan CC, Davis RB, Coffman GA, Iezzoni LI. Costs of potential complications of care for major surgery patients. Am J Med Qual. 1995;10(1):48–54.
66. Kaafarani HM, Mavros MN, Hwabejire J, Fagenholz P, Yeh DD, Demoya M, et al. Derivation and validation of a novel severity classification for intraoperative adverse events. J Am Coll Surg. 2014;218(6):1120–8.
67. Bohnen JD, Mavros MN, Ramly EP, Chang Y, Yeh DD, Lee J, et al. Intraoperative adverse events in abdominal surgery: what happens in the operating room does not stay in the operating room. Ann Surg. 2017;265(6):1119–25.
68. Han K, Bohnen JD, Peponis T, Martinez M, Nandan A, Yeh DD, et al. The surgeon as the second victim? Results of the Boston intraoperative adverse events surgeons' attitude (BISA) study. J Am Coll Surg. 2017;224(6):1048–56.
69. Peponis T, Baekgaard JS, Bohnen JD, Han K, Lee J, Saillant N, et al. Are surgeons reluctant to accurately report intraoperative adverse events? A prospective study of 1,989 patients. Surgery. 2018;164(3):525–9.
70. Hashimoto DA, Rosman G, Rus D, Meireles OR. Artificial intelligence in surgery: promises and perils. Ann Surg. 2018;268(1):70–6.
71. Szeliski R. Computer vision: algorithms and applications. Philadelphia: Springer Science & Business Media; 2010.
72. Kenngott H, Wagner M, Nickel F, Wekerle A, Preukschas A, Apitz M, et al. Computer-assisted abdominal surgery: new technologies. Langenbecks Arch Surg. 2015;400(3):273–81.
73. Volkov M, Hashimoto DA, Rosman G, Meireles OR, Rus D, editors. Machine learning and coresets for automated real-time video segmentation of laparoscopic and robot-assisted surgery. 2017 IEEE International Conference on Robotics and Automation (ICRA); Piscataway: Institute of Electrical and Electronics Engineers; 2017.
74. Grenda TR, Pradarelli JC, Dimick JB. Using surgical video to improve technique and skill. Ann Surg. 2016;264(1):32.
75. Bonrath EM, Gordon LE, Grantcharov TP. Characterising 'near miss' events in complex laparoscopic surgery through video analysis. BMJ Qual Saf. 2015;24(8):516–21.
76. Natarajan P, Frenzel JC, Smaltz DH. Demystifying big data and machine learning for healthcare. Boca Raton: CRC Press; 2017.

Simulation Technical Training to Improve Safety in the OR

13

Rana M. Higgins and Marc A. de Moya

Introduction

Simulation is an invaluable part of training and continued professional development in health care, especially within surgery. It provides helpful training for both technical and non-technical skills. Through the development of skills, patient safety and efficiency in the operating room can be optimized [1]. The purpose of simulation is to recreate real-world scenarios through an external device or setup. Through this system, the trainer controls the learning environment by establishing specific goals of the simulation training and providing feedback [2]. This leads to deliberate practice, which is necessary for skill acquisition and mastery even as it applies to teams.

Within the simulation environment, fidelity represents the realism of the simulation model. Fidelity is multi-dimensional, incorporating environment, equipment, and psychological components [2]. Environment fidelity addresses the extent to which the simulator replicates the various senses, such as motion and vision, of the actual environment. Equipment fidelity addresses the extent to which the appearance of the simulator replicates the actual environment. Psychological fidelity highlights the extent to which the trainee perceives the simulated environment to be realistic and representative of the actual environment. These three components can overlap to varying degrees within each simulation environment.

Three primary categories of simulation vary in the degree to which they incorporate environment, equipment, and psychological fidelity (Table 13.1) [2]. The first category of simulation is case studies and role plays, which serve as fictional examples in an attempt to reinforce specific training material. This type of simulation is

R. M. Higgins
Department of Surgery, Medical College of Wisconsin, Milwaukee, WI, USA

M. A. de Moya (✉)
Division of Trauma and Acute Care Surgery, Medical College of Wisconsin, Milwaukee, WI, USA
e-mail: mdemoya@mcw.edu

J. J. Hoballah et al. (eds.), *Principles of Perioperative Safety and Efficiency*, https://doi.org/10.1007/978-3-031-41089-5_13

Table 13.1 Categories of simulation-based training

Simulation type	Teamwork competencies	Primary strengths	Primary weaknesses
Case studies/ role plays	Knowledge, attitudes	Low cost, positive trainee reactions	Few opportunities for skills practice
Part-task trainers	Knowledge, skills	Low cost, distraction-free environment	No opportunity for dual task practice
Full-mission simulations	Knowledge, skills	Can simulate rare (but critical) tasks in a safe environment	High cost, currently limited to a few medical specialties

typically low cost, with low environment, equipment, and psychological fidelity. A second category of simulation is partial-task trainers, which include examples such as standardized patients and laparoscopic trainers. The purpose of this type of simulation is to break down a complex task into parts. The equipment, environment, and psychological fidelity for this type of simulation are all medium. The final type of simulation is full-mission simulation, which mimics all the environmental complexities at once. All types of fidelity are high for this simulation, given that trainees can practice skills under the most realistic of scenarios, but it does require the highest cost of all three types. Each type of simulation has its role, depending on the goals of training identified, the purpose of the simulated environment, the available resources, and the number of people being trained.

Simulation is used to develop both technical and non-technical skills in the operating room. The skills that must be trained and developed vary depending on the role of the provider in the operating room. Surgeons, anesthesiologists, nurses, scrub techs, residents, and medical students all play a different role in the operating room, and therefore simulation training should vary depending on the skill and provider being trained. The five primary skills that improve surgical outcomes that can be trained in a simulated environment are:

1. Team-based competency
2. Operating room fire safety
3. Infection prevention and control
4. Crisis resource management (CRM)
5. Technical skills training

Team-Based Competency

Team-based competency is a critical skill in the high-risk environment of the operating room. A team is defined as a group of individuals who perform a work-related task, interact with one another in a dynamic fashion, and share a common goal [3]. It is critically important that all members of the teamwork together to achieve the common goal, and teamwork is defined as the behaviors that allow for effective and efficient achievement of this goal. The five most important behaviors that facilitate teamwork are: (1) team leadership, (2) team orientation, (3) mutual performance monitoring, (4) backup behaviors, and (5) adaptability [2]. Ensuring these behaviors are optimized in the operating room environment can be challenging, with various team members and their differing roles, training, and responsibilities. Mill et al. [4] identified discrepancies between surgeons' perception of the team operating room environment in comparison to nurses and anesthesiologists. Surgeons perceived a stronger culture of safety, communication, and teamwork than either nurses or anesthesiologists. These discrepancies highlight that optimizing teamwork is important to ensure a safe and efficient operating room environment for patients.

On a national level, the Department of Defense and the Agency for Healthcare Research and Quality developed a program to improve the quality, safety, and efficiency of health care through teamwork. The Team Strategies and Tools to Enhance Performance and Patient Safety (TeamSTEPPS™) is the program that was developed and released in 2006 and has been implemented in numerous hospitals across the United States [5]. The curriculum focuses on four competencies including leadership, situational monitoring, mutual support, and communication. Although available as a national program, many facilities have adopted their own institution-based training programs, focusing on simulation and the development of team-based competency. When applied specifically within the operating room environment, the application of TeamSTEPPS™ has led to a reduction in the occurrence of retained foreign bodies. Prior to the application of the program, retained foreign bodies were occurring every 16 days, an interval which increased to an average of 69 days after its implementation [6]. Additional implementation sites of TeamSTEPPS™ identified improvements in the quantity and quality of presurgical procedure briefings, as well as teamwork behaviors during operative cases [7].

One institutional simulation approach to develop team-based competency focuses on case studies and role plays. Stewart-Parker et al. [8] developed Surgical Teamworking in Emergency and Acute Medical Situations (S-TEAMS), a one-day course consisting of lectures, case studies, and simulated patient scenarios focusing on communication strategies and situational awareness. The three learning objectives of the course are situational awareness, anticipation and planning, and effective communication strategies. The individuals participating in this course are typically nurses, scrub techs, surgeons, and anesthesiologists. Self-assessments identified that after the course, 55% of participants felt an increased confidence to speak up in difficult situations. Six months after the course, 94% of course participants felt the course directly improved patient safety. This study highlights that a course focusing on case studies in conjunction with simulated scenarios provides a strong foundation of skills for operating room staff regarding team communication and, ultimately, patient safety.

Another case study-based simulation training from Man et al. [9] focused on crew resource management (CRM). CRM was a workshop from the National Aeronautics and Space Administration (NASA) that was created in 1979 to promote and improve air safety. This concept has expanded across teams in various specialties, including medicine. The pillars for CRM focus on six areas: (1) managing fatigue, (2) creating and managing teams, (3) recognizing adverse situations, (4) cross-checking and communication, (5) decision-making, and (6) program feedback. This study highlighted a CRM course that was piloted at two hospitals, in which various operating room staff participated, including surgeons, nurses, anesthesiologists, and scrub techs. This one-day course focused on classroom case-based studies, video training and, ultimately, a simulation experience. Overall, from 45 workshops and 712 participants, 99% felt the program was applicable to their daily practice, and 96% found the simulation to be more useful than the classroom-based case studies. Additionally, participants felt an overall improvement in satisfaction with regard to goal setting and communication within their departments. This study, similar to the previous one, highlights that case-based courses can be an effective means for participants to learn the importance of communication in the operating room.

A surgical team-simulation training model from Weldon et al. [10] is a type of partial-task training simulation for team-based competency and communication. Through the Video-Supported Simulation of Interactions in the Operating Theater (ViSIOT), operating room teams participating in the simulation training observed actual video footage from the operating room and identified improvements in communication techniques. In the second phase of the simulation training, the teams implemented the strategies. This study took place in both the United States and United Kingdom. Participants found the course to be very beneficial, rating course objectives and simulation activity higher than debriefing and course evaluations. This study highlights that through a specific task of video assessment, the environment of team communication in the operating room can be simulated.

A full-mission simulation focusing on team-based competency and communication completely recreates a clinical experience for trainees that they can participate in, as opposed to observe. Paige et al. [11] conducted a 2-h dual-scenario simulation involving a full-scale computer-operated human patient simulator mannequin and inanimate torso procedural training model. Prior to the simulation experience, there were no didactic sessions provided. The two scenarios included a life-threatening intra-abdominal hemorrhage from a stab wound, and local anesthetic toxicity from a regional upper arm block. Participants included both nursing and medical students, and they demonstrated improved self-efficacy and team-based behaviors when comparing pre- to post-session scores. Therefore, this study demonstrates that full-mission simulation can provide trainees the opportunity to improve team-based attitudes and behaviors, ultimately impacting the operating room culture and patient safety.

Operating Room Fire Safety

Team-based competency and communication is one aspect of efforts to improve patient safety in the operating room as it pertains to fire safety. The Emergency Care Research Institute (ECRI) identified operating room fires as one of the top 10 health technology hazards in 2019 [12]. In the operating room, a surgical fire is one that occurs on or in a patient. The components of a "fire triad" that are necessary for a fire to occur include an oxidizer, an ignition source, and fuel [13]. An oxidizer includes gases such as oxygen and nitrous oxide, which exist within the closed or semi-closed ventilation system of the patient's airway. An ignition source includes products such as electrocautery devices, lasers, heated probes, coagulators, and light cables. Finally, examples of fuel sources include drapes, gauze, alcohol-containing skin preparation materials, and oxygen masks. Given this high-risk environment in the operating room, a focus on fire safety is critically important through institutional and national fire safety protocols and educational opportunities. To prevent operating room fires, staff must be aware of minimizing or avoiding an oxidized-enriched atmosphere near the operative site, and safely managing ignition and fuel sources. One of the most effective ways to educate staff on fire safety in the operating room is through simulation.

On an institutional level, Sankaranaryanan et al. [14] developed the Virtual Electrosurgery Skill Trainer (VEST©), which is a simulator that trains participants in the cognitive and motor skills for safely operating electrosurgical devices, in an attempt to minimize operating room fires. The simulator is a three-dimensional display with a tissue pad that provides force feedback and simulates the physics of electrosurgery, such as smoke and electrical spark. Through simulating the effects of electrosurgery, surgeons can learn to avoid injury, and therefore increase patient safety. Though VEST© is a partial-task trainer, those who have used the VEST© simulator have found it to be visually realistic and reproducible of live tissue [15].

When the VEST© simulator was applied to a team-training module focusing on operating room fire prevention and response, 67% of participants chose the VEST© simulator over traditional textbook or animal models [15]. This extension of the prior partial-task trainer of the VEST© simulator itself was applied to a full-mission simulation, where a virtual operating room environment was created including anesthesia, electrosurgical equipment, nurses, a virtual patient, and a fire extinguisher. Through a head-mounted display, participants were able to fully interact with this virtual environment with the goal of identifying the "fire triad" elements and then successfully containing a fire (Fig. 13.1). Participants reported that this

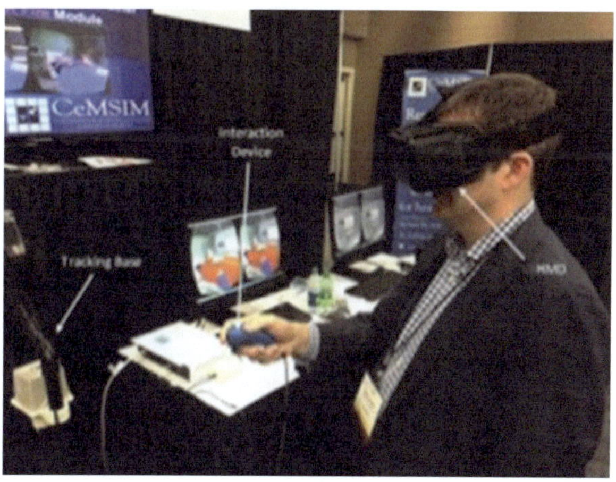

Fig. 13.1 Operating room fire training simulator interface. Used with permission of Springer Nature BV from OR fire virtual training simulator: design and face validity; Society of American Gastrointestinal Endoscopic Surgeons, European Association for Endoscopic Surgery. Vol. 31:9; copyright ©1987; permission conveyed through Copyright Clearance Center, Inc

virtual reality simulator was useful and effective, increasing their comfort with managing operating room fires compared to how they felt prior to the training (Fig. 13.2).

Classroom-based training is also a potential adjunct method to simulation for managing operating room fires. Kishiki et al. [16] randomized 14 groups of participants into either receiving classroom training alone prior to testing, or practice simulation followed by classroom training. The full-mission simulation environment consisted of a patient simulator mannequin with a fog machine in an operating room that was manipulated in an adjacent control room to produce smoke. The participants were exposed to two clinical scenarios, first of which was a cervical lymph node biopsy where oxygen from the nasal cannula was ignited by monopolar cautery; the second was a laparoscopic fiber optic cable resting on a surgical drape. Competency and confidence scores in the simulation group were significantly higher than those who underwent classroom training alone.

The significance of surgical energy and its influence on the risk of operating room fires has been championed by the Society of American Gastrointestinal and Endoscopic Surgeons (SAGES) through the Fundamental Use of Surgical Energy™ (FUSE) program. This program is an educational resource with a web-based multimedia curriculum and a certification examination, all focused on the competencies required to safely use energy-based surgical devices [17]. Prior to the initial post-graduate course piloted for this curriculum, a survey of 27 participants on surgical energy safety had a median percent of 59% correct, compared to 90% after the course [18].

The simulation application of the FUSE curriculum was conducted by Madani et al. [19] through a randomized, controlled trial of 56 surgical trainees. Trainees were randomized into either an unstructured (control) or goal-directed (simulation) hands-on session with electrosurgery devices. Control group trainees were provided no predefined tasks or objectives, in addition to electrosurgical equipment and raw meat. Simulation group trainees had four structured, goal-directed workstations using electrosurgical equipment and raw meat, consistent with part-task trainer

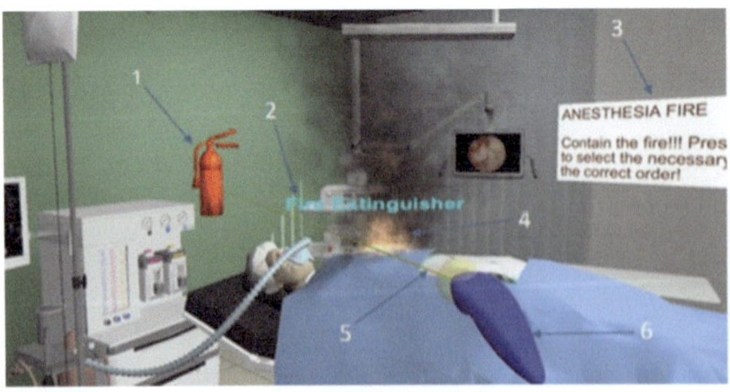

Fig. 13.2 Simulated operating room fire caused by a gas enrichment area under the surgical drape. Used with permission of Springer Nature BV from OR fire virtual training simulator: design and face validity; Society of American Gastrointestinal Endoscopic Surgeons, European Association for Endoscopic Surgery. Vol. 31:9; copyright ©1987; permission conveyed through Copyright Clearance Center, Inc

simulation. The four workstations included: setup of the electrosurgical circuit, electrosurgical tissue effects, electrosurgery-related adverse events in open surgery, and electrosurgery-related adverse events in laparoscopic surgery. Immediate post-curriculum scores were higher in the simulation group compared to control group (89% vs. 83%, $p = 0.02$), as well as at 3 months (77% vs. 60%, $p < 0.01$). Through a standardized curriculum that incorporates simulation, trainees and surgeons can learn how to safely operate electrosurgical devices, which is critically important for patient safety in the prevention of operating room fires. For more on preventing and managing fire and smoke hazards in the OR, see Chap. 21.

Infection Prevention and Control

Infection prevention and control is a critical part of a patient's safety within the hospital environment. Ten components have been identified as crucial in hospital infection control [20]. Organization of infection control at the hospital level requires an infection-control program, nursing staff, dedicated physicians, microbiology support, and data management. Ward occupancy cannot exceed the capacity in regard to rooms or workload by the healthcare provider staff, as methicillin-resistant *Staphylococcus aureus* has been associated with bed occupancy and low nurse staffing. Materials and equipment must be compliant, such as hand-washing dispensers, isolation precautions, and dedicated central venous catheter kits. The use of guidelines, education, and training are another significant component of infection control. Optimizing these components can be challenging, but simulation-based training can aid in emphasizing the significance and importance of infection control.

Breckwoldt et al. [21] provided a 2-h teaching module in a simulated operating room setting for students, consistent with a case study and role play type of simulation. In this module, students were provided four workstations: operating room entry, surgical hand disinfection, dressing for surgery with disinfection of the surgical field and applying surgical drapes, and a debriefing. The debriefing focused on the safety culture in the operating room. Overall, trainees rated the teaching module with high overall satisfaction and teaching quality. Therefore, it is important to provide training in infection control and prevention regardless of training level and has been effective through simulation-based teaching modules.

Operating Room Crisis Resource Management

Surgical crises in the operating room are rare, but when they occur, require immediate and efficient intervention to minimize harm to the patient. Emergency manuals, or crisis checklists, have been found to be helpful, given that stressful situations can significantly impair individuals' ability to think clearly and efficiently [22]. Four vital elements for implementing emergency manuals include create, familiarize, use, and integrate. These manuals must be created appropriately for the context, familiar to those who will use them, accessible and effectively used, and supported by the institution's safety and quality culture [23]. However, the mere presence of these manuals does not guarantee their utilization in crisis situations. Therefore, the role of simulation and training becomes important to train staff about the utility of these emergency manuals.

Through a full-mission simulation, 126 participants were involved in a 50-min simulation-based training session on how to use emergency manuals, integration into teamwork and communication, and simulated scenarios of critical events [24]. The critical events that were simulated included malignant hyperthermia and massive hemorrhage. A cardiopulmonary mannequin with externally controlled vitals was used for the simulation. By fully immersing the participants in the operating room, they were able to simulate a realistic operating room environment. A total of nine training sessions were conducted over 5 months. After the simulation, participants reported significantly increased awareness of and familiarity with the emergency manual, willingness to use it for educational review, and suggest its use in crisis situations although no data has yet been provided for its use in practice.

Another institutional study used an operating room comprehensive unit-based safety program (CUSP) team to evaluate instituting surgical crisis checklists, specifically in regard to cardiac arrest [25]. The purpose of the checklists was to provide appropriate steps, medication dosages and treatments, and role assignments during emergencies. Initially, small-scale case study and role play simulations were conducted outside the operating room environment, where team members assumed the roles of the surgical team and practiced responding to a cardiac arrest using a checklist. This smaller scale simulation was then expanded to a full-mission simulation with a mannequin in the operating room, where there was also a defibrillator and emergency cart present. During and after the simulation, 80% of participants were comfortable with caring for a cardiac arrest patient. Therefore, simulation training provides a strong foundation for operating room staff in the management of a surgical crisis.

The importance of simulation in surgical crises has also been identified in a multi-institutional study. Arriaga et al. [26] conducted a study across three institutions that participated in surgical-crisis scenarios in an operating room, consistent with full-mission simulation. A total of 17 operating room teams participated in 106 surgical crisis scenarios. Of those scenarios, half were randomized to be managed with crisis checklists, and the other half only from memory. When checklists were available, only 6% of steps were missed, compared to 23% when the crisis was managed from memory alone ($p < 0.001$). Overall performance was improved when the crisis checklists were used. Of the participants, 97% stated they would want the checklist used if they were undergoing an operation. This simulation demonstrated that the use of checklists provides an opportunity to optimize patient care in surgical crisis scenarios.

Technical Skills Training

Simulation that provides the opportunity for surgeons and trainees to practice technical skills undoubtedly improves confidence and competence [27–29]. The correlation of competence gained from simulators and improvement in patient safety and outcomes has not yet been identified in the literature. However, it is certainly a reasonable assumption that improved training paradigms with simulators can lead to earlier competence in training, and therefore improved patient safety in the operating room. Specifically, simulators with assessment components that provide trainees and surgeons with feedback about their performance and goals toward achieving competence are important in achieving this goal.

Partial-task trainers, focusing on endoscopic, laparoscopic, and robotic skills, have been the most commonly used simulators for technical skill training in the operating room. Laparoscopic skill simulation trainers include both virtual reality and box trainers [30]. Virtual reality trainers allow for repeated practice without the cost or risk of practicing on an animal, cadaver, or human patient [31]. These established virtual reality systems include procedure simulation for bronchoscopy, colonoscopy, gastroscopy, and laparoscopy. These virtual reality platforms have demonstrated a significant transfer of skills in performance of a laparoscopic cholecystectomy by residents in regard to operative time, injury rate, and progress through the operation [32]. Through technical skill competence, undoubtedly patient safety is affected as a result.

The fundamentals of laparoscopic surgery (FLS) uses box trainers for simulation. Through these box trainers, residents are trained in five tasks: (1) peg transfer, (2) precision cutting, (3) loop ligation, and suturing with both (4) extracorporeal and (5) intracorporeal tying [33]. The American Board of Surgery now requires that all residents pass the FLS assessment examination to become board eligible. This assessment includes web-based didactic, hands-on skills training, and an examination. This is a similar requirement for the fundamentals of endoscopic surgery (FES). However, unlike using a box trainer as in FLS, residents use a virtual reality simulator in FES to mimic skills needed for colonoscopy and gastroscopy through various training modules.

Technical skill simulation for robotic surgery involves a partial-task trainer using the daVinci skills simulator (dVSS). This is a simulator backpack that sits on the back of the robotic surgeon console. Exercises on the simulator include camera manipulation, energy transmission, dexterity, range of motion, fourth arm control, and needle driving. Scores on each of these exercises are tracked, and trainees are provided feedback and assessment reports on their performance after completing each task. Robotic procedural simulation is being introduced in certain specialties but has yet to become prevalent in general surgery [34]. A standardized robotic skills assessment has yet to be established, unlike in laparoscopic and endoscopic surgery [35].

Conclusion

Simulation in the operating room is critically important to provide an opportunity for learning and training in a well-controlled environment. All types of simulation have their role and can be applied in various training paradigms. Through simulation training in team-based competency, fire safety, infection prevention and control, crisis management, and technical skills training, all providers and staff within the operating room can work together to maximize patient safety.

References

1. Milburn JA, Khera G, Hornby ST, Malone PS, Fitzgerald JE. Introduction, availability and role of simulation in surgical education and training: review of current evidence and recommendations from the Association of Surgeons in Training. Int J Surg. 2012;10(8):393–8.
2. Beaubien JM, Baker DP. The use of simulation for training teamwork skills in health care: how low can you go? Qual Saf Health Care. 2004;13(Suppl 1):i51–6.
3. Salas E, Cannon-Bowers JA, Blickensderfer EL. Team performance and training research: emerging principles. J Wash Acad Sci. 1993;83:81–106.
4. Mills P, Neily J, Dunn E. Teamwork and communication in surgical teams: implications for patient safety. J Am Coll Surg. 2008;206(1):107–12.
5. King HB, Battles JB, Baker DP, Alonso A, Salas E, Webster J, et al. TeamSTEPPS™: team strategies and tools to enhance performance and patient safety. In: Henriksen K, Battles JB, Keyes MA, Grady ML, editors. Advances in patient safety: new directions and alternative approaches. Rockville, MD: Agency for Healthcare Research and Quality; 2008.
6. Cima RR, Kollengode A, Storsveen AS, Weisbrod CA, Deschamps C, Koch MB, et al. A multidisciplinary team approach to retained foreign objects. Jt Comm J Qual Patient Saf. 2009;35(3):123–32.
7. Weaver SJ, Rosen MA, DiazGranados D, Lazzara EH, Lyons R, Salas E, et al. Does teamwork improve performance in the operating room? A multilevel evaluation. Jt Comm J Qual Patient Saf. 2010;36(3):133–42.
8. Stewart-Parker E, Galloway R, Vig S. S-TEAMS: a truly multiprofessional course focusing on nontechnical skills to improve patient safety in the operating theater. J Surg Educ. 2017;74(1):137–44.
9. Man APN, Lam CKM, Cheng BCP, Tang K, Tang P. Impact of locally adopted simulation-based crew resource management training on patient safety culture: comparison between operating room personnel and general health care populations pre and post course. Am J Med Qual. 2019;35:79. https://doi.org/10.1177/1062860618824863.
10. Weldon SM, Korkiakangas T, Calzada J, Korndorffer JR, Kneebone RL. A surgical team simulation to improve teamwork and communication across two continents: ViSIOT proof-of-concept study. J Surg Educ. 2019;76:1413. https://doi.org/10.1016/j.surg.2019.03.016.
11. Paige JT, Garbee DD, Kozmenko V, Yu Q, Kozmenko L, Yang T, et al. Getting a head start: high-fidelity, simulation-based operating room team training of interprofessional students. J Am Coll Surg. 2014;218:140–9.
12. ECRI Institute: 2019 top 10 health technology hazards executive brief: a report from health devices. www.ecri.org/2019hazards. Accessed 20 Jul 2019.
13. Practice advisory for the prevention and management of operating room fires: an updated report by the American Society of Anesthesiologists Task Force on Operating Room Fires. Anesthesiology. 2013;118(2):271–90.
14. Sankaranarayanan G, Li B, Miller A, Wakily H, Jones SB, Schwaitzberg S, et al. Face validation of the Virtual Electrosurgery Skill Trainer (VEST©). Surg Endosc. 2016;30:730–8.
15. Dorozhkin D, Olasky J, Jones DB, Schwaitzberg SD, Jones SB, Cao CGL, et al. OR fire virtual training simulator: design and face validity. Surg Endosc. 2017;31:3527–33.
16. Kishiki T, Su B, Johnson B, Lapin B, Kuchta K, Sherman L, et al. Simulation training results in improvement of the management of operating room fires—a single-blinded randomized controlled trial. Am J Surg. 2019;218(2):237–42.
17. Feldman LS, Brunt LM, Fuchshuber P, Jones DB, Jones SB, Mischna J, et al. Rationale for the fundamental use of surgical energy™ (FUSE) curriculum assessment: focus and safety. Surg Endosc. 2013;27:4054–9.
18. Feldman LS, Fuchshuber P, Jones DB, Mischna J, Schwaitzberg SD. Surgeons don't know what they don't know about the safe us of energy in surgery. Surg Endosc. 2012;26:2735–9.

19. Madani A, Watanabe Y, Vassiliou MC, Fuchshuber P, Jones DB, Schwaitzberg SD, et al. Impact of a hands-on component on learning in the Fundamental Use of Surgical Energy™ (FUSE) curriculum: a randomized-controlled trial in surgical trainees. Surg Endosc. 2014;28:2772–82.
20. Zingg W, Holmes A, Dettenkofer M, Goetting T, Secci F, Clack L, et al. Hospital organization, management, and structure for prevention of health-care-associated infection: a systematic review and expert consensus. Lancet Infect Dis. 2015;15(2):212–24.
21. Brackwoldt J, Knecht M, Massée R, Flach B, Hofmann-Huber C, Kaap-Fröhlich S, et al. Operating room technician trainees teach medical students—an inter-professional peer teaching approach for infection prevention strategies in the operation room. Antimicrob Resist Infect Control. 2019;8:75.
22. Goldhaber-Fiebert SN, Lei V, Nandagopal K, Bereknyei S. Emergency manual interpretation: can brief simulation-based OR staff trainings increase familiarity and planned clinical use? Jt Comm J Qual Patient Saf. 2015;41(5):212–20.
23. Goldhaber-Fiebert SN, Howard SK. Implementing emergency manuals: can cognitive aids help translate best practices for patient care during acute events? Anesth Analg. 2013;117(5):1149–61.
24. Goldhaber-Fiebert SN, Lei V, Jackson ML, McCowan K. Simulation-based team training: crisis resource management and the use of emergency manuals in the OR. MedEd PORTAL Publications; 2014. http://www.mededportal.org
25. Dagey D. Using simulation to implement an OR cardiac arrest crisis checklist. AORN J. 2017;105(1):67–72.
26. Arriaga AF, Bader AM, Wong JM, Lipsitz SR, Berry WR, Ziewacz JE, et al. Simulation-based trial of surgical-crisis checklists. N Engl J Med. 2013;368(3):246–53.
27. Miller S, Shipper E, Hasty B, Bereknyei Merrell S, Lee EW, Lin D, et al. Introductory surgical skills course: technical training and preparation for the surgical environment. MedEdPORTAL. 2018;14:10,775.
28. Kim SC, Fisher JG, Delman KA, Hinman JM, Srinivasan JK. Cadaver-based simulation increases resident confidence, initial exposure to fundamental techniques, and may augment operative autonomy. J Surg Ed. 2016;73:e33–41.
29. Vedula SS, Ishii M, Hager GD. Objective assessment of surgical technical skill and competence in the operating room. Annu Rev Biomed Eng. 2017;19:301–25.
30. Brinkmann C, Ritz M, Pankratius U, Bahde R, Neumann P, Schlueter S, et al. Box- or virtual-reality trainer: which tool results in better transfer of laparoscopic basic skills?—A prospective randomized trial. J Surg Ed. 2017;74:724–35.
31. Palter VN, Grantcharov TP. Virtual reality in surgical skills training. Surg Clin N Am. 2010;90:605–17.
32. Seymour NE, Gallagher AG, Roman SA, O'Brien MK, Bansal VK, Andersen DK, et al. Virtual reality training improves operating room performance: results of a randomized, double-blinded study. Ann Surg. 2002;236(4):458–63.
33. Zendejas B, Ruparel RK, Cook DA. Validity evidence for the fundamental of laparoscopic surgery (FLS) program as an assessment tool: a systematic review. Surg Endosc. 2016;30:512–20.
34. Bric DJ, Lumbard DC, Frelich MJ, Gould JC. Current states of virtual reality simulation in robotic surgery training: a review. Surg Endosc. 2016;30(6):2169–78.
35. Chen J, Cheng N, Cacciamani G, Oh P, Lin-Brande M, Remulla D, et al. Objective assessment of robotic surgical technical skill: a systematic review. J Urol. 2019;201(3):461–9.

14 Teamwork and Communication Simulation to Improve Safety in the OR

Jamie L. Sparling and Jeffrey B. Cooper

Introduction

The Society for Simulation in Healthcare (SSH) defines simulation as, "the imitation or representation of one act or system by another." [1] In healthcare, simulation is generally thought of as an educational and training tool, especially in surgical disciplines. Importantly, however, simulation is also highly leveraged as a tool to improve patient safety, as well as for research and performance assessment. In the current healthcare system, where basic science education and individual skills are prioritized, simulation offers an opportunity to enhance the performance of clinical teams working as a cohesive unit [2].

In this chapter, we will describe the historical context of simulation use in healthcare, detail the role for simulation in patient safety, compare medical simulation with other industries, review various forms of simulation, explore its specific use in the perioperative context, and discuss implementation.

J. L. Sparling (✉)
Department of Anesthesia, Critical Care, & Pain Medicine, Massachusetts General Hospital, Boston, MA, USA

Department of Anesthesia, Harvard Medical School, Boston, MA, USA
e-mail: jlsparling@mgh.harvard.edu

J. B. Cooper
Department of Anesthesia, Critical Care, & Pain Medicine, Massachusetts General Hospital, Boston, MA, USA

Department of Anesthesia, Harvard Medical School, Boston, MA, USA

Center for Medical Simulation, Boston, MA, USA

J. J. Hoballah et al. (eds.), *Principles of Perioperative Safety and Efficiency*,
https://doi.org/10.1007/978-3-031-41089-5_14

History of Simulation in Medicine

Simulation is widely used in high-risk fields including aviation, nuclear power, and chemical plants, where it is often required by regulations. For example, the Federal Aviation Administration (FAA) established the National Simulator Program (NSP) to administer its safety simulations and has expanded since the 1970s to now include certification of flight simulation training devices (FSTDs) [3]. Similarly, the U.S. Nuclear Regulatory Commission (NRC) requires that nuclear power plant operators complete ongoing simulation, and it certifies simulation facilities and ensures their continued fidelity [4]. It is only more recently, and in part from the lessons of those other industries, that simulation is used for healthcare education and patient safety. This may be, in part, due to the overall under-regulation of healthcare, and the sense of autonomy among healthcare practitioners. Moreover, as compared with the aforementioned industries, safety events in healthcare tend to cause harm to one patient at a time rather than mass casualties. And, because many errors in healthcare cannot be easily separated from the underlying disease process "taking its course," actions on the part of healthcare teams that may be remedied are more easily overlooked.

Although widespread use of simulation in healthcare is relatively recent, there is a history of simulation dating back more than a hundred years, with many uses in the nineteenth century. For example, as far back as 1740, simulators or "obstetric machines" were used to teach obstetric skills. The first known doctoral thesis on simulation was published in 1797 titled, "A short account of likenesses or devices for practicing obstetric skills also called phantoms." [5] Modern healthcare simulation, however, has its roots in the 1960s [6, 7]. There was a large leap forward, driven by patient safety, starting in the late 1980s [6, 8]. Anesthesiology was among the first specialties to use critical-incident analysis to examine patient safety events [9]. The concern for safety led to the development of many interventions, including simulation, to avoid preventable harm. Further, medical education began to incorporate computer-based simulation during the 1970s as computers became more widespread. In a 1984 report, the Association of American Medical Colleges (AAMC) urged medical schools to "require students to be active, independent learners and problem solvers" and to "lead in the application of information science and computer technology and promote their effective use." [10, 11] This was an indirect encouragement for simulation.

As a specialty, anesthesiologists began to incorporate simulation as a component of the patient safety movement. The Anesthesia Patient Safety Foundation (ASPF) was formed in 1985 under the leadership of Dr. Ellison C. (Jeep) Pierce, Jr., and early on reinforced the concept of simulation as a tool to improve the delivery of safe anesthetic care [12]. The APSF was the first multidisciplinary organization to include not only anesthesia practitioners, but also equipment and drug manufacturers and other professionals in a broad collaboration to improve perioperative safety. At the time of its inception, anesthesia was thought to contribute to a mortality rate of 1–2/10,000 anesthetics, reflecting the time period from the 1950s–1970s. Additionally, media coverage in the early 1980s reported harshly on anesthesia events that contributed to patient harm. By the late 1980s, the APSF provided grant funding to develop high-fidelity patient simulators for use in education, teamwork, and critical event training, and human factors research. Since then, medical simulation has expanded to virtually all medical specialties and to all allied health professions.

Simulation in surgical specialties has been used largely for training and educational purposes; its growth has been driven not only by the patient safety movement, but also by technological advances in imaging, computing, virtual reality, and three-dimensional printing [13]. These changes have happened concurrently with restrictions placed on resident and fellow work hours in 1999 for ACGME (Accreditation Council for Graduate Medical Education)-based training programs, which reduced surgical case experience [14]. In part due to these factors, the American Residency Review Committee for Surgery has mandated skills training labs for surgical residency programs since 2008 [15]. In neurosurgery, simulators are available for general surgical techniques, life-saving emergency procedures (e.g., ventriculostomy, decompressive craniectomies), critical care emergencies (e.g., spinal shock, cerebral vasospasm), vascular neurosurgery, and minimally invasive neurosurgery [13]. Plastic surgery similarly has developed simulators for vascular anastomosis microsurgery, as well as sophisticated simulators for specific procedures such as craniosynostosis repair, which can simulate surgical bleeding and may even be imaged pre- and post-operatively. A children's hospital-based simulation program has developed an extensive two-day-long simulation experience for their residents featuring 11 of the most common pediatric orthopedic procedures, using a combination of cadavers and synthetic bones. (See https://www.youtube.com/watch?v=7fG_-hRrBjE). While not used for teaching directly, computer simulation is also used extensively to predict a desired outcome and establish surgical planning for cosmetic plastic surgery uses [16].

Simulation has similarly grown in its role in nursing education and in interdisciplinary team training involving nurses, physicians, and other healthcare practitioners. In 2009, the Carnegie Foundation for Advancement of Teaching's National Nursing Education Study launched *Educating Nurses: A Call for Radical Transformation* prompting curricular and pedagogic changes to nursing education programs nationwide, including increased incorporation of simulation [17]. The International Nursing Association for Clinical Simulation and Learning (INACSL) publishes standards of best practices for nursing simulation, for a variety of simulation types from task trainers (e.g., IV placement) to high-fidelity, in situ simulators [18, 19].

Applying Simulation to Patient Safety Issues

Numerous patient safety concerns may be addressed by simulation exercises:

- Communication failures
- Teamwork inadequacy
- Infrequency of critical event practice
- Patient risk in practicing technical skills
- Cognitive load during critical events (use of cognitive aids)
- Poor patient safety culture
- Identifying risks of new facilities and processes
- Root cause analysis

Communication

Cross-disciplinary communication is essential for the delivery of safe patient care and has been shown to be enhanced by simulation exercises [20]. Conversely, communication failures are a common contributing cause to patient harm [21]. Simply providing a safe environment for practice can reduce barriers in communication between nursing, anesthesiology, and surgery practitioners, reducing dependence on situation factors or individual personalities. Further, specific communication practices such as closed-loop communication can be taught. Standardized communication tools are increasingly being developed and utilized in the perioperative environment, and training on these handoff tools is enhanced by simulation [20, 22–24].

Teamwork

Teamwork concepts adapted from the aviation industry are critical to both preventing and rescuing from unanticipated critical events. Crisis resource management (CRM), also adapted from aviation, is now widely recognized as a process that can enable effective teamwork in such events [25]. Effective teamwork requires that there is clearly defined leadership, that team members have mutual respect, for one another and that tasks, goals, and key information are shared to enable each member to do their job well. Simulation-based CRM and teamwork training have been shown to improve teamwork behaviors and reduce the rate of errors during event management [26]. For example, a recent study of a post-operative OR-to-ICU handoff bundle in the cardiac surgical ICU, consisting of a four-hour handoff simulation and debriefing session, reported improvements in team leadership, communication, coordination, and cooperation that were sustained 2.3 years following their initial deployment [27].

Critical Event Practice

In the perioperative environment, harmful critical events happen infrequently, yet they demand our best performance and the utilization of many specialized resources. Simulation aids in preparing for these events by allowing clinicians to practice and to familiarize themselves with appropriate resources. Simulation-based practice aims to make instinctive personal and team-based behaviors that will be essential during a stressful, high-risk situation [28]. For example, pediatric OR staff, who were largely untrained in pediatric advanced life support (PALS), were studied in a two-part high-fidelity simulation experience. They underwent an initial high-fidelity simulation with an intraoperative pediatric emergency involving airway management and recognition of an arrhythmia requiring defibrillation. They subsequently underwent an educational debriefing and hands-on training session with the defibrillator. One month later, they again participated in a similar simulation session where objective improvements in performance were achieved, including time to obtain the code cart and time to defibrillation [29]. Similarly, early simulation-based training for recognizing and treating hypoxemia and hypotension among novice anesthesiology residents resulted in improved performance on a standardized checklist over a

6-week time period. Thus, simulation can play a role not only in ongoing training for critical events, but also in accelerating the acquisition of specific management skills in learners new to the perioperative environment [30].

Technical Skills

Perioperative medicine involves procedures with inherent risk to the patient. Simulation allows practitioners to practice these skills in a controlled environment, of fidelity appropriate to the learning objectives, without exposing patients to risk. Studies have shown improved outcomes with simulation-based placement of peripheral and central venous lines, [31, 32] sterile technique, [33] airway management, [34–36] open and laparoscopic surgical skills, [37, 38] and blood pressure measurement [39]. In one surgical residency program, new interns participate in a day-long simulation boot camp with hands-on practice in endoscopy, laparoscopy, bronchoscopy, and abdominal surgical access. After the one-day session, both mean skill assessment and self-confidence ratings improved significantly across all four topics [40]. Similarly, surgical personnel of different levels (medical student through attending) used a simulated model for preperitoneal mesh repair of an umbilical hernia; they were assessed by blinded raters using a competency assessment tool (CAT). Participation in the simulation experience was associated with statistically significant learning increase from the first to the second surgery among beginners [41] (Fig. 14.1).

Use of Cognitive Aids

Discussed elsewhere in Chap. 4, the use of checklists and cognitive aids, often adapted from other high-risk industries such as nuclear power and aviation, has been shown to improve patient outcomes in numerous environments. They can be

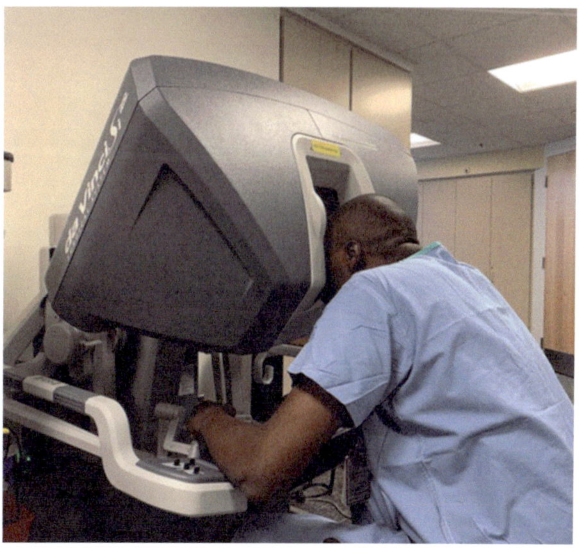

Fig. 14.1 A surgical trainee practices robotic knot-tying, courtesy of the Massachusetts General Hospital Surgical Skills Laboratory

applied for crisis management and for routine tasks. Perioperative cognitive aids are increasingly being used as a tool to help manage acute situations, especially those not commonly encountered. However, familiarity with the tool is necessary in order for it to be useful during an emergency, and simulation using the tools helps to achieve this. It is well known that cognition and memory may be blurred during times of stress and can be degraded by distractions during emergent perioperative events. An emergency manual consisting of numerous checklists for relatively infrequent, but still likely to be encountered, events has been demonstrated via simulation to be effective in improving event management, for example, reducing the number of errors or missed critical steps [42, 43]. The Emergency Manual Implementation Collaborative has assembled examples of such manuals and advice for effective implementation [44]. The Stanford Emergency Manual contains guides for management of 25 critical events in the OR, as well as tips for crisis resource management. While these and other such cognitive aids are similar in concept, they differ in the way they are organized and presented. It is not clear which approach is optimal, but there is mounting evidence of the value of such tools (Fig. 14.2).

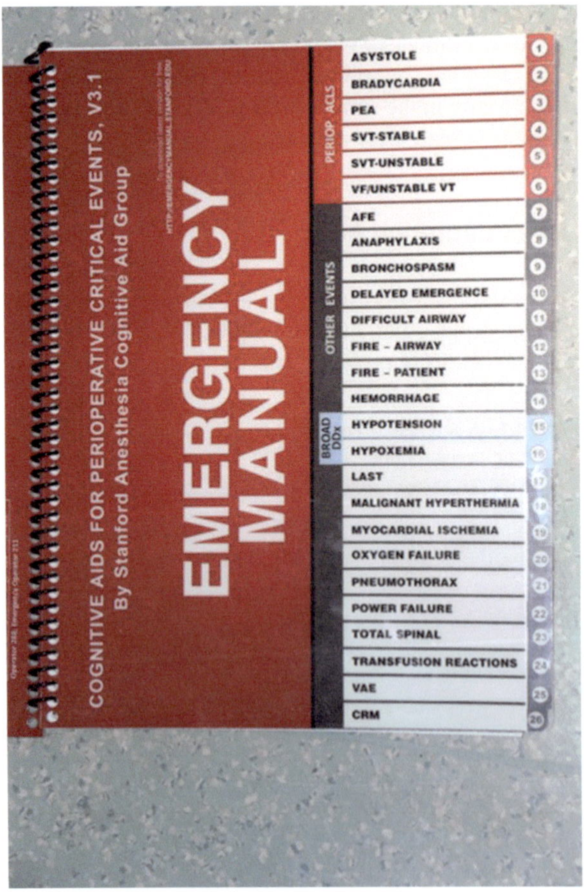

Fig. 14.2 Cover and index page for the Stanford Emergency Manual, used with permission from D. Gaba, Stanford Anesthesia Cognitive Aid Group

Cognitive aids have also been implemented for the many different situations where responsibility for a patient is transferred from one provider or team to another, the process known as a handover or handoff. Many different forms of handoffs and cognitive aids for enabling them have been developed [45–47]. There is evidence that the use of a standardized handoff tool decreases technical errors and handoff omissions [48, 49]. Yet there is not yet good evidence for what format of cognitive aid is best, nor have many other questions about the use of handoff processes or tools been answered. A recent consensus process reported recommendations for many aspects of handoff practices [50].

Research, evaluation, and training for the use of cognitive aids and processes like handoffs are enabled, and greatly benefit from the use of simulation.

Developing a Patient Safety Culture

Patient safety culture is defined as "an organization's shared perceptions, beliefs, values, attitudes, and competencies that combine to create a commitment to safety and an effort to minimize harm." [51] While safety culture is difficult to measure, surveys of safety attitudes have been correlated with important outcomes such as professional burn-out and engagement. Further, hospitals with better scores on patient safety climate, as demonstrated on surveys, have better scores on patient safety indicators, specifically among frontline personnel [52].

It serves to reason that simulation enhances safety culture, for example, by emphasizing an organization's commitment to improvement and practicing for emergencies; yet, to date little research has been performed examining the relationship between safety attitudes and participation in simulation [53]. Interdisciplinary surveys have shown opportunity for improvement in safety culture through the use of CRM simulation [54].

Forms of Simulation

Medical simulation exists in many forms to meet diverse goals and suit difference audiences. Gaba describes 11 dimensions of simulation applications which may be tweaked to optimize outcomes and to derive maximal benefit from the simulation experience [2]. These 11 dimensions are described in Fig. 14.3. Some of these dimensions represent a spectrum from one extreme to another, while other dimensions are simply categorical distinctions. While many permutations of options across different dimensions have been described, many more options remain to be explored.

For example, simulation may serve any of a number of different purposes, including education, training, performance assessment, clinical rehearsal, and human factors research. Medical students may participate in simulation as an initial learning exercise for procedural skills, such as intubation, arterial line placement, lumbar puncture, and central line insertion, [55] while surgical residents

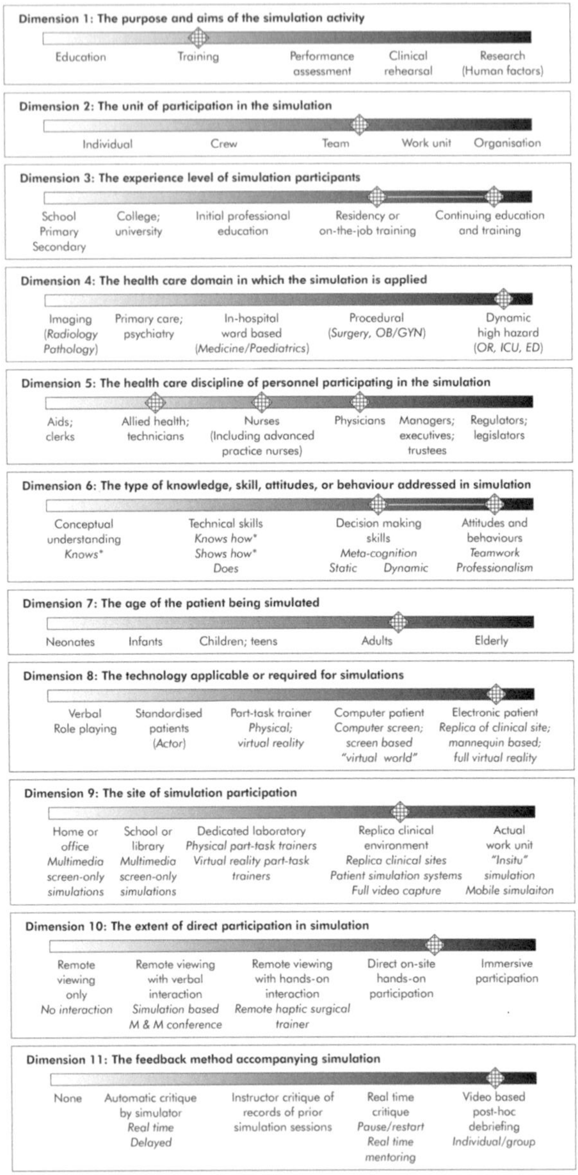

Fig. 14.3 The 11 dimensions of simulation application. Used with permission from *Gaba* [2]

may use simulation as training to hone technical surgical skills (Fig. 14.4) [15]. Various medical organizations now use simulation as means of performance assessment for licensure and board accreditations. The United States Medical Licensing Exam (USMLE) Step 2 clinical skills (CS) exam was one such assessment that is required for physicians to gain initial licensure in the United States, wherein medical students interviewed and examined standardized patients in

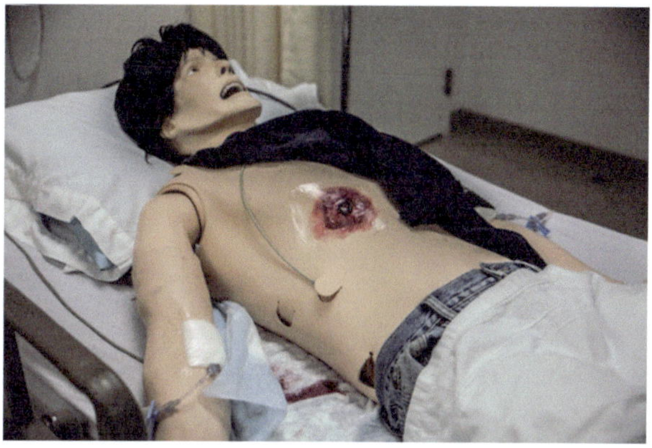

Fig. 14.4 A simulation mannequin, illustrating a thoracoabdominal gunshot wound. Courtesy, Center for Medical Simulation

order to demonstrate clinical skills and come to a diagnosis and treatment plan [56]. The USMLE Step 2 CS exam was discontinued during the COVID-19 pandemic, and replaced by computer-based case simulations in the Step 3 exam. Clinical rehearsal includes simulations geared toward practicing use of emergency manuals and critical events [44]. Finally, simulation has been used broadly in human factors research. For example, simulation experiences based on previously experienced real-life adverse events, including errors in drug infusion pump programming, have been used to discern factors contributing to errors during the simulation debrief sessions [57].

The unit of participation in simulation also varies from individual use through a crew, team, or other work unit, all the way up to an entire organization. These units may represent a single discipline focused on skills or behaviors specific to their purview, such as a surgeon training to tie knots laparoscopically [58]. Alternatively, a unit may include several different disciplines working together to optimize team performance and response to critical events as a team [26, 59–63].

The site of simulation is another dimension across which experiences can vary in order to suit particular needs. Simple simulations may be presented as a computer program-based case where the participant steps through clinical decisions in a progression; indeed, some of the earliest medical simulations were of this type [11]. In the surgical specialties, simulation tends to focus on technical skills and thus may be more likely to take place in a skills lab. In a 2017 systematic review, 41.9% of the simulation programs studied took place in a skills lab, while only 6.5% took place in a dedicated simulation center [15]. However, the earliest modern simulation was conducted in a replica of an OR, and today simulation centers have developed high-fidelity simulators where participants train together in a realistic replica of an operating room or in situ in a real operating or procedure room. Fig. 14.5 is an example of one such simulator. Successful simulation interventions may be conducted in a number of different sites; however, it is not clear that training in a simulation center enhances outcomes compared with hospital-based simulations [59]. Fig. 14.6 illustrates simulation in an out-of-OR environment.

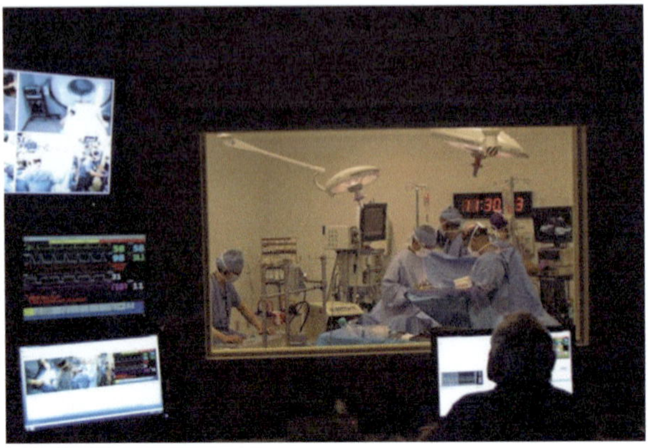

Fig. 14.5 View of a high-fidelity simulated operating room, from the control room. Courtesy, Center for Medical Simulation

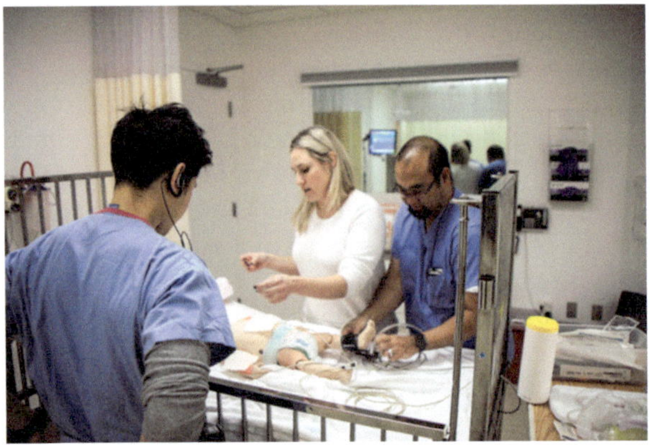

Fig. 14.6 Typical out-of-OR simulation environment and illustrative pediatric mannequin. Courtesy, Center for Medical Simulation

Debriefing

Debriefing is a, or perhaps *the*, critical element of simulation exercises. Debriefing had its origins in the military where individuals reported back following a mission, and the report was analyzed and strategy for ongoing missions developed. It was further developed for psychological reasons as a way to defuse following a traumatic event [64]. Since then, critical incident stress debriefing (CISB) was developed as a facilitator-led approach to review facts, experiences, and reactions among emergency first responders [65]. The skill used in debrief simulation scenarios is easily extended into debriefing following a critical event, both for the purpose of identifying causative factors, as well as for the purpose of supporting clinicians affected as second victims [64]. Debriefs typically occur following the conclusion of a simulation session, but a "time-out" during the scenario may also provide an opportunity for debriefing (see Table 14.1). The conventional wisdom is that debriefings should be led by a trained facilitator, but it has also been advocated that participants can debrief themselves via self-reflection using various conversational structures [66].

Table 14.1 Overview of Healthcare Simulation Debriefing Methods. Used with permission from Sawyer et al. [66]

		Process elements		
Timing and facilitation	Conversational structure	Essential elements	Conversational techniques/ Educational strategies	Debriefing adjuncts
Facilitator-guided postevent debriefing	• 3-phase • Multiphase	• Psychological safety • Debriefing stance or basic assumption • Establish debriefing rules • Shared mental model • Address learning objectives • Open-ended questions • Using silence	• Learner self-assessment • Directive feedback • Circular questions • Advocacy inquiry • Guided team self-correction	• Codebriefer • Debriefing script • Video review
Self-guided postevent debriefing	Cognitive aid driven	• Psychological safety • Debriefing stance or basic assumption • Establish debriefing rules • Shared mental model • Address learning objectives • Open-ended questions • Using silence	• Learner self-assessment • Guided team self-correction	• Debriefing script • Video review
Facilitator-guided within-event debriefing	Event/ performance focused	• Psychological safety • Debriefing stance or basic assumption • Establish debriefing rules • Shared mental model • Address learning objectives • Open-ended questions • Using silence	• Learner self-assessment • Directive feedback • Circular questions • Advocacy inquiry	• Codebriefer • Video review

There are numerous approaches to debriefing [9]. There is no solid empirical evidence for what method is best in general, nor exactly when to use each approach. Yet there are generally accepted suggestions for what situations call for what type of debriefing. Debriefing is a skill that requires great self-awareness of the debriefer and for which many training programs are offered around the world. For example, the Debriefing Assessment for Simulation in Healthcare (DASH) program is used to develop debriefing skills and evaluate debriefing effectiveness; it takes into account the evidence and theory behind adult experiential learning, and it provides frameworks that may be used across disciplines and courses [67].

Simulation in Perioperative Care

Perioperative care has many opportunities for improvement in patient safety through simulation. All of the elements listed in previously (see "Applying Simulation to Patient Safety Issues") have application in the perioperative environment, from when a patient first enters the pre-operative preparation space to leaving from recovery or intensive care.

Crisis resource management (CRM) refers to the skills that contribute to effective leadership, teamwork, communication, resource utilization, task management, situational awareness, problem-solving and decision-making used in a crisis [68–71]. High-acuity settings such as perioperative medicine and emergency medicine benefit from practicing these skills in a simulated environment, as critical events are rare. The goals of these simulations are to improve patient safety, and thus patient outcomes. In a recent systematic review, simulation-based CRM training was more effective than didactic sessions or no intervention in transferring CRM principles to clinical care. Further, several studies have shown improved patient outcomes and mortality with CRM simulation training [69]. One such example is Gallagher's Anesthesia Resident Emergency Scenarios Series (see https://www.youtube.com/watch?v=IeObjHh5M7g). This video series is designed for anesthesia residents to improve their capability to handle critical anesthesia emergencies in clinical practice and in preparation for the OSCE exam for primary anesthesia certification. Once residents have prepared for sessions via watching the video, they complete a live simulation session, demonstrating competence on that particular anesthesia emergency. Another such example is the American Society of Anesthesiology's SimSTAT virtual reality training, which is available online to fulfill MOCA® 2.0 requirements. SimSTAT is a high-fidelity, virtual operating room scenario in a gaming environment, focusing specifically on management of anesthesia emergencies [72]. It features virtual patients and operating theaters, interactive anesthesia equipment with live physiological data and performance tracking to allow the learner to receive feedback and identify areas for improvement. An example video is available at https://www.youtube.com/watch?v=cktrth6ejO0.

Teamwork is critical in the high-stakes perioperative setting, and team-based simulation exercises are increasingly being used [60]. Studies have shown an improvement in participant-reported post-simulation performance assessments

[61]. By virtue of a shared experience, barriers to communication among team members break down. Rehearsing working together and recognizing one another's contributions in a simulation environment translates readily into clinical practice. Indeed, studies in obstetrics and elsewhere have shown improved objective team performance following multidisciplinary simulation [59].

The acquisition and practice of technical skills in the perioperative environment come with inherent procedural risks. Surgical personnel, and anesthesia providers and nurses each have opportunities to improve their skills in the simulation laboratory prior to and in parallel to clinical practice. As mentioned previously, simulation studies have shown improvement in both open and laparoscopic surgical skills by surgical trainees [37, 38]. Anesthesia medical students and residents improve their advanced airway management skills using both hands-on and computerized simulation [34, 36]. Novice and veteran scrub nurses have benefitted from a virtual reality simulator to improve procedural skills [73]. Perfusionists may utilize simulation software to improve technical skills related to volume management, vasopressor titration, and warming/cooling kinetics [74].

Simulation can also be used for assessment of performance at all levels of experience. This has a clear patient safety relationship by ensuring competence of trainees, continuing competence of providers at intervals along their career, and for re-entry of providers who have left practice for various reasons and now wish to return. Assessment of performance itself is a complex topic. Simulation-based assessments have been examined for many years [75, 76]. Developing an assessment that is psychometrically robust, appropriately realistic and salient, and practical to implement is challenging. Recent studies have demonstrated that such simulations can be employed, but that many repeat scenarios are required to ensure test reliability [77]. Still, as noted earlier, simulation-based, high-stakes (passing required to obtain a license or to practice) are now used at some stage of training or practice for most perioperative healthcare providers.

Another less widely used application of simulation in healthcare is as a part of root cause analysis (RCA) or a failure mode and effect analysis (FMEA). [78] RCA and FMEA are processes adapted from other industries. RCA is now applied widely in healthcare to learn about the causes of adverse events. More recently, another A, for action, has been added (RCA^2) to focus the process on creating interventions that will at least reduce, if not eliminate, the occurrence of future events that are similar to the one being studied [79, 80]. RCA is now widely practiced in healthcare. FMEA is less widely employed.

There are various structured guidelines for conducting an RCA. The general idea is straightforward: Assemble a team of appropriately experienced people, conduct interviews with the people involved in the event, plot out the elements of the event (using one or more of various tools, for example, flowcharting, fishbone diagram, asking "5 whys"), consider various ways in which it could have been prevented, suggest and take action to implement specific interventions, and then follow through to ensure changes have been made for the positive. Simulation has great potential utility as part of the RCA^2 process, but it is now only rarely utilized in healthcare for this purpose [81].

On the surface, using simulation to investigate an event is not complicated. A reenactment of the event can be created in an existing simulation facility or in situ. Ideally, the actual cast of participants in the event would be assembled. They would previously have been prepared and given assurance of confidentiality and psychological safety. They would discuss antecedent factors and then step through, reenact, the events that actually took place, pausing to discuss their various views on what happened. Reenactment may be video recorded for re-analysis. Ideally, this process would reveal aspects of the causes and, hopefully, future prevention of the event that otherwise would not be discovered by the normal process.

In reality, this process is not so simple. Having the original team reenact the event together could cause psychological harm and exacerbate any conflict about what happened or placing blame. The possibility of this must be considered and explored before conducting the reenactment. The logistics and scheduling of people and place to conduct a reenactment can be challenging. Facilitating such an event requires skill and insight of the investigation leader and team. And, the time and expense of this additional process can be substantial. Thus, it should only be done when the normal process is not likely sufficient to intensify critical causes that could add to the prevention strategy or tactics.

Failure mode and effect analysis (FMEA) is similar to RCA but is applied before potential events, preferably before any new patient care process is implemented. In FMEA, the new process is mapped out, for example, in a flow chart of the steps, and potential failure points are identified, with each point being assigned an estimated value for its likelihood of occurrence and potential severity of outcome. The team will then work on ameliorating those potential failure modes that are of highest priority.

Similar to an RCA, simulation can be—but to date is rarely—used to test out processes, including to identify what are called "latent safety threats" [62, 82]. So doing almost invariably identifies potential failure modes that were not identified in the pseudo-simulation conducted only with the imagination of the process designers, even when actual clinicians are involved. Like RCA, FMEA requires time and money and can delay implementation of a new process. So, it should be used selectively. And it can be used for existing processes that are known to have failure modes. This has been demonstrated successfully in labor and delivery [83]. Simulation is also used to train in the use of RCA and could be used for FMEA training as well [84].

Measuring Success

Simulation programs have been evaluated in a number of ways; these metrics largely fall into process metrics, outcomes metrics, and balance metrics [85]. Process metrics measure whether the simulation program is proceeding as planned. This could be a measure of how many clinicians have participated in a given program. Outcome metrics assess the impact of a given simulation program. For example, simulation for technical skills can be evaluated with a pre- and post-simulation standardized assessment; however, these assessment tools should be validated and have high inter-rater reliability. In addition to these objective measures, participants are often asked to rate their confidence with specific scenarios or skills before versus after a simulation. Finally, the ultimate outcome of simulation is an improvement in patient safety, so measures could include a reduction in adverse events or objective measures of improved teamwork during actual crises. Balance metrics assess whether an improvement in one part of the system causes new problems in another area of the system. For simulation, balance metrics may look at the cost effectiveness of implementing a new program or may measure time spent away from the operating room or other educational endeavors.

Implementation

Implementation of a medical simulation program requires leadership and structural elements to be put into place. Kotter's 8-Step Process for Leading Change can be used as a model for implementing change, as in developing a new simulation program [86]. One of the first steps entails the building of a "guiding coalition" which translates to developing a multidisciplinary team of invested clinicians across different disciplines and specialties to lead the implementation efforts. It is important in this coalition to have the commitment of senior leadership to have the power to dedicate resources, as well as the political capital to inspire others to "buy-in" to the simulation program. While some types of simulation may be implemented with little upfront capital costs, the time commitment is warranted in all scenarios, and senior leadership must invest in this to demonstrate institutional support for the program. Capital investment may be required in other types of simulation, from building or adapting a dedicated facility to the purchase of simulator mannequins and other equipment. Retired or expired clinical equipment often can be utilized to minimize the cost of implementation and reduce clinical waste.

Building a simulation facility is the relatively easier part of building an effective program. Operations, instructor, and other personnel must be selected and trained to run and facilitate simulations. The process and issues in hiring and training operations staff is not dissimilar to other types of hospital or healthcare educational school programs. Identifying and training instructors usually presents a greater challenge. Clinical acumen and educational skills are required, as they are for any healthcare professional educator. Simulation-based education has some unique aspects that make it more difficult to attract and sufficiently train educators to use simulation effectively. Much of simulation-based training calls for creating a non-threatening environment, presenting students with direct, objective evidence of their performance, and doing so in the presence of their colleagues. Furthermore, since simulation often requires a commitment, sometimes unpaid or less highly paid than clinical work, attracting clinicians to work in a simulation environment can be difficult. And not all are well suited to doing it.

Fortunately, numerous training courses exist for simulation educators at all levels of experience and directed to the various types of healthcare simulation; these are detailed below. Ongoing commitment by the institution requires that participants have dedicated time away from clinical care to engage in simulation in a focused fashion—this may form an element of both upfront training and ongoing certification. Finally, metrics, including those above, must be tracked over time to ensure ongoing adherence to the program and quality of the simulations delivered.

Role of Simulation in Healthcare Regulation

With the growing body of evidence for the success of simulation in improving patient safety, it is natural for simulation to become incorporated into regulatory and certification requirements for healthcare providers [87]. Physicians in both general surgical and anesthesiology training are required to complete simulation exercises in order to become board-eligible. The American College of Surgeons (ACS) requires surgery residents to complete the Resident Skills Curriculum, which includes simulations to teach Core Surgical Skills (16 modules), Advanced Procedures (15 modules), and Team-Based Skills (10 modules) [88]. The American Board of Anesthesiology (ABA) requires simulation activities for both initial certification and maintenance of certification. The initial certification requires completion of an Objective Structured Clinical Exam (OSCE) with standardized patient actors and simulated technical skills. Simulation for MOCA® (Maintenance of Certification in Anesthesiology) is only optional but offers 3 h of credit for each hour of participation, which is an incentive, versus some other options for attaining the required points every 5 years [89, 90]. The MOCA® simulation only requires participation; there is no assessment of performance. Additional points can be claimed for providing a self-determined performance improvement plan and reporting back about the progress in achieving it.

Further, malpractice insurers may provide incentives for providers to participate in team-based simulation for the purpose of patient safety [87, 91]. CRICO, the malpractice insurance program for all Harvard Medical School-affiliated hospitals and physicians, offers substantially lower malpractice insurance premiums for anesthesiologists, surgeons, and obstetricians who participate in a program that includes multidisciplinary, team-based high-realism simulations that focus on communication, assertiveness, and the use of the World Health Organization surgical safety checklist. Each simulation involves at least one attending surgeon, one attending anesthesiologist, and one operating room nurse [63].

Current Status of Simulation in Perioperative Care

Simulation is increasingly being used for both task and team training worldwide, and the number of medical simulation centers is growing. The Society for Simulation in Healthcare (SSH), established in 2004, is an international organization of physicians, nurses, allied health personnel, researchers, and educators dedicated to the use of simulation to improve performance and reduce errors in healthcare [1]. The SSH has certification for individuals and for simulation programs. For individuals, certification allows for specializing either in simulation education, for which there are different levels of certification, or in operations. Certification of various types is available for simulation programs, an opportunity to evaluate and build on the program's outcomes, research, education, and systems integration. The SSH website lists 493 centers in the United States alone, and more than 600 worldwide. More than 2000 individuals have completed certification and more than 100 programs have been accredited [92].

Several other organizations also support simulation in healthcare, including the Association for Simulated Practice in Healthcare (ASPiH), the Association of Standardized Patient Educators (ASPE), the International Nursing Association for Clinical Simulation (INACSL), and the International Pediatric Simulation Society (IPSS) [93–96].

The American Society of Anesthesiologists (ASA) has a Simulation Education Network (SEN), which offers endorsement for programs seeking to teach courses for Maintenance of Certification in Anesthesiology® (MOCA®; an optional element of the required Part IV recertification), hosts an annual simulation summit, and has other initiatives and programs to foster simulation in that specialty [97]. Similarly, the American College of Surgeons (ACS) founded the Accredited Education Institutes (AEIs) with the goal of educating and training surgeons and trainees using simulation [97, 98]. The ACS-AEI offers accreditation of surgical education programs that use simulation and hosts an annual Surgical Simulation Summit. The ACS-AEI and the ASA-SEN had their first joint meeting in 2020, and meet annually. In 2023, their focus was specifically on using simulation to improve quality and safety.

Simulation instructor training is widely available, through both in-person courses and online programs [99]. Through programs like these, instructors gain valuable skills in creating safe learning environments, teaching teamwork skills and critical thinking, debriefing, developing simulation scenarios, and in implementing simulation programs at their own institution. Participation and ongoing practice in simulation facilitation and teaching can lead to certification as a Certified Healthcare Simulator Educator (CHSE) through the Society for Simulation in Healthcare (SSH), as above. Certification requires an application including a confidential assessment of the candidates' performance, and completion of a structured, computerized examination [100].

Conclusion

In the future, we expect simulation to grow in the perioperative field, fueled by enthusiasm and demands for improved healthcare safety from the public, government payors, accrediting organizations, and others. Ideally, not only will we reach a point where all healthcare providers train and certify prior to entering clinical practice, but simulation will also likely become "embedded in the fabric of care." [69] Simulation will be embraced by clinical educators and practicing clinicians and will increasingly become a component of certification and accreditation. We will regularly train for teamwork, focusing not on individual performance, but on cohesive function as a team.

As simulation becomes further integrated into healthcare, we expect the literature base to support its ongoing use. In the meantime, we rely on the growing evidence referenced in this chapter to inform the propagation of simulation, as well as the high face-value validity.

References

1. Society for Simulation in Healthcare. About simulation 2019. https://www.ssih.org/About-SSH/About-Simulation. Accessed 8 Aug 2019.
2. Gaba DM. The future vision of simulation in health care. Qual Saf Health Care. 2004;13(Suppl 1):i2–10.
3. Federal Aviation Administration. Flight simulation training device qualification guidance. 2019. https://www.faa.gov/about/initiatives/nsp/ac/. Accessed 8 Aug 2019.
4. Nuclear Regulatory Commission. Simulation facilities. https://www.nrc.gov/reading-rm/doc-collections/cfr/part055/part055-0046.html. Accessed 8 Aug 2019.
5. Owen H. Simulation in healthcare: an extensive history. Cham, Switzerland: Springer International Publishing; 2016.
6. Cooper JB, Taqueti VR. A brief history of the development of mannequin simulators for clinical education and training. Qual Saf Health Care. 2004;13((Suppl 1):i11–8.
7. Denson JS, Abrahamson S. A computer-controlled patient simulator. JAMA. 1969;208(3):504–8.
8. Jones FP-NC, Braghiroli OF. Simulation in medical education: brief history and methodology. Principles Pract Clin Res. 2015;1(2):56–63.
9. Cooper JB, Newbower RS, Long CD, McPeek B. Preventable anesthesia mishaps: a study of human factors. Anesthesiology. 1978;49(6):399–406.
10. Rosen KR. The history of medical simulation. J Crit Care. 2008;23(2):157–66.
11. Piemme TE. Computer-assisted learning and evaluation in medicine. JAMA. 1988;260(3):367–72.
12. Anesthesia Patient Safety Foundation. About APSF. https://www.apsf.org/about-apsf/foundation-history/. Accessed 8 Aug 2019.
13. Rehder R, Abd-El-Barr M, Hooten K, Weinstock P, Madsen JR, Cohen AR. The role of simulation in neurosurgery. Childs Nerv Sys. 2016;32(1):43–54.
14. Beall DP. The ACGME institutional requirements: what residents need to know. JAMA. 1999;281(24):2352C.
15. Kurashima Y, Hirano S. Systematic review of the implementation of simulation training in surgical residency curriculum. Surg Today. 2017;47(7):777–82.
16. Kazan R, Cyr S, Hemmerling TM, Lin SJ, Gilardino MS. The evolution of surgical simulation: the current state and future avenues for plastic surgery education. Plast Reconstr Surg. 2017;139(2):533e–43e.
17. Benner P. Educating nurses: a call for radical transformation-how far have we come? J Nurs Educ. 2012;51(4):183–4.
18. Aebersold M, Tschannen D. Simulation in nursing practice: the impact on patient care. Online J Issues Nurs. 2013;18(2):6.
19. Aebersold M. The history of simulation and its impact on the future. AACN Adv Crit Care. 2016;27(1):56–61.
20. Leonard M, Graham S, Bonacum D. The human factor: the critical importance of effective teamwork and communication in providing safe care. Qual Saf Health Care. 2004;13(Suppl 1):i85–90.
21. Arriaga AF, Sweeney RE, Clapp JT, Muralidharan M, Burson RC 2nd, Gordon EKB, et al. Failure to debrief after critical events in anesthesia is associated with failures in communication during the event. Anesthesiology. 2019;130(6):1039–48.

22. Farnan JM, Paro JA, Rodriguez RM, Reddy ST, Horwitz LI, Johnson JK, et al. Hand-off education and evaluation: piloting the observed simulated hand-off experience (OSHE). J Gen Intern Med. 2010;25(2):129–34.
23. Filichia L, Halan S, Blackwelder E, Rossen B, Lok B, Korndorffer J, et al. Description of web-enhanced virtual character simulation system to standardize patient hand-offs. J Surg Res. 2011;166(2):176–81.
24. Elgin KW, Poston RD. Optimizing registered nurse bedside shift report: innovative application of simulation methods. J Nurs Prof Dev. 2019;35(2):E6–e14.
25. Gaba DM, Howard SK, Fish KJ, Smith BE, Sowb YA. Simulation-based training in anesthesia crisis resource management (ACRM): a decade of experience. Simul Gaming. 2001;32(2):175–93.
26. Morey JC, Simon R, Jay GD, Wears RL, Salisbury M, Dukes KA, et al. Error reduction and performance improvement in the emergency department through formal teamwork training: evaluation results of the MedTeams project. Health Serv Res. 2002;37(6):1553–81.
27. Keebler JR, Lynch I, Ngo F, et al. ECHO ICU collaborative. Leveraging the science of teamwork to sustain handoff improvements in cardiovascular surgery. Jt Comm J Qual Patient Saf. 2023;49(8):373–83. https://doi.org/10.1016/j.jcjq.2023.05.006. Epub 2023 Jun 1. PMID: 37357132.
28. Gaba DM, DeAnda A. A comprehensive anesthesia simulation environment: re-creating the operating room for research and training. Anesthesiology. 1988;69(3):387–94.
29. Willie C, Chen F, Joyner BL, Blasius K. Using high-fidelity simulation for critical event training. Med Educ. 2016;50(11):1161–2.
30. Park CS, Rochlen LR, Yaghmour E, Higgins N, Bauchat JR, Wojciechowski KG, et al. Acquisition of critical intraoperative event management skills in novice anesthesiology residents by using high-fidelity simulation-based training. Anesthesiology. 2010;112(1):202–11.
31. Jung EY, Park DK, Lee YH, Jo HS, Lim YS, Park RW. Evaluation of practical exercises using an intravenous simulator incorporating virtual reality and haptics device technologies. Nurs Educ Today. 2012;32(4):458–63.
32. Laack TA, Dong Y, Goyal DG, Sadosty AT, Suri HS, Dunn WF. Short-term and long-term impact of the central line workshop on resident clinical performance during simulated central line placement. Simul Healthc. 2014;9(4):228–33.
33. Gerolemou L, Fidellaga A, Rose K, Cooper S, Venturanza M, Aqeel A, et al. Simulation-based training for nurses in sterile techniques during central vein catheterization. Am J Crit Care. 2014;23(1):40–8.
34. Kennedy CC, Cannon EK, Warner DO, Cook DA. Advanced airway management simulation training in medical education: a systematic review and meta-analysis. Crit Care Med. 2014;42(1):169–78.
35. Kovatch KJ, Harvey RS, Schechtman SA, Healy DW, Malloy KM, Prince MEP, et al. Integrated otolaryngology-anesthesiology clinical skills and simulation rotation: a novel 1-month intern curriculum. Ann Otol Rhinol Laryngol. 2019;128(8):715–20.
36. Pastis NJ, Tobin CD, Wolf BJ, Reves JG, Schaefer JJ. A pilot study of simulation training in difficult bag mask ventilation using a computerized patient simulator. J Med Educ Curric Dev. 2019;6:2382120519834327.
37. Macfie RC, Webel AD, Nesbitt JC, Fann JI, Hicks GL, Feins RH. "Boot camp" simulator training in open hilar dissection in early cardiothoracic surgical residency. Ann Thorac Surg. 2014;97(1):161–6.
38. Gawad N, Zevin B, Bonrath EM, Dedy NJ, Louridas M, Grantcharov TP. Introduction of a comprehensive training curriculum in laparoscopic surgery for medical students: a randomized trial. Surgery. 2014;156(3):698–706.
39. Ballard G, Piper S, Stokes P. Effect of simulated learning on blood pressure measurement skills. Nurs Stand. 2012;27(8):43–7.
40. Nakazato T, Callahan Z, Kuchta K, Linn JG, Joehl RJ, Ujiki MB. A 1-day simulation-based boot camp for incoming general surgery residents improves confidence and technical skills. Surgery. 2019;166(4):572–9.

41. Friedrich U, Backhaus J, Zipper CT, Konig S, Mavroveli S, Wiegering A, et al. Validation and educational impact study of the NANEP high-fidelity simulation model for open preperitoneal mesh repair of umbilical hernia. Hernia. 2020;24(4):873–81.
42. Haynes AB, Weiser TG, Berry WR, Lipsitz SR, Breizat AH, Dellinger EP, et al. A surgical safety checklist to reduce morbidity and mortality in a global population. New Engl J Med. 2009;360(5):491–9.
43. Hepner DL, Arriaga AF, Cooper JB, Goldhaber-Fiebert SN, Gaba DM, Berry WR, et al. Operating room crisis checklists and emergency manuals. Anesthesiology. 2017;127(2):384–92.
44. Howard SK, Goldhaber-Fiebert SN, Gaba DM, Harrison TK. Emergency manual implementation collaborative. Creative Commons BY-NC-ND; 2019. http://emergencymanual.stanford.edu/emic.html. Accessed 8 Aug 2019.
45. Methangkool E, Tollinche L, Sparling J, Agarwala AV. Communication: is there a standard handover technique to transfer patient care? Int Anesthesiol Clin. 2019;57(3):35–47.
46. Barbeito A, Agarwala AV, Lorinc A. Handovers in perioperative care. Anesthesiol Clin. 2018;36(1):87–98.
47. Segall N, Bonifacio AS, Schroeder RA, Barbeito A, Rogers D, Thornlow DK, et al. Can we make postoperative patient handovers safer? A systematic review of the literature. Anesth Analg. 2012;115(1):102–15.
48. Petrovic MA, Martinez EA, Aboumatar H. Implementing a perioperative handoff tool to improve postprocedural patient transfers. Jt Comm J Qual Patient Saf. 2012;38(3):135–42.
49. Joy BF, Elliott E, Hardy C, Sullivan C, Backer CL, Kane JM. Standardized multidisciplinary protocol improves handover of cardiac surgery patients to the intensive care unit. Pediatr Crit Care Med. 2011;12(3):304–8.
50. Agarwala AV, Lane-Fall MB, Greilich PE, Burden AR, Ambardekar AP, Banerjee A, et al. Consensus recommendations for the conduct, training, implementation, and research of perioperative handoffs. Anesth Analg. 2019;128(5):e71–e8.
51. DiCuccio MH. The relationship between patient safety culture and patient outcomes: a systematic review. J Patient Saf. 2015;11(3):135–42.
52. Singer S, Lin S, Falwell A, Gaba D, Baker L. Relationship of safety climate and safety performance in hospitals. Health Serv Res. 2009;44(2 Pt 1):399–421.
53. Cooper JB, Blum RH, Carroll JS, Dershwitz M, Feinstein DM, Gaba DM, et al. Differences in safety climate among hospital anesthesia departments and the effect of a realistic simulation-based training program. Anesth Analg. 2008;106(2):574–84, table of contents.
54. Hicks CM, Bandiera GW, Denny CJ. Building a simulation-based crisis resource management course for emergency medicine, phase 1: results from an interdisciplinary needs assessment survey. Acad Emerg Med. 2008;15(11):1136–43.
55. Toy S, McKay RS, Walker JL, Johnson S, Arnett JL. Using learner-centered, simulation-based training to improve medical students' procedural skills. J Med Educ Curric Dev. 2017;4:2382120516684829.
56. United States Medical Licensing Examination—Step 2 CS. https://www.usmle.org/step-2-cs/ [cited 8 August 2019].
57. Lobos AT, Ward N, Farion KJ, Creery D, Fitzgibbons C, Ramsay C, et al. Simulation-based event analysis improves error discovery and generates improved strategies for error prevention. Simul Healthc. 2019;14(4):209–16.
58. Bilgic E, Alyafi M, Hada T, Landry T, Fried GM, Vassiliou MC. Simulation platforms to assess laparoscopic suturing skills: a scoping review. Surg Endosc. 2019;33(9):2742–62.
59. Merien AE, van de Ven J, Mol BW, Houterman S, Oei SG. Multidisciplinary team training in a simulation setting for acute obstetric emergencies: a systematic review. Obstet Gynecol. 2010;115(5):1021–31.
60. Cumin D, Boyd MJ, Webster CS, Weller JM. A systematic review of simulation for multidisciplinary team training in operating rooms. Simul Healthc. 2013;8(3):171–9.
61. Meeker K, Brown SK, Lamping M, Moyer MR, Dienger MJ. A high-fidelity human patient simulation initiative to enhance communication and teamwork among a maternity care team. Nurs Womens Health. 2018;22(6):454–62.

62. Rodriguez-Paz JM, Mark LJ, Herzer KR, Michelson JD, Grogan KL, Herman J, et al. A novel process for introducing a new intraoperative program: a multidisciplinary paradigm for mitigating hazards and improving patient safety. Anesth Analg. 2009;108(1):202–10.
63. Arriaga AF, Gawande AA, Raemer DB, Jones DB, Smink DS, Weinstock P, et al. Pilot testing of a model for insurer-driven, large-scale multicenter simulation training for operating room teams. Ann Surg. 2014;259(3):403–10.
64. Fanning RM, Gaba DM. The role of debriefing in simulation-based learning. Simul Healthc. 2007;2(2):115–25.
65. Mitchell JT, Everly GS Jr. Critical incident stress debriefing (CISD): an operations manual for the prevention of traumatic stress among emergency services and disaster workers. Ellicott City, MD: Chevron Publishing Cooperation; 1993. Dyregrov A, editor.
66. Sawyer T, Eppich W, Brett-Fleegler M, Grant V, Cheng A. More than one way to debrief: a critical review of healthcare simulation debriefing methods. Simul Healthc. 2016;11(3):209–17.
67. Center for Medical Simulation. Debriefing Assessment for simulation in Healthcare© (DASH). https://harvardmedsim.org/debriefing-assessment-for-simulation-in-healthcare-dash/. Accessed 12 Aug 2019.
68. Parsons JR, Crichlow A, Ponnuru S, Shewokis PA, Goswami V, Griswold S. Filling the gap: simulation-based crisis resource management training for emergency medicine residents. West J Emerg Med. 2018;19(1):205–10.
69. Boet S, Bould MD, Fung L, Qosa H, Perrier L, Tavares W, et al. Transfer of learning and patient outcome in simulated crisis resource management: a systematic review. Can J Anaesth. 2014;61(6):571–82.
70. Howard SK, Gaba DM, Fish KJ, Yang G, Sarnquist FH. Anesthesia crisis resource management training: teaching anesthesiologists to handle critical incidents. Aviat Space Environ Med. 1992;63(9):763–70.
71. David MG. Crisis management in anesthesiology. 2nd ed. Philadelphia, PA: Elsevier/Saunders; 2015.
72. American Society of Anesthesiologists. Anesthesia SimSTAT. https://www.asahq.org/education-and-career/educational-and-cme-offerings/simulation-education/anesthesia-simstat?gclid=Cj0KCQjw-b7qBRDPARIsADVbUbUKL7er5e6vnCW06lp9qsOdJOCwrM-CWkwSUK2vjPGbrfpFBb9xPLUaAnUfEALw_wcB&ct=09d97253771lf8c1f49a46af8282e3dbd72a10961bd67c585d76a1afd5e7869eae166213b21cf9dc55821e36827a7115bd6cda6cb61e0a9f4b764d61a8b3560c. Accessed 12 Aug 2019.
73. Bracq MS, Michinov E, Arnaldi B, Caillaud B, Gibaud B, Gouranton V, et al. Learning procedural skills with a virtual reality simulator: an acceptability study. Nurs Educ Today. 2019;79:153–60.
74. Morris RW, Pybus DA. "Orpheus" cardiopulmonary bypass simulation system. J Extra Corpor Technol. 2007;39(4):228–33.
75. Murray DJ, Boulet JR, Avidan M, Kras JF, Henrichs B, Woodhouse J, et al. Performance of residents and anesthesiologists in a simulation-based skill assessment. Anesthesiology. 2007;107(5):705–13.
76. Mudumbai SC, Gaba DM, Boulet JR, Howard SK, Davies MF. External validation of simulation-based assessments with other performance measures of third-year anesthesiology residents. Simul Healthc. 2012;7(2):73–80.
77. Weinger MB, Banerjee A, Burden AR, McIvor WR, Boulet J, Cooper JB, et al. Simulation-based assessment of the management of critical events by board-certified anesthesiologists. Anesthesiology. 2017;127(3):475–89.
78. Shaqdan K, Aran S, Daftari Besheli L, Abujudeh H. Root-cause analysis and health failure mode and effect analysis: two leading techniques in health care quality assessment. J Am Coll Radiol. 2014;11(6):572–9.
79. Charles R, Hood B, DeRosier JM, Gosbee JW, Bagian JP, Li Y, et al. Root cause analysis and actions for the prevention of medical errors: quality improvement and resident education. Orthopedics. 2017;40(4):e628–e35.

80. Institute for Healthcare Improvement. RCA2: improving root cause analyses and actions to prevent harm. http://www.ihi.org/resources/Pages/Tools/RCA2-Improving-Root-Cause-Analyses-and-Actions-to-Prevent-Harm.aspx
81. Slakey DP, Simms ER, Rennie KV, Garstka ME, Korndorffer JR Jr. Using simulation to improve root cause analysis of adverse surgical outcomes. Int J Qual Health Care. 2014;26(2):144–50.
82. Jafri FN, Yang CJ, Kumar A, Torres RE, Ahmed ST, Seneviratne N, et al. In Situ Simulation as a Tool to Longitudinally Identify and Track Latent Safety Threats in a Structured Quality Improvement Initiative for SARS-CoV-2 Airway Management Simulation in Healthcare: The Journal of the Society for Simulation in Healthcare. 2023;18(1):16–23. https://doi.org/10.1097/SIH.0000000000000633.
83. Ventre KM, Barry JS, Davis D, Baiamonte VL, Wentworth AC, Pietras M, et al. Using in situ simulation to evaluate operational readiness of a children's hospital-based obstetrics unit. Simul Healthc. 2014;9(2):102–11.
84. Quraishi SA, Kimatian SJ, Murray WB, Sinz EH. High-fidelity simulation as an experiential model for teaching root cause analysis. J Grad Med Educ. 2011;3(4):529–34.
85. Institute for Healthcare Improvement. Science of improvement: establishing measures. www.ihi.org. Accessed 12 Aug 2019.
86. Kotter JP. Leading change: why transformation efforts fail. Harvard Bus Rev. 1995:59–67.
87. Holmboe E, Rizzolo MA, Sachdeva AK, Rosenberg M, Ziv A. Simulation-based assessment and the regulation of healthcare professionals. Simul Healthc. 2011;6(Suppl):S58–62.
88. American College of Surgeons. ACS/APDS surgery resident skills curriculum. https://www.facs.org/education/program/resident-skills. Accessed 8 Aug 2019.
89. American Board of Anesthesiology. About APPLIED (staged exams). https://www.theaba.org/TRAINING-PROGRAMS/APPLIED-(Staged-Exam)/About-APPLIED-(Staged-Exam). Accessed 8 Aug 2019.
90. The American Board of Anesthesiology. About MOCA. https://www.theaba.org/MOCA/Physician-s-Requirements. Accessed 8 Aug 2019.
91. Hanscom R. Medical simulation from an insurer's perspective. Acad Emerg Med. 2008;15(11):984–7.
92. Society for Simulation in Healthcare. Center directory. https://www.ssih.org/Home/SIM-Center-Directory. Accessed 8 Aug 2019.
93. Association for Simulated Practice in Healthcare. https://aspih.org.uk/. Accessed 8 Aug 2019.
94. Association of Standardized Patient Educators. https://www.aspeducators.org/. Accessed 8 Aug 2019.
95. International Nursing Association for Clinical Simulation and Learning. https://www.inacsl.org/. Accessed 8 Aug 2019.
96. International Pediatric Simulation Society. https://www.ipssglobal.org/. Accessed 8 Aug 2019.
97. American Society of Anesthesiologists. Simulation education network summit. https://www.asahq.org/meetings/sen-summit. Accessed 8 Aug 2019.
98. American College of Surgeons. Surgical simulation summit. https://www.facs.org/education/accreditation/aei/surgical-simulation-summit. Accessed 8 Aug 2019.
99. Center for Medical Simulation. Simulation instructor training. https://harvardmedsim.org/training/simulation-instructor-training/. Accessed 8 Aug 2019.
100. Society for Simulation in Healthcare. Certification. https://www.ssih.org/Credentialing/Certification. Accessed 9 Aug 2019.

15 Implementing Crew Resources Management Principles to Improve Perioperative Safety

Abdulelah Alhawsawi and M. Sofia Macedo

It is estimated that more than 230 million surgeries are performed globally every year [1]. According to the World Health Organization (WHO), the significant complications rate could reach up to 16% of all surgical procedures, with mortality rates ranging between 0.4% and 0.8% [2]. However, a recent study has found the rates of surgical complications to be much higher [3]. This was a prospective study of more than 46,000 surgical patients across 498 European hospitals that found a mortality rate as high as 4% for all non-cardiac, obstetric, or neurosurgical inpatient surgical admissions. With almost 7 million people worldwide harmed annually due to perioperative surgical complications, and a mortality rate of up to 10% in developing countries, it has become evident that improving perioperative patient safety is an essential requirement for all healthcare systems globally [2].

Safe Operating Room

The operating room (OR) is one of the most essential and dynamic units within the hospital. The level of complexity, speed, and culture has a direct impact on patient safety. In its efforts to improve safety in this high-stakes and potentially high-risk unit, the Saudi Patient Safety Center (SPSC) issued a publication as a guideline to hospitals for establishing safe operating rooms (SOR).

The following components are needed to establish an SOR while keeping the focus on the patient:

A. Alhawsawi (✉)
Novo Genomics, Riyadh, Saudi Arabia
e-mail: a.alhawsawi@novo-genomics.com

M. S. Macedo
Center for National Health Insurance, Ar Rabi, Riyadh, Saudi Arabia

J. J. Hoballah et al. (eds.), *Principles of Perioperative Safety and Efficiency*,
https://doi.org/10.1007/978-3-031-41089-5_15

1. **Competent Leadership.** Operating room director and specialized nursing manager with experience and focus on safety (patients, staff).
2. **Competent operating room staff.** Nursing staff, anesthesia technicians, respiratory technicians, and biomedical engineers.
3. **Competent operating room support staff.** Biomedical engineers, infection control, histopathology lab technicians, CSSD, housekeeping.
4. **Safe Processes:**
   (a) Proper handover between clinical unit staff and operating room staff.
   (b) Implementation of the WHO Surgical Safety Checklist.
   (c) Proper infection control measures: proper scrubbing, proper attire, especially around the aseptic field, adequate administration of prophylactic antibiotics (e.g., right antibiotics within 60 min of skin incision), proper handling of isolation patients.
   (d) Preventative periodic maintenance (PPM) of all equipment/devices and periodic inspection of HVAC/air exchanges.
   (e) Postoperative plan of care: communicated among the surgical team, recovery room (RR) staff, and receiving clinical unit staff.
5. **Periodic Fire Safety Plan training.**
6. **Safe multidisciplinary team.** Surgeons, anesthesiologist, nurses.

What Do We Mean By a Safe Healthcare Professional (Surgeon, Anesthesiologist, Scrubbed Nurse Circulating Nurse)?

Safe Surgeon

(PRE-OP Phase)

- Listens carefully to the patient and answers his/her questions.
- Involved personally in making the diagnosis.
- Performs proper "informed consent": indications, description, potential complications, and provides an alternative treatment.
- Prepares well: pre-anesthesia consultation, reviews the images, reviews the anatomy, reviews the OR readiness (instruments, equipment, sutures, blood products availability).
- Meets the patient in the pre-op (holding area) for reassurance, answers any questions the patient and/or family might have, reviews the appropriateness of documentation.

(INTRA-OP Phase)

- Performs the WHO Surgical Checklist.
- Discusses the effective plan with the team: anesthesia, surgical, and nursing.
- Scrubs well: the operative site, his/her hands/arms, and his/her assistants.
- Performs proper surgical techniques: handles tissues well, adequate hemostasis, good exposure, good illumination, aseptic technique (right operative theater attire), safe handling of sharps.

- Effective communication: with an assistant (explaining What, How, Why When, Who), with anesthesia (proactive communication, especially consequential steps in the procedure, for example, any steps that might result in physiological/hemodynamics changes); with the nursing staff: clear and proactive communication with both scrubbed and circulating nurses.
  - **Divides the Procedure into Three Phases:**

    Beginning (starts with the skin incision): incision and opening.

    Middle (starts with getting access to the surgical field): the actual procedure.

    End (starts with the onset of closure): restoration of anatomic barriers, for example, closing fascia and skin.

(POST-OP Phase)

- Proper documentation: operative note, labeling of the specimen (histopathology, microbiology).
- Leaves the OR with the patient to recovery room (RR) to observe for any immediate postoperative complications.
- Discusses (open and transparent communication) the outcome of the procedure with the patient family shortly after the procedure.
- Observes the patient for any late postoperative complications (until discharge from hospital).
- Available for any emergency or assign another competent surgeon in case he/she is not available.

Safe Anesthesiologist

(PRE-OP Phase)

- Establishes pre-anesthesia clinic (PAC).
- Listens carefully to the patient and answers his/her questions in PAC.
- Performs proper preoperative risk assessment and/or optimization at PAC: ASA classification, airway assessment.
- Discusses the risks and benefits of anesthetic option and pain management strategy at PAC.
- Performs final patient assessment in the pre-op (holding area) to rule out any reasons for cancellations and/or postponement.
- Prepares well: makes sure anesthesia machines are safe, the anesthesia team and medications are ready, blood products available, appropriate IV (lines, fluid) available.

(INTRA-OP Phase)

- Performs the WHO Surgical Checklist.
- Discusses the anesthesia plan with the team: anesthesia, surgical, and nursing.
- Proper procedures techniques: aseptic technique, ultrasound-assisted catheter (central line—arterial line) insertion, difficult airway set in OR (if needed).

- Continuously monitors and documents the physiological/hemodynamics status of the patient.
- Effective communication: with an assistant (explaining What, How, Why, When, Who), with the surgical team (proactive communication, especially consequential steps in the procedure, for example, any actions that might result in physiological/hemodynamics changes); with the nursing staff: clear and proactive communication with circulating nurse.

(POST-OP Phase)
- Proper airway management.
- Leaves the OR with the patient to recovery room (RR) to observe for any immediate postoperative complications.
- Proper handover of the patient to the RR staff.
- Continuously observe the patient in the RR for airway, hemodynamics, and pain management.
- Assures proper documentation and safe discharge of patients from RR.

Safe OR Nurse

(PRE-OP Phase—Holding Room OR)
- Performs proper handover with the clinical unit nursing staff.
- Insures proper pre-op documentation: patient identification, informed consent, PAC forms.
- Participates in the WHO Surgical Checklist.
- Reassurance to patients and family.
- Prepares the OR table, instruments (surgical team), and meds (anesthesia team).
- Coordinates with the surgical staff, anesthesia staff, and OR nursing staff to ensure patient safety.

(INTRA-OP Phase—Scrubbed Circulating)
- Performs the WHO Surgical Checklist.
- Maintains sterile field and aseptic instruments/OR table/surgical field.
- Safe handling of instruments (scrubbed nurse) and prompt OR circulation (circulating nurse).
- Effective communication: with surgical team (proactive communication, especially consequential steps in the procedure, for example, any actions that might result in physiological/hemodynamics changes); with the nursing staff: clear and proactive communication with circulating nurses.
- Effective implementation of counting policy (sponges, instruments, etc.).

(POST-OP Phase—Scrubbed Circulating)
- Maintenance of the surgical field sterility until the patient is extubated and/or leaves the room.
- Leaves the OR with the patient to recovery room (RR) to observe for any immediate postoperative complications.

- Proper labeling and documentation.
- Proper handover of the patient to RR staff.
- Proper handling of instruments with CSSD staff.

In addition to the above traits and competencies that OR team members should observe to maintain patient safety, the following are common safety competencies that are instrumental to be part of the conduct of OR multidisciplinary team members:

1. Patient advocacy: patient safety is first, second, third … and last!
2. Clinical risk management.
3. Speak–up. Responsibility to speak up and inform the OR leadership, in case of any risky behavior by any of the team members.

In 2006, the American College of Surgeons (ACS) published an article about the seven main crew resource management (CRM) principles that the OR environment should learn from the aviation industry. These seven CRM Principles are:

1. **Command.** Even though the OR should have a teamwork environment, in the end, one final person must be the decision-maker who should accept responsibility and accountability for their team's actions.
2. **Leadership.** Leaders must be willing to allow team members to exercise their rights and responsibilities to ensure a safe and positive outcome. Although there is only one commander, any member of a team can show leadership. Surgeons who encourage teamwork are MORE respected.
3. **Communication.** Many studies have shown that poor communication is implicated as a root cause for many medical errors.
4. **Situational awareness.** A safe and effective leader understands the fluidity and complexity of the OR and is always thinking ahead (What if … happened?) and involving the entire team members.
5. **Workload management.** Staffing and working hours could lead to stress/overwork and consequently, could jeopardize patient safety.
6. **Resource management.** Making sure ALL resources (human, financial, equipment, medications) are used toward improving quality and patient safety.
7. **Decision-making.** Collaborative, unilateral, and consultative, which is the most effective in high-performance teams. A leader must avoid analysis paralysis.

Crew Resource Management Approach, Human Factors, and Resilience

The main goal of CRM training is to enhance cognitive and interpersonal skills that are crucial to maintain situational awareness, solve problems, and make decisions within a team, in addition to a set of communication skills and a variety of behavioral approaches. The focus is on how to apply these skills to effectively manage resources within an organized system that will enhance the safety of related operations, with less focus on the team's technical skills. In this approach, a flat hierarchy should be promoted; not by dismissing the role of the operations' leader, but by, respectfully, questioning authority, in a timely, specific, and constructive manner. This is a critical aspect considering the number of incidents reported where crew-members tried, unsuccessfully, to bring the captain's attention to vital information, resulting in disasters.

Even though CRM has been introduced by the aviation industry in response to the Tenerife airport disaster in 1977, the principles that encompass this concept have been widely applied in other industries where time-sensitive and crucial decisions must be made constantly, such as nuclear, oil and gas, ship handling, railways transportation, healthcare, and others. The reason lies in the fact that CRM recognizes that human errors, leader's decision-making and leadership styles and communication failures are at the root of major errors, which is applicable to several areas other than aviation.

To truly understand how the human-to-human interaction and the human-to-environment interaction impacts safety and, thus, chances for error (be it patients or workforce), CRM training is rooted on human factors engineering (HFE). HFE is a scientific discipline that studies humans' interactions with each other, and among organizations and systems, in order to optimize personal well-being and system performance [4]. The understanding of human factors and its dynamics within safety will promote *resilience* within healthcare, which is the "intrinsic ability of a system to adjust its functioning prior to, during, or following changes/disturbances in order to sustain required operations under expected or unexpected conditions." [5] Until recently, the focus of healthcare institutions that were committed to increasing levels of patient safety would be to identify processes that would fail at some point, allowing for errors to happen. Their focus is, therefore, on "what are the things that could go wrong." With this approach, institutions would fix these gaps and decrease errors. Building a culture of resilience within healthcare allows for a mindset shift from focusing on what goes wrong into focusing on "what goes right and works well." One must appreciate that in addition to the average 10% of cases that result in adverse events, the remaining 90% of cases result in safe care. *So, what happens within healthcare that ensures safe care?* The key is the capacity of healthcare professionals to be resilient and focus on what works well instead of stressing over what went wrong. This mindset can reduce stress and emotional fatigue, which will positively impact patient care [6]. This daily mental exercise, where clinicians strive to understand on how the provision of care succeeds most of the time rather than on why it occasionally fails, is an important facilitator for CRM principles implementation, where the understanding of human factors engineering impact on patient safety is at its root.

> *"The human brain is a complex organ with the wonderful power of enabling man to find reasons for continuing to believe whatever it is that he wants to believe"*—Voltaire

Additionally, healthcare professionals must appreciate the impact of cognitive errors, originated by cognitive biases, in the clinical decision-making process (diagnosis and treatment) so that strategies can be developed to mitigate the cognitive deficits that are intrinsic to the human nature. These can be inherent to the human evolutionary condition but could also be acquired throughout the person's cognitive development, with the additional impact of the working environment [7]. Regardless, the source of biases, if not recognized, may have a negative impact on the decision-making process, which can lead to errors. Moreover, work conditions such as cognitive overload, sleep deprivation, and stress are factors commonly found among operating room staff, which may compromise safe clinical-related decisions. To this point, cognitive bias avoidance training has been suggested as a key strategy in reducing diagnostic errors, [8] where its main goal is to mitigate the adverse effects of cognitive biases in patient outcomes.

Flying is very safe. According to IATA, in 2018, 4.3 billion passengers (the equivalent of more than half the world's population), traveled safely on 46.1 million flights. Out of those 46.1 million flights, there were only 62 aircraft accidents, which led to 523 fatalities.

Compare these remarkable safety stats to healthcare, and you will understand how challenging the patient safety situation is. At a global level, 64 million disability-adjusted life years (estimated) are lost in the world, annually, because of unsafe care, bringing patient harm related to adverse events as one of the top 10 leading causes of death and disability in the world. Moreover, evidence suggests that 134 million adverse events occur in low- and middle-income countries' (LMIC) hospitals, contributing to 2.6 million deaths (the equivalent of 1 death per 11 seconds!). In high-income countries, approximately 1 in 10 patients is harmed while receiving medical care, and about two-thirds of the global burden of adverse events occur in LMIC. In the USA, 251,000 Americans die from medical errors each year. This is equivalent to more than 680 patients dying each day from medical errors, making adverse events the third leading cause of death, preceded only by cardiovascular diseases and cancer [9]. In England, 3.6% of deaths in acute hospitals happen due to the wrong provision of care, while one incident of patient harm is reported every 35 s.

There are many similarities shared between the operating room (OR) and an airplane cockpit: both pilots and surgeons require advanced skill sets to perform their duties, hierarchy is important in both environments, and safe outcomes are dependent on effective communication among various team members. Because aviation is known as an ultra-safe industry, it has been an inspiration to many in healthcare to look at some of the analogies between the two sectors and try to draw some lessons learned to improve patient safety. One of the areas that received much attention lately is crew resource management (CRM).

The concept of CRM originated in 1979 within the U.S. National Aeronautics and Space Administration (NASA), which underwent a workshop to understand the root causes of aviation accidents [10]. The overall conclusion was that human factors, not technical ones, played a pivotal role in air traffic accidents. CRM focuses on three primary measures, or the error troika: (1) Avoidance of errors (prevention). (2) Trapping of errors before they are committed (early recognition). (3) Mitigation of consequences emanating from errors [11]. It is noteworthy that 2 years before the establishment of CRM, in 1977, the world's worst aviation disaster to date (Tenerife accident) took place. That accident involved the collision of two Boeing 747 airplanes and claimed the lives of 583 people. One of the many factors that resulted in that preventable tragedy was the absence of flat hierarchy in the cockpit, as it was evident that the First Officer of one of the Boeing 747 airplanes (KLM Airlines) was aware of the situation but could not challenge the Pilot in Command.

CRM is about empowering all crew members to promote flight safety. Due to the ongoing efforts in the healthcare system to improve patient safety, CRM received more interest by healthcare safety experts as an attempt to learn from other industries. The efforts to apply CRM principles in healthcare started in the early 1980s (a few years after the establishment of CRM in aviation), in anesthesia as a crisis resource management tool [1].

Given the similarities between the conditions in the airplane cockpit (aviation) and the operating room (healthcare), there is growing interest recently among some surgical leaders to adopt CRM principles to improve the safety of patients in the preoperative phase.

Here Is Our Suggested Approach to Improving Perioperative Safety

At the Saudi Patient Safety Center, we firmly believe that the sterility of the operating room should not only refer to its degree of germs-free physical environment, but also to its degree of *cleanliness* of distractions and interruptions that may impact the safety of the procedure being performed, and thus the safety of patients and the healthcare team. While several reports apply the "sterile cockpit" principles from aviation into specific isolated procedures in healthcare, such as medication delivery, [12] little has been found regarding the mapping of the "sterile cockpit" concept to the journey through which patients and surgical teams flow while performing an invasive procedure; be it in the operating room or any other related invasive procedural setting. Considering the high risk for communication errors, misunderstanding of individuals' roles within a team, noise, and mishandling of safe transitions within the perioperative phase, SPSC proposes the following mapping of the "sterile cockpit" concept throughout the intraoperative journey, where the CRM principles are applied, with the main focus on communication levels to ensure higher levels of safety in OR (Fig. 15.1).

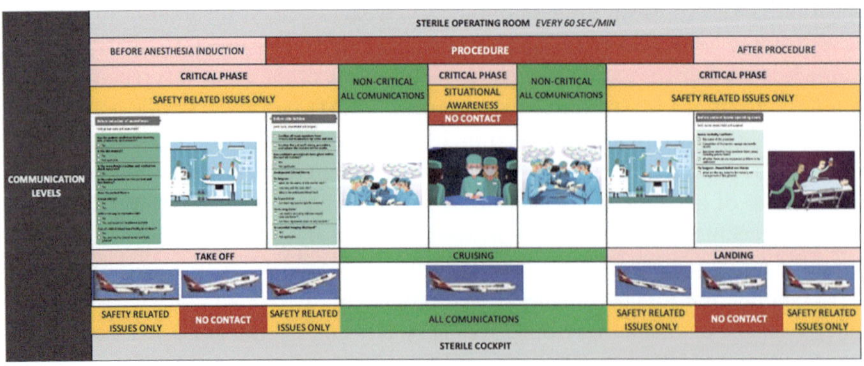

Fig. 15.1 Sterile Operating Room—a framework aligned with the Sterile Cockpit concept

In this proposed framework, we acknowledge that, within healthcare (as in aviation), communication failures have a high chance to occur, making it one of the leading causes for adverse events in the health industry, as reported by the Joint Commission 2004–2011, where it highlights that 70% of sentinel events were due to communication errors [13]. These failures may be presented more often within the healthcare industry, as there is a higher variety of staff with specific skills, disruptions, and noise in addition to a higher rate of transitions of care within the patient's journey, making *safe transitions,* within OR, a focus to ensure patient safety, safeguarding, thereby, a positive experience from the point of admission, throughout the surgical procedure until discharge. Teamwork and culture to open communication are, therefore, vital elements within the OR setting.

The *Sterile OR* framework and CRM Principles

The Crew Resource Management main principles are *command, leadership, communication, situation awareness, workload management, resource management, and decision-making.* In order to ensure high levels of safety in OR, these principles must be present at all times, *every 60 s/min.* Similar to what is applied in aviation, the intraoperative journey has been divided into three phases: before anesthesia induction (*take-off*), procedure (*cruising*), and after procedure (*landing*). In the same way that there are clear periods of restricted communication throughout these phases in aviation, it is proposed that similar periods of restricted communication are applied within the OR setting according to the level of criticalness. In view of this, an extra layer was added to highlight areas that are more critical and thus, prone to higher degrees of errors and link these to the levels of communication *allowed* during these periods.

The Sterile Cockpit

In aviation, during the phases of *take-off* and *landing* there are three periods (below 10,000 feet) of restricted communication: during taxiing (before takeoff and after landing), where only safety-related issues are to be communicated. On departure, the *sterile cockpit* starts when all doors are closed and ends when the seat belt sign is switched off after takeoff. On arrival, the *sterile cockpit* period starts with the cabin preparation for landing and it ceases when the aircraft arrives at the terminal. These periods are characterized by restricted communication, where the cockpit can only have safety-related communications. Some examples of issues that can be communicated are, but not limited to, smoke or fire anywhere in or outside the aircraft, seat belt related info and/or turbulence situation, problems related to securing the cabin for landing, and any other issues that may prevent a safe takeoff or landing procedure (Figs. 15.2 and 15.3).

Within these *"safety-related issues only"* periods, are *"no contact"* periods, characterized by a complete communication restriction. These periods are very critical and coincide with the highest workload/risk segments of takeoff and landing and operate between the commencement of the takeoff roll to gear-up and during

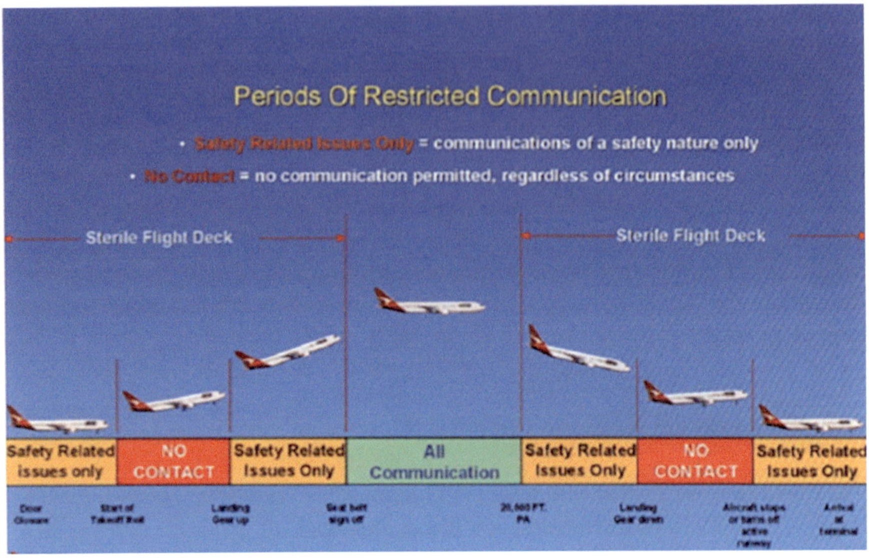

Fig. 15.2 Communications during the Sterile Cockpit is restricted to safety-related communications only

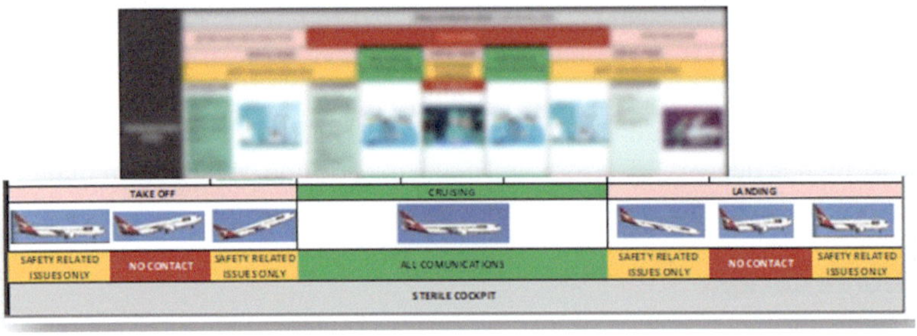

Fig. 15.3 Take off and landing phases are considered "Sterile Cockpit" phase whereas cruising altitude is considered non-Sterile Cockpit phase

landing, between gear-down until the runaway is vacated or the aircraft has stopped on the runaway. Contact with the cockpit crew during this period is not permitted, as distractions may disrupt the crew at a critical time. During these critical flight phases, no crewmember should perform or ask to perform any non-essential activities other than those required for the safe operation of the plane. During cruising flight phase, all type of communications is permitted (Fig. 15.4).

Before Anesthesia Induction phase: This is the OR phase that immediately precedes the procedure and is considered a *critical* phase. During this period, only safety-related issues should be communicated (similarly to what is seen during *taxiing* in aviation) and is when the first component of the WHO Surgical Safety Checklist (WHO SSC) is applied by at least the nurse and the anesthetist (Fig. 15.5).

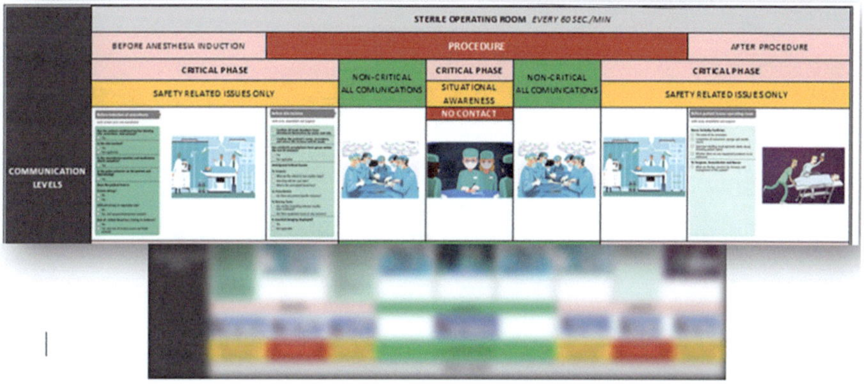

Fig. 15.4 "Sterile Operating Room" Concept: Before, during, and after the procedure

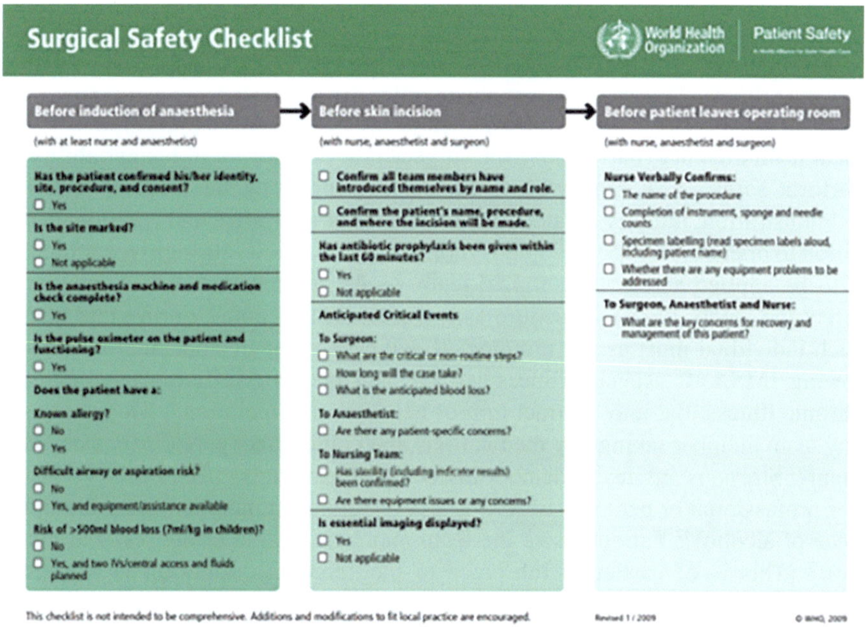

Fig. 15.5 WHO Surgical Safety Checklist

Once the patient is under anesthesia and the surgical team initiates the procedure phase, the critical phase continues as the second component of the WHO SSC is applied just before skin incision. Here, the team composed by the nurse, the anesthesiologist, the surgeon, and other allied healthcare professionals performs *time out*. *Time out* reflects the CRM briefing and debriefing, incorporated by WHO, while developing the SSC. During this briefing period, the elements of CRM (*command, leadership, communication, situation awareness, workload management, resource management, and decision making*) are determined (Fig. 15.6).

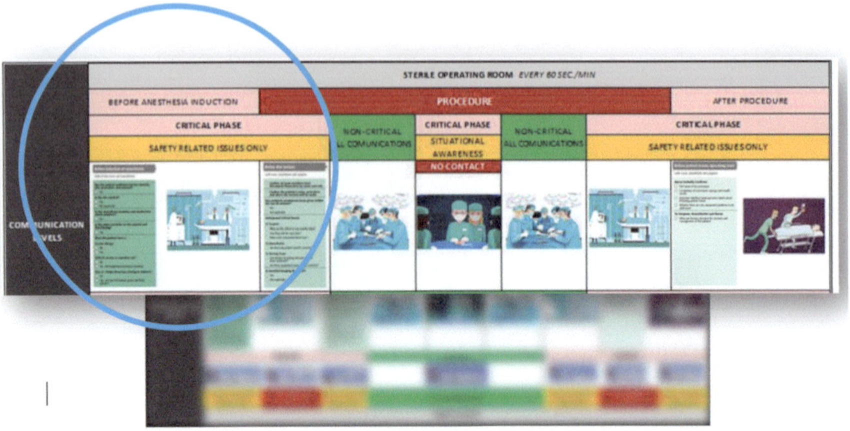

Fig. 15.6 The phase before anesthesia induction

Furthermore, it is known that factors such as substance abuse, mental illness, physical illness, fatigue, exhaustion, and other related issues are associated with medical errors [14]. During this segment of the perioperative journey, every surgical team member (particularly the surgeon) must be aware of his/her ability to perform safely. The mnemonic IMSAFE developed by the Federal Aviation Administration, initially created to assess the pilot's physical and emotional condition to operate, has been adopted among surgeons. SPSC strongly recommends it to be applied across the surgical team, as the unfitness of one member will affect the safety of the procedure as a whole. At this point, during this phase, each individual must assess him/herself and each other by checking on the following **IMSAFE** aspects: **I**llness–is any team member suffering any acute or chronic illness that may distract him or her from the operation?; **M**edication–is any team member taking any medications that could affect performance or judgment?; **S**tress–is any team member under significant stress from events in his or her professional or personal life?; **A**lcohol–is any team member under the influence of alcohol?; **F**atigue–have the team members had adequate rest and nutrition? (This is of particular relevance to the surgeon.); **E**motion–is any team member emotionally competent to operate? There might be occasions where an individual person may not be able to recognize that he or she is not fit to carry out related duties, and therefore it is vital that the team members feel empowered to raise concerns.

Similar to what occurs within aviation, it is important that every team member of the surgical team understands and is aware of what situations are considered "safety-related issues." Due to the variety and complexity of cases, it is up to the surgical team to decide and agree upon what defines "safety-related issues." Unless all the surgical team members are in the loop regarding this point, effective responses to raised concerns won't be possible, thereby posing a risk to patient safety.

Procedure phase: This phase is further divided into sub-phases that are considered *non-critical* and *critical*. The Procedure phase corresponds to the *"cruising phase"* of the sterile cockpit concept. During *non-critical* phases, all kinds of communications are allowed. The definition of which procedural phases are non-critical and critical should be determined, as much as possible, during the briefing phase, where the surgical team should be aware (*situational awareness*) of potential risks that are associated with the interventions within the procedure. Situational awareness is highly important, as it guarantees that the team members *share a mental model* of the procedure and its potential risks, allowing for effective decisions and actions that may eventually have to take place in a short period of time. In addition, it helps to determine what crucial moments are expected within the procedure phase that may require full attention from the surgeon where no contact should be made, and the team is aware in which exceptional situations the "*no contact*" rule may be overridden. Once again, in order for the shared mental model to be created, adequate communication is key. The operating room staff, regardless of their role or their hierarchal position, are empowered to *say something if they see something*. A "speak up" culture, where each team member feels comfortable to raise concerns, is vital and must be encouraged at all times, as postoperative complications and fatal errors have been associated with lack of sharing vital information. This fact highlights the impact of effective teamwork within the surgical team for safe care (Fig. 15.7).

After-procedure phase: This phase is characterized by debriefing, and, similarly to the "*take off*" period (*sterile cockpit*) and the *before anesthesia induction phase* (*sterile OR*), only safety-related issues should be communicated. During this period, the last component of the WHO Surgical Safety Checklist (WHO SSC) is applied by at least the nurse, the surgeon, and the anesthetist. Before the patient leaves the operating room, the debriefing will allow for team members to raise safety concerns, if any.

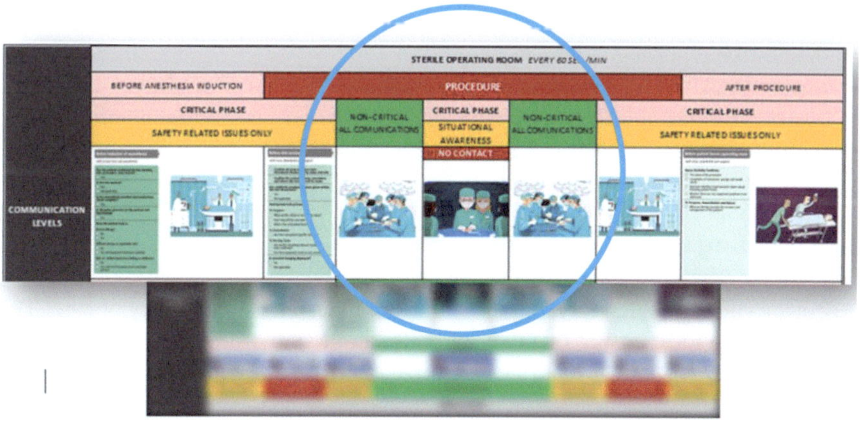

Fig. 15.7 The phase during the surgical procedure

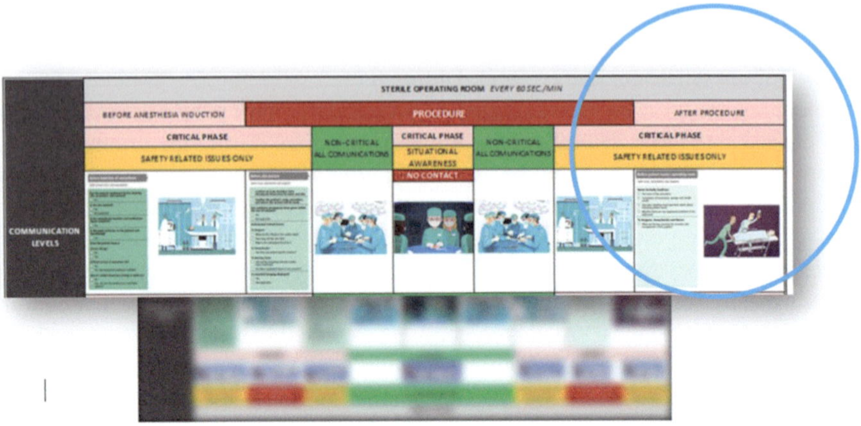

Fig. 15.8 The phase after the surgical procedure

Suggested Strategies from CRM

In a nutshell, and additionally to what was previously suggested, operating rooms and other settings where invasive interventions take place will benefit from implementing aviation strategies such as:

- cross-checks
- readback
- "two-challenge rule," when a person has been challenged twice and has failed to respond accordingly, anyone from the team can override this person
- peer monitoring
- briefings, defining operating procedures and standards
- recognition of fatigue as a factor in performance
- regular "check rides" in the form of assessment in a simulator
- blame-free reporting culture
- use of checklists for the team to stand back and appraise procedures
- direct eye contact, introducing each other, using non-judgmental words
- putting safety before self-esteem [14] (Fig. 15.8).

Safe Staffing in the Operating Room

Adequate staffing in the operating room is vital to ensure safe delivery of care. The OR leadership must ensure that the right number of staff with the right skill mix is assigned to each surgical team at all times. International and national regulatory bodies across the globe recognize the need to establish minimum acceptable nursing and other allied healthcare professionals' ratio standards to provide safe patient care. Hospitals with poor patient outcomes are found to have unsafe work environments, with insufficient nursing and allied healthcare staff. The estimation of the appropriate number of staff and proper skill mix must be based on evidence and is usually informed by the professional associations of each specialty. The Association of periOperative Registered Nurses (AORN) [15] recognizes that the primary focus of the perioperative nurses and other healthcare professionals within OR is patient safety. Thus, adequate personal staffing plan must be developed to meet the safety needs of both the patient and the healthcare professional. SPSC in collaboration with the International Council of Nurses released a White paper on Nurse Staffing Levels For Patient Safety And Workforce Safety in 2019, [16] which is a high-level advisory framework on the regulatory landscape, and recommendations that must be in place for optimal nurse-staffing ratios and skill mix that will serve as the foundation for a culture of safety. Moreover, it is important to take into consideration factors that have a direct impact on the safe provision of care within the OR. The AORN establishes evidence-based calculation methodologies that facilitate the decision on adequate staffing for the OR. Factors to take into consideration while establishing OR staff ratios are hours of operation (defined by the department), hours required to cover off-shift schedules (holidays, nights, weekends), urgent procedures, the number of OR rooms, historical data regarding minutes and hours of service, procedure volumes, and mix and technology requirements, in addition to the effect that extended shift hours have in staff performance and consequently in-patient safety.

To ensure safe nursing and other allied healthcare professionals care, one must recognize that there's no "one size fits all" approach to this. The nurse-to-patient ratio may vary across OR suites as well as within the same OR suit throughout the same procedure and are thereby not rigid. Also, while determining safe nurse-to-patient ratios, one must consider the overall availability of ancillary staff/allied health professionals such as nursing aids, licensed practice nurses (LPNs), and technicians. Often, the recommended ratios are put forward based on the premise that a full complement of ancillary and support staff is present at all times during each shift within a unit. The bottom line to determine nurse-to-patient ratios or other healthcare professionals must be always the safety of patient care and the safety of the professionals providing care, and not the number of staff available.

Given this, SPSC put forward recommendations for RN-patient ratios in OR as follows (Fig. 15.9):

** Additional staff members (technicians, ancillary staff), with suitable and adequate competencies, must be used to meet safe staffing [15].

Patient Care Area	RN-to-Patient Limit
Intensive/critical care (adult and pediatric)	1:2 or 1:1*
Neonatal intensive care	1:2 or 1:1*
Step Down/intermediate care	1:4
Operating room	1:1**
Post anesthesia recovery	1:2
Labor & Delivery (active labor)	1:2
Antepartum	1:4
Post-partum	1:6
Post-partum with "mother-baby set" model of care	1:4
Well-Baby Nursery	1:8
Pediatrics unit	1:4
Emergency Room	1:2
ICU patients in the ER	1:2*
Trauma patients in the ER	1:1
Acute Respiratory Care	1:2
Burn Unit	1:2*
Non-urgent patients	1:4
Medical, surgical	1:4
Telemetry/ cardiac care unit	1:4*
Oncology	1:3
Hemodialysis	1:2*
Observation/Outpatient	1:4
Rehabilitation/transitional care	1:5
Home Care	1:6
Special Care Unit	1:4*
Psychiatric	1:6*
Forensic centers (clinic)	1:2*

Fig. 15.9 Safe Nurse: Patient Ratios

Conclusion

In the healthcare industry, near misses and actual adverse events may go underreported due to the premise that errors are "part of the business." Moreover, healthcare professionals may not feel comfortable reporting, due to an institutionalized blaming culture where errors are seen as consequences of individual malpractice as opposed to a system failure, and also due to an inflated sense of pride as well as fear of legal consequences. To shift this trend, it is vital that healthcare professionals understand the value of reporting errors as much as near misses as a valuable learning tool. Similar to the aviation industry that implemented the Confidential Human

Factors Incident Reporting Programme, surgical teams introduced the Confidential Reporting System in Surgery. Reporting and learning systems such as this have been proven to not only bring to light errors and near misses that are analyzed so they won't happen again, but also to promote a just culture.

Another method proven to be efficient in identifying behaviors and actions with high potential for errors is to involve expert observers in the surgical rooms during procedures. This approach was established by the aviation industry known as "Line Operations Safety Audit" or LOSA. It identifies not only the actions that may put patient safety at risk, but also the risk factors or the sources for these potential errors. LOSA is thereby a valuable strategy to identify conscious or unconscious protocol violations, failures in communication, and poor decision-making processes, by direct observation of the surgical team, allowing for focused implementation strategies aimed at managing human-error factors of the identified risks.

The failures found in the perioperative journey are not only highly prone for serious or fatal adverse events, but also highly preventable. Any approach that aims at preventing the gaps and/or failures in the process will improve the reliability of surgical care and consequently improve safety levels for surgical patients and surgical teams [17].

***Sterile OR* Made Easy—Supporting Framework for Surgical Teams**

Given the relation between aviation concepts and healthcare industry, SPSC proposes the following framework to be used as a guiding tool by each surgical team before commencing a procedure:

1. Divide your intervention into segments: before (*takeoff*), during (*cruising*), and after (*landing*).
2. Identify which tasks belong to each segment for clarity.
3. Insert CRM principles as: briefing, debriefing, flat hierarchy, situation awareness.
4. For each segment, identify:
   (a) Critical phases: where safety-related issues only take place. Here identify what are considered safety-related issues.
   (b) Non-critical phases: where any type of communication can take place
   (c) No-contact phases, if any: where no communication of any kind is allowed

References

1. Weiser TG, Regenbogen SE, Thompson KD. An estimation of the global volume of surgery: a modelling strategy based on available data. Lancet. 2008;372(9633):139–44.
2. WHO guidelines for Safe Surgery, 1st ed. Geneva: World Health Organisation; 2008.
3. Pearse RM, Moreno RP, Bauer P. Mortality after surgery in Europe: a 7 day cohort study. Lancet. 2012;380(9847):1059–65.
4. Crew Resource Management, LLC. https://www.criticalcrm.com/topics
5. Hollnagel E, Braithwaite J, Wears R. Resilient Health care. Boca Raton, FL: CRC Press; 2013.
6. UNCHealth. Enhancing resilience, building a stronger patient safety culture. http://news.unchealthcare.org/empnews/2015/oct-1/enhancing-resilience-building-a-stronger-patient-safety-culture

7. Croskerry P, Singhal G, Mamede S. Cognitive debiasing 1: origins of bias and theory of debiasing. BMJ. 2013;22(Suppl 2):ii58–64. https://doi.org/10.1136/bmjqs-2012-001712.
8. Kapur N, Parand A, Soukup T, Reader T, Sevdalis N. Aviation and healthcare: a comparative review with implications for patient safety. JRSMed Open. 2015;7(1):2054270415616548. https://doi.org/10.1177/2054270415616548.
9. Makary MA, Daniel M. Medical error–the third leading cause of death in the US. BMJ. 2016;353:i2139.
10. Helmreich RL, Merritt AC, Wilhelm JA. The evolution of crew resource management training in commercial aviation. Int J Aviat Psychol. 1999;9:19–32. https://doi.org/10.1207/s15327108ijap0901_2.
11. Howard SK, Gaba DM, Fish KJ, Yang G, Sarnquist FH. Anesthesia crisis resource management training: teaching anesthesiologists to handle critical incidents. Aviat Space Environ Med. 1992;63(9):763–70.
12. Federwisch M, Ramos H, Adams S. The sterile cockpit: an effective approach to reducing medication errors? Am J Nurs. 2014;114:47–55.
13. Joint Commission. Improving patient and worker safety: opportunities for synergy, collaboration and innovation. Oakbrook Terrace, IL: The Joint Commission; 2012. p. 171.
14. Stripe SC, Best LG, Cole-Harding S, Fifield B, Talebdoost F. Aviation model cognitive risk factors applied to medical malpractice cases. J Am Board Fam Med. 2006;19:627–32.
15. AORN. AORN position statement on perioperative safe staffing and on-call; 2014. https://www.aorn.org/-/media/.../posstat-personnel-safe-staffing-on-call-practices.pdf. Accessed May 2019.
16. Saudi Patient Safety Center; International Council of Nurses. Nurse staffing levels for patient safety and workforce safety. SPSC and ICN white paper. Riyadh, Saudi Arabia; 2019. spsc.gov.sa and icn.ch.
17. Symons NR, Almoudaris AM, Nagpal K, Vincent CA, Moorthy K. An observational study of the frequency, severity, and etiology of failures in postoperative care after major elective general surgery. Ann Surg. 2013;257(1):1–5. https://doi.org/10.1097/SLA.0b013e31826d859b.

Peer Review of Perioperative Adverse Events

16

Lydia R. Maurer, Elizabeth Mort, and Haytham M. A. Kaafarani

Introduction

> "Every surgeon carries about him a little cemetery, in which from time to time he goes to pray, a cemetery of bitterness and regret, of which he seeks the reason for certain of his failures."—*René Leriche* [1]

> "To effect improvement, the first step is to admit and record the lack of perfection."—*Ernest A. Codman* [2]

By taking a patient to the high-risk environment of the operating room, the surgeon often develops a special and personal bond of trust with the patient. As such, patient mishaps often take a personal toll on surgeons. Critically analyzing complications and adverse events to prevent their reoccurrence has become a key part of training and is central to the discipline of surgery. While there are many described and practical ways that perioperative adverse events could be analyzed, a peer review discussion in the morbidity and mortality (M & M) conference is the standard in almost all surgical specialties. The profession's commitment to learn from adverse outcomes has evolved over time and is incorporating tools from safety science and is encouraging quality improvement. These advances should both accelerate needed improvements and give surgeons the tools to provide better care and to contribute more effectively with systems improvements.

L. R. Maurer
Department of Surgery, Massachusetts General Hospital, Boston, MA, USA

E. Mort (✉)
Department of Medicine, Massachusetts General Hospital, Boston, MA, USA
e-mail: emort@partners.org

H. M. A. Kaafarani
Department of Surgery, Division of Trauma, Emergency Surgery and Surgical Critical Care, Massachusetts General Hospital, Boston, MA, USA

J. J. Hoballah et al. (eds.), *Principles of Perioperative Safety and Efficiency*,
https://doi.org/10.1007/978-3-031-41089-5_16

Morbidity and Mortality Conference

The history of the M & M conference is often traced back to Dr. Ernest Emory Codman, a surgeon at the Massachusetts General Hospital in the late nineteenth and early twentieth centuries [3]. He created the "end result" concept, or the idea that surgeons should follow their patients to determine the outcome of their treatment and/or any adverse effects or complications that occurred as a result of the operation. He was a controversial figure who also believed in public reporting of outcomes, an unpopular concept back then among surgeons and hospital leaders. However, despite the resistance to public reporting, analyzing adverse events, or what he termed as the "end result" idea, was adopted in many hospitals and eventually evolved into what is now known as M & M. An additional sentinel text on error and the culture of surgical practice was Charles Bosk's book *Forgive and Remember*, in which he dissects the role of error in surgical culture. He refers to the M & M conference as a place where the responsible parties take responsibility for the error, and other clinicians offer comment and often forgiveness, and do so in a way that everyone will remember and not repeat the error [4]. M & M provides an environment where errors can be addressed and analyzed directly among peers in a memorable way that all can learn from them, but in the end the surgeon gains the support of his or her peers to move forward, learn from it, and keep treating patients safely.

The M & M conference is currently a well-established feature for quality assurance in most surgery and anesthesia departments, but its structure remains variable. Essential components of the M&M conference format are confidentiality and the allowance of candid discussion away from fear of medicolegal repercussions. This so-called peer review privilege is legislated at the state level and its intent is to promote candid conversations among peers without fear of the content of the conversations being discovered in the context of medical malpractice proceedings [5]. Any individuals involved in managing these sessions should familiarize themselves with the laws in their state and ensure that the proceedings are managed in keeping with their institution's policies. While the existence of a regular M & M conference is a required feature for accreditation by professional societies, there is no set format that must be followed. There is often one central M & M conference for the department of surgery, and in many cases individual divisions (i.e., trauma, transplant, thoracic) will have their own division-specific conferences. Surgeons voluntarily submit their perioperative complications, and these are discussed in a peer feedback-and-review format to identify what went wrong and opportunities for improvement. For example, in an academic training setting, senior residents and fellows might present a brief synopsis of the case of interest and will field questions regarding the operation and/or the management of the patient from the other faculty and trainee surgeons in the audience. In some institutions, a select number of M & M presentations (a small number of the total submitted per week) are presented for group discussion, while in other institutions every complication is presented. The format of the discussion varies among institutions from an informal discussion led by the faculty surgeon responsible for the patient to more formalized discussions including presentation of relevant literature and, occasionally, more formal root cause analyses.

Complications are often categorized into preventable and unpreventable, or gradations of preventability. Lessons learned and opportunities for improvement are emphasized and highlighted. An example that may be considered unpreventable is the death of an elderly trauma patient arriving hypotensive and unconscious to the hospital, who eventually succumbs to the severity of her injury despite best efforts by the team. While discussions happen surrounding the perioperative management of this patient to ensure it was consistently appropriate, most surgeons would classify it as unpreventable. On the other hand, there are a vast range of complications that would be considered "preventable." Technical complications are often labeled as such. Another example would be a patient who was not started on deep vein thrombosis (DVT) prophylaxis after an elective operation, and then subsequently developed a DVT. This would be considered preventable and would likely be subject to considerably more scrutiny and criticism as to the decision of not initiating prophylaxis.

Traditionally, the benefit of discussing these cases was to help all faculty surgeons and trainees to avoid making the same mistakes, when appropriate. The extent to which systemic change or broader policy is implemented as a result of M & M can vary and is generally more limited. One of the criticisms of the M & M conference is that the lens of adjudication is often narrow, where the discussion focuses on diagnosis, surgical technique, and perioperative management. Bosk describes it best in his book: "When the patient of an internist dies, the natural question his colleagues ask is, 'What happened?' When the patient of a surgeon dies, his colleagues ask, 'What did you do?'." [4] We know, however, there are many other systems factors that can contribute to perioperative adverse events. Potential solutions are often discussed under the lens of changing decision-making, with the classic question, "What would you have done differently?" While considering personal responsibility for patient outcomes is imperative, patients exist in a sociodemographic context and hospital system, which should be considered when discussing adverse events and interventions.

Consider the hypothetical example of a young, female, Spanish-speaking patient who undergoes elective, open ventral hernia repair, with extensive lysis of adhesions, and mesh placement. An abdominal binder is placed. The evening of the operation she spikes a fever. The intern on overnight is covering multiple patients and does not see the patient, but reassures the nurse that fevers are very common the night of surgery. The patient also tells the nurse that she saw some green staining on the binder. The team does not use an interpreter on rounds and misses this history. On post-op day 3, she then becomes tachycardic and hypotensive, the abdominal binder is removed and she has green liquid coming out of the incision. She is taken back to the OR urgently where a missed enterotomy is found. The complication reported at M & M conference would likely be presented in a more streamlined fashion, for example: "35 y/o female with a history of a ventral hernia underwent open ventral hernia repair with component separation, lysis of adhesions, and retrorectus mesh. On post-op day 0 she developed a fever but was otherwise hemodynamically stable. On post-op day 3 she became hemodynamically unstable and was found to have green fluid coming out of her wound. At this point, given concern for a missed enterotomy she was taken back to the OR urgently."

The discussion for a case like this could go multiple ways but would likely focus on the operation itself—how the lysis of adhesions was performed, what type of mesh was placed, and how it was secured. Some may ask whether the complication could have been identified sooner with a better physical exam. What is often omitted, however, is how this patient's language status, and the team's lack of interpreter use, may have contributed to delays in recognizing what was really going on. She was not able to tell them that she saw green staining on the abdominal binder the day before she became unstable, a critical piece of information that could have led to earlier diagnosis and treatment. What might also go undiscussed are the system barriers that prevented the intern from seeing the patient the first night (covering a large number of patients overnight) that may have affected this patient's care. In some cases, M & M conference is an effective venue for experts in the field to discuss perioperative adverse events and give important advice to their peers and trainees. In other cases, it can miss more nuanced system factors that should be addressed to avoid similar adverse events in the future.

Some have argued that this lack of standardized procedures and limited scope diminishes the effectiveness of the M & M conference and limits the potential for actionable change. Sacks et al. published in 2015 on changes they made in their department to make their M & M conference more actionable [6]. After identification by leadership of three to four cases per conference, the resident presenting is encouraged to pursue a root cause analysis to more thoroughly evaluate the factors that may have contributed to the complication. This encouraged residents to look at more systemic factors that may have influenced the outcome. Concerns that emerge from these discussions then create the fodder for future quality improvement (QI) projects pursued in the department. Many institutions have moved toward a more formalized M & M structure that incorporates root cause analysis and explicit discussion of contributing factors as QI and is emphasized by the Accreditation Council for Graduate Medical Education (ACGME) [7]. Incorporating root cause analysis [8] into M & M reviews will allow a more comprehensive understanding of what happened, and identify the contributing factors, while still allowing for discussion of technical skills and other clinical errors.

Additionally, there has been some concern that because the faculty surgeons select cases, there is a risk of under-reporting of complications. In 2002, Hutter et al. compared complications presented at M & M conference to data collected via American College of Surgeons National Surgical Quality Improvement Program® (ACS-NSQIP) in the general surgery division and found that considerably fewer deaths and complications were presented in M & M conference than were collected via ACS-NSQIP. [9] As a result, they changed the M & M reporting system to include discrete and well-defined complication categories to improve reporting. This chapter illustrates the challenge with the peer review M & M conference format—that ultimately the faculty surgeon decides what is presented, and what constitutes a "complication," despite concerted efforts to better define and report complications.

In cases with particularly negative outcomes, there are additional more formal review procedures the hospital pursues to examine the event, and that we will not discuss in this chapter. Additionally, in certain types of cases, there is mandatory reporting of adverse events, which goes beyond the peer review format to a regulatory review. The National Quality Forum (NQF) has established and maintained a list of 27 serious, preventable adverse events deemed "never events" that require "mandatory reporting" (Table 16.1). This will be discussed in more depth in another chapter of this text.

Table 16.1 NQF's never events

Surgical or invasive procedures	
1A.	Surgery or other invasive procedure performed on the wrong site
1B.	Surgery or other invasive procedure performed on the wrong patient
1C.	Wrong surgical or other invasive procedure performed on a patient
1D.	Unintended retention of foreign object in a patient after surgery or other invasive procedure
1E.	Intraoperative or immediately postoperative/postprocedure death in an ASA Class 1 patient
Product or device events	
2A.	Patient death or serious injury associated with the use of contaminated drugs, devices, or biologics provided by the healthcare setting
2B.	Patient death or serious injury associated with the use or function of a device in patient care, in which the device is used or functions other than intended
2C.	Patient death or serious injury associated with intravascular air embolism that occurs while being cared for in a healthcare setting
Patient protection events	
3A.	Discharge or release of a patient/resident of any age, who is unable to make decisions, to other than an authorized person
3B.	Patient death or serious injury associated with patient elopement (disappearance)
3C.	Patient suicide, attempted suicide, or self-harm that results in serious injury, while being cared for in a healthcare setting
Care management events	
4A.	Patient death or serious injury associated with a medication error (e.g., errors involving the wrong drug, wrong dose, wrong patient, wrong time, wrong rate, wrong preparation, or wrong route of administration)
4B.	Patient death or serious injury associated with unsafe administration of blood products
4C.	Maternal death or serious injury associated with labor or delivery in a low-risk pregnancy while being cared for in a healthcare setting
4D.	Death or serious injury of a neonate associated with labor or delivery in a low-risk pregnancy
4E.	Patient death or serious injury associated with a fall while being cared for in a healthcare setting
4F.	Any Stage 3, Stage 4 or unstageable pressure ulcers acquired after admission/presentation to a healthcare setting
4G.	Artificial insemination with the wrong donor sperm or wrong egg
4H.	Patient death or serious injury resulting from the irretrievable loss of an irreplaceable biological specimen
4I.	Patient death or serious injury resulting from failure to follow up or communicate laboratory, pathology, or radiology test results
Environmental events	
5A.	Patient or staff death or serious injury associated with an electric shock in the course of a patient care process in a healthcare setting
5B.	Any incident in which systems designed for oxygen or other gas to be delivered to the patient contains no gas, the wrong gas, or are contaminated by toxic substances
5C.	Patient or staff death or serious injury associated with a burn incurred from any source in the course of a patient care process in a healthcare setting
5D.	Patient death or serious injury associated with the use of physical restraints or bedrails while being cared for in a healthcare setting
Radiologic events	
6A.	Death or serious injury of a patient or staff associated with the introduction of a metallic object into the MRI area

Voluntary Reporting Systems

While the peer review format of the M & M conference in a department of surgery has many benefits for analyzing and learning from adverse events, a downside of this venue is that the decision to bring forward a specific adverse event is often reliant on the surgical staff.

To address this, the Joint Commission has required that hospitals implement voluntary incident reporting systems to capture adverse events and "near miss" potential errors picked up by other perioperative staff members. At our institution, the Massachusetts General Hospital (MGH), a "safety report" can be filed by anyone in the Mass General Brigham system, and every safety report is reviewed and triaged to the appropriate person or group for peer review in a peer review protected setting. This process is managed by skilled nurses, trained in safety science at root cause analysis. These nurses review the reports for both severity and specialty, and then work with departmental staff safety champions, who may be either nurses or physicians, to conduct the investigations. At MGH each clinical department has a designated Chair of Quality and Safety who is assigned by the service chief to oversee the review of safety events as well as many other quality and safety functions in the department. Each clinical department also has a designated trainee who represents the department on the quality and safety committee for trainees. Safety events undergo investigation and, at times, these investigations are extensive, particularly if there is an unexpected adverse outcome or when there is a significant event that had no harm, but was considered a near miss and well worth investigating to prevent an adverse event from occurring. In this peer review format, adverse events can be investigated in a collegial way by initiating a conversation with the other providers involved, and trying to identify the factors leading to the event and a root cause analysis can be performed [10]. This system utilizes a very different approach than the in-person M & M conference format, and supplements additional data and well-rounded review of adverse events. In our institution, we have held cross-departmental M & Ms. to share learnings across disciplines. This work continues to evolve as we promote more transparency, and appreciate more that teamwork and communication across groups is often an important contributing factor in adverse events.

Conclusion

Reviewing performance with the goal of improving outcomes has been embedded in professional surgical activities for most of the last century. The M & M conference offers a confidential venue for candid discussion of perioperative complications and mortality where surgeons can learn from each other to avoid similar complications. Over time, our methods and procedures have changed and migrated from focusing on the accountability of the individual surgeon to considering a range of contributing factors and systems issues that impact the quality of care we, as surgeons, deliver. We believe that the M & M conference offers an important learning environment for faculty and trainees alike and are working to refine and improve these processes.

References

1. La LR. Philosophie de La Chirurgie [The philosophy of surgery]. Paris: Flammarion; 1951.
2. Codman EA. The classic: a study in hospital efficiency: as demonstrated by the case report of first five years of private hospital. Clin Orthop Relat Res. 2013;471(6):1778–83. https://doi.org/10.1007/s11999-012-2751-3.
3. American College of Surgeons. Ernest A. Codman, MD, FACS (1869–1940). https://www.facs.org/about-acs/archives/pasthighlights/codmanhighlight. Accessed 27 July 2019.
4. Bosk CL. Forgive and remember: managing medical failure. 2nd ed. Chicago: University of Chicago Press; 2003.
5. Peer Review Protection Act. 63 Pa. Stat. § 425.1. 1974.
6. Sacks GD, Lawson EH, Tillou A, Hines OJ. Morbidity and mortality conference 2.0. Ann Surg. 2015;262(2):228–9. https://journals.lww.com/annalsofsurgery/Fulltext/2015/08000/Morbidity_and_Mortality_Conference_2_0.6.aspx.
7. ACGME. ACGME program requirements for graduate medical education in general surgery. https://www.acgme.org/globalassets/pfassets/programrequirements/440_generalsurgery_2020.pdf.
8. National Patient Safety Foundation. RCA2 improving root cause analyses and actions to prevent harm.; 2016.
9. Hutter MM, Rowell KS, Devaney LA, Sokal SM, Warshaw AL, Abbott WM, et al. Identification of surgical complications and deaths: an assessment of the traditional surgical morbidity and mortality conference compared with the American College of Surgeons-National Surgical Quality Improvement Program. J Am Coll Surg. 2006;203(5):618–24. https://doi.org/10.1016/j.jamcollsurg.2006.07.010.
10. Aaronson EL, Brown D, Benzer T, Natsui S, Mort E. Incident reporting in emergency medicine: a thematic analysis of events. J Patient Saf. 2019;15(4):E60–3. https://doi.org/10.1097/PTS.0000000000000399.

Enhanced Recovery After Surgery Protocols

17

Timothy E. Newhook and Thomas A. Aloia

Enhanced Recovery After Surgery

Fast-track surgery as a concept is almost 30 years old, as streamlining perioperative care to reduce intensive care stay following cardiac surgery was initially reported in the 1990s [1]. However, at a time when the length of stay (LOS) following colon surgery was 10 days or more in most European countries, Kehlet and Mogensen reported that most patients had recovered enough for discharge 2 days after sigmoid resection by following a multimodal approach to recovery [2]. After initial skepticism, what resulted from this was a complete paradigm shift, emphasizing best practices and evidence-based approaches to the perioperative care of the surgical patient, and that this care was as important to outcomes as the surgical technique [3, 4]. In an effort to promote these principles throughout Europe and beyond, as well as develop further research opportunities and present implementation guidelines, the ERAS® Society (http://www.erassociety.org) was created, and its members represent various disciplines involved in the perioperative care of the surgical patient.

The application of ERAS principles to the care of patients following surgery began more than 20 years ago, originally focusing on fast-track recovery of patients following colorectal surgery [2]. Protocols involving ERAS concepts have now been applied to the perioperative care of patients within most surgical specialties, and contemporary management of most patients undergoing surgery involves at least some ERAS concepts. These fundamental perioperative care principles, or "four pillars," including early feeding, early ambulation, goal-directed fluid therapy,

T. E. Newhook
Department of Surgical Oncology, Division of Surgery, MD Anderson Cancer Center, Houston, TX, USA

T. A. Aloia (✉)
Oncology Services, Maternal Health and Perinatal Medicine, Ascension, Houston, TX, USA
e-mail: thomas.aloia@ascension.org

J. J. Hoballah et al. (eds.), *Principles of Perioperative Safety and Efficiency*,
https://doi.org/10.1007/978-3-031-41089-5_17

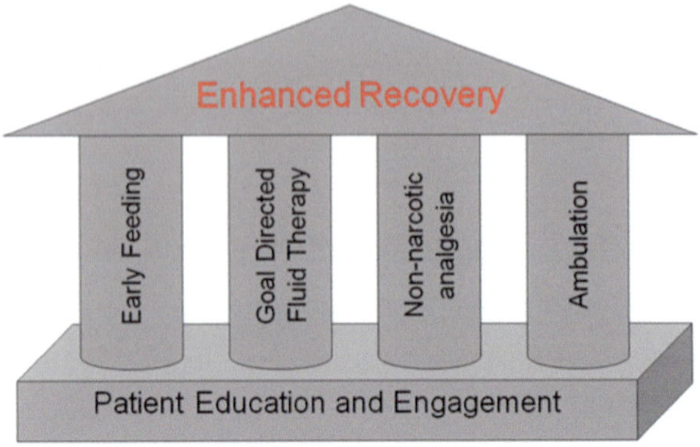

Fig. 17.1 The four pillars of perioperative care, essential multidisciplinary components of modern ERAS

and opiate-sparing analgesia, rest upon a foundation of effective patient education and engagement (Fig. 17.1). These are the essential multidisciplinary components of modern ERAS.

Initial reports on ERAS principles were focused on colorectal surgery beginning with Kehlet, subsequently igniting many reports on multimodal approach to perioperative care and reduced length of stay (LOS) [2]. Use of epidural analgesia, early enteral nutrition, and early mobilization reduced what was a 6–12-day LOS to 5 days [5–8]. The inclusion of laparoscopic techniques further improved reported LOS to 2–3 days following colon surgery [9]. However, the major goal of ERAS is not just the rapidity of recovery, but also the quality of recovery [4]. Great efforts have been made by the ERAS® Society and surgical community in general to improve the quality of perioperative care via these protocols, now being applied across many disciplines including colorectal, hepato-pancreato-biliary, gastric, bariatric, gynecologic, and head and neck surgery [10–16].

Perioperative Safety and Efficiency

As the overarching theme of ERAS evidence-based approaches is to create perioperative care pathways that reduce stress associated with surgery, patients may recover faster with reduced complications and delays in planned postoperative therapies [4, 17, 18]. Further results following implementation have supported both the safety and efficiency of this approach as compared to traditional perioperative care strategies.

Safety

Adoption of ERAS has been shown to reduce complications rates and to reduce hospital LOS without increasing readmission rates after surgery [18, 19]. These outcomes are a result of coordinated, multimodal, and multidisciplinary approaches to the care of a patient undergoing surgery.

Regarding oncology surgery, evaluation of the safety of ERAS has been limited. As enhanced recovery principles were largely initiated for patients undergoing colorectal surgery, much of the experience in the oncologic space has been in protocols for patients with colorectal cancer. Randomized clinical trials of patients undergoing colorectal surgery along with ERAS principles have resulted in a decrease in complication rates of 50% [20, 21]. However, efforts have been made to define the impact of ERAS on both short-term and long-term outcomes for patients undergoing oncologic surgery. In an evaluation of more than 1200 patients cared for along ERAS pathways across multiple surgical specialties from 2011 to 2016 at a large-volume cancer center, complication rates and LOS were significantly reduced as compared to patients cared for along non-ERAS pathways [18]. Specifically, patients managed on ERAS pathways had significantly reduced rates of surgical site infections (SSIs), wound complications, urinary tract infections (UTIs), and any severe complications [18]. Conclusions from many of these studies support a lower rate of perioperative complications following surgery if managed according to ERAS principles. In none of these studies did ERAS pose a risk of harm. In fact, ERAS may be one of the most impactful perioperative therapies, based largely on the fact that its strategies produce tremendous benefit without the risk of harm.

The reduction in surgical stress afforded by following ERAS principles allows patients to recover more rapidly and effectively; however, beyond endpoints such as LOS and complication rates is patient functional recovery [22]. Unfortunately, benchmarks for measuring the rapidity of recovery are lacking. An effective measure of functional recovery is to decipher the efficiency with which patients are moving onto planned adjuvant therapies, further interventions, or resumption of chronic therapies following surgery [23]. An example from oncologic surgery is the return to intended oncologic therapy (RIOT) concept, which is not only a valuable midterm quality metric in oncologic surgery, but also an effective measure to evaluate ERAS and rates of recovery [22–24]. Initial investigations into the RIOT concept in patients undergoing hepatic resection revealed a RIOT rate of 75% and a median time to RIOT of 42 days, which was improved to 86% and 36 days after internal quality improvement [23, 24]. After introduction of ERAS after liver surgery at our institution (termed ERILS), we found an astounding improvement in the rate of RIOT readiness to 95% at 21 postoperative days, which reinforced the ability of ERAS principles to return patients to functional baseline and beyond following surgery [25].

Efficiency

The benefits observed for patients managed according to ERAS principles translate to more efficient care, with reduced LOS and decreased complications, resulting in cost reductions. A systematic review and meta-analysis by Visioni and colleagues found that length of stay and complication rates were significantly reduced across 39 studies of non-colorectal abdominal surgical procedures, and that this translated to cost savings of over $5000 (USD) per patient [26]. Implementation of an ERAS for elective colorectal surgery across an entire provincial healthcare system in Canada resulted in a cost saving of between $2806 and $5898 (USD) per patient, largely due to decreased rates of complications and readmissions [27]. Further, Thiele and colleagues reported that implementation of an ERAS following colorectal surgery at a single academic center resulted in over $7000 (USD) direct cost saving per patient, translating to over $777,000 (USD) total savings across 109 patients. Moreover, patient-reported satisfaction scores improved significantly throughout the protocol implementation period [28]. The ability to deliver superior outcomes as previously described in this chapter, while decreasing costs, identifies ERAS as a major driver of improved surgical efficiency and overall value.

Maintaining adherence to protocols once implemented, as well as regular audit to allow for dynamic changes to optimize care pathways, is important for realization of the full potential of ERAS [29, 30]. Many aspects of ERAS are vulnerable to omission, likely due to the multidisciplinary approach to care, and compliance rates of many components of these pathways are incompletely reported in the surgical literature [31, 32]. Increasing protocol compliance was correlated with fewer complications and shorter LOS following elective colorectal cancer operations in more than 1500 patients from an international registry [31]. The benefit of adherence to increasing components of an ERAS following elective colorectal surgery was demonstrated in the Postoperative Outcomes Within Enhanced Recovery After Surgery Protocol (POWER) study, where an increase in adherence was associated with decreases in postoperative complications [33]. Specifically, patients with the highest adherence rates incurred approximately 65% less moderate-to-severe complications, overall complications, and almost 75% less risk of mortality as compared to low adherence rates [33]. It is possible that individual components of ERAS are not as effective in isolation, and that a synergistic response occurs with high adherence, thus highlighting the importance of protocol compliance.

Principles of Enhanced Recovery After Surgery Protocols

As previously mentioned, a modern ERAS approach to the surgical patient consists of four fundamental perioperative care principles underpinned by a foundation of effective patient education and engagement [34]. These "four pillars" include early feeding, early ambulation, goal-directed fluid therapy, and opiate-sparing analgesia, as seen in Fig. 17.1. Further considerations for inclusion within ERAS are discussed below.

Foundation: Patient Evaluation, Education, and Engagement

As with every patient being considered for operative intervention, a thorough preoperative evaluation is imperative. A complete history and physical examination are compulsory, including review of all comorbid conditions, prior surgical history, and current medications. If patients are undergoing surgery for oncologic indications, a thorough oncologic history and review of multimodal therapies, such as radiation, systemic cytotoxic/targeted/immunologic chemotherapies, and adjuvant therapy plans, should be reviewed and communicated in a multidisciplinary fashion.

Review of chronic comorbid conditions and potential intervention to correct medical deficits prior to planned surgery are important for quality of recovery. Particular attention should be paid to optimization of conditions leading to borderline operability. Using data from the American College of Surgeons National Surgical Quality Improvement Program, Kim and colleagues demonstrated that patients with borderline operability (age >75 years, dependent function, lung disease, ascites/varices, myocardial infarction, stroke, steroids, weight loss >10%, and/or sepsis) have a threefold higher mortality following hepatectomy [35]. Patient functional status should be evaluated and graded via reported outcome tools [36–40]. Identification of conditions that can be modified may be part of a coordinated "prehabilitation" program prior to elective surgery, such as smoking cessation, physical activity, and nutritional counseling. This allows for a greater preoperative "starting point" prior to undergoing a potentially stressful surgery (Fig. 17.2). In fact, prehabilitation as part of an operative plan along with ERAS is the subject of an ongoing clinical trial for patients undergoing surgical management of colorectal cancer [41].

Patient education and engagement are essential to the successful implementation of ERAS and for realization of maximal benefits of this approach to perioperative care. Patients should receive materials describing their proposed operations and expectations for inpatient care and length of hospital stay, including pain control and physical activity. Moreover, educational literature should be provided on ERAS principles and goals to ensure time for the patient and caregivers to align themselves with their expected recovery, as well as allow for ample time for questions. As with core ERAS principles, a multimodal approach to patient education reduces anxiety and improves compliance [42]. Consistent language and communication regarding expectations are important, including use of scripted telephone calls and education materials to improve outcomes [43].

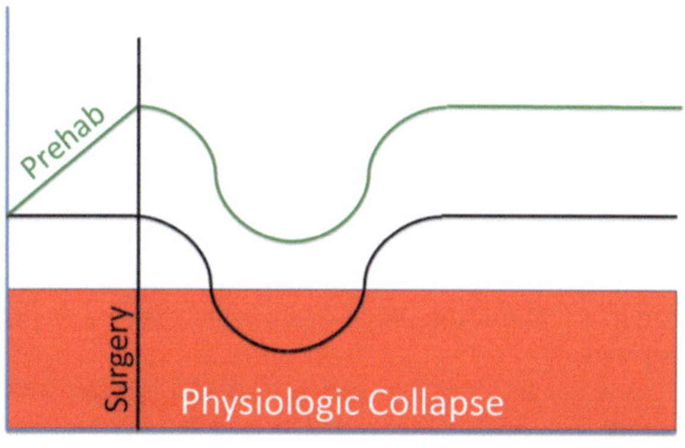

Fig. 17.2 Identification of conditions that can be modified may be part of a coordinated "prehabilitation" program prior to elective surgery, such as smoking cessation, physical activity, and nutritional counseling. This allows for a greater preoperative "starting point" prior to undergoing a potentially stressful surgery

Perioperative Nutrition and Early Feeding

A nutritional assessment prior to any elective surgery is extremely important to postoperative outcomes, and screening for nutritional detriments is imperative prior to any major surgery [44, 45]. Recent weight loss as well as obesity may need to be addressed prior to intervention. Measurement of nutritional indices, such as albumin, prealbumin, and ferritin, may give some indication as to the chronicity of malnutrition. In fact, an albumin <3.5 g/dL and prealbumin <18 mg/dL are associated with postoperative morbidity [46, 47]. Interestingly, the concepts of both sarcopenia and sarcopenic obesity are accepted contemporary measures of frailty and are associated with both postoperative morbidity and mortality [48]. Preoperative optimization of the patient's nutritional status is clearly associated with outcomes and may be an integral part of prehabilitation programs.

A key element of ERAS programs is the maintenance of homeostasis in efforts to limit the stress response after surgery and avoid catabolism. This, in turn, prevents protein degradation, preserves muscle function, and maintains cellular metabolism [49]. This reduces insulin resistance after tissue injury, allowing for adequate cellular function. Preoperative nutritional support helps achieve this; however, patients have historically endured prolonged periods of fasting immediately prior to elective operations (i.e., nil per os after midnight). Patients increasingly consume clear liquids up to 2 h prior to induction of anesthesia in accordance with the American Anesthesiologist's Association (ASA) guidelines, provided that there is no gastroduodenal impairment that would raise the risk for aspiration [50]. In fact, fasting for no more than 2 h for liquids and 6 h for solids preoperatively has been shown to be safe, and thus currently recommended prior to gastrointestinal surgery, provided that there is no gastroesophageal pathology [51]. Maintenance of euvolemia and prevention of fluid shifts begin in the preoperative setting and should continue.

Carbohydrate loading before surgery, such as consumption of carbohydrate-containing clear liquids up to 2 h prior to anesthesia induction, is a strong recommendation by the ERAS® Society [49, 52]. A systematic review of more than 1400 patients undergoing surgery in 17 randomized clinical trials found that preoperative carbohydrate loads significantly improved patient measures of comfort prior to surgery, as well as improved insulin resistance, while finding no adverse events related to the preoperative carbohydrate drink [53]. By maintaining the "fed" state, lipolysis and protein breakdown are suspended, energy stores are optimized, and thus glycogen storage is initiated, and thus the anabolism is initiated [52]. Benefits of preoperative carbohydrate loading include the aforementioned decrease in postoperative insulin resistance, patient discomfort, and improved healing [54–56]. A solution of 100 g of carbohydrates should be administered the evening prior to surgery and an additional 50 g solution given the morning of surgery, or alternatively complex commercial products are available (i.e., maltodextrin content and immune adjuvants).

A major factor in the success of ERAS is a fast-track return to a patient's preoperative diet. Most patients undergoing surgery will have no contraindications to at least clear liquids per os in the immediate postoperative period, and inclusion of protein-rich liquid drinks or shakes is recommended. For example, ERAS for patients undergoing complex operations such as liver resections or colorectal surgeries should be started on clear liquids upon return from the operating room [34, 57]. Patients should then advance their diets to regular by the second or third postoperative day; however, we do not recommend full-liquid diet as an intermediate because as many as 30% of patients may be lactose intolerant [34]. Further, we recommend that intravenous fluid replacement be only used if patients are unable to maintain euvolemia by oral intake and that maintenance intravenous fluids be discontinued once the patient consumes 600 mL of oral intake. Recently, use of the highly selective μ-receptor antagonist alvimopan (Entereg) has been incorporated into fast-track protocols for complex operations such as colorectal surgery. Although the evidence is mixed, some studies have shown improved recovery of intestinal function while not impacting analgesia [58]. Integration of the use of alvimopan into ERAS may be considered in select circumstances.

Goal-Directed Fluid Therapy

Historically, fluid management during complex operations involved the liberal use of fluids in all phases of care. Proponents of ERAS principles believe that this superfluous volume results in increased interstitial fluid, thus impeding recovery via decreased ambulation, weaning of supplemental oxygen, and tissue oxygenation [57]. Interestingly, one study has demonstrated that improvement in fluid administration practices alone decreased morbidity following major abdominal surgery by 50% [59]. Fluid administration on ERAS is best approached as goal directed on a continuum from preoperative to intraoperative and postoperative periods, with each being important to ensuring optimal outcomes.

Maintenance fluids are intended to replace urine output and insensible losses (i.e., perspiration, evaporation), and these must be limited in order to prevent fluid shift to the interstitium [60]. Hypervolemia results in increased hydrostatic pressure, leading to endothelial damage and release of endogenous mediators that alter vascular permeability, and thus fluid shifts to the interstitium [61]. This is commonly realized as increases in rates of postoperative ileus, likely as a result of edema of the gut wall, and results in increased rates of morbidity and length of hospital stay [62]. To prevent this, administration of maintenance fluid should focus on preserving preoperative patient weight in a "zero-balance" approach, thus eliminating excess salt and water [60].

There may be periods during complex operations when maintenance fluid approaches may not be sufficient to maintain euvolemia, such as during blood loss or acute volume loss. This results in a physiologic response with splanchnic vasoconstriction, leading to conservation of core tissue and organ perfusion. Traditional hemodynamic measurements such as heart rate and blood pressure are only indicators of potential need for fluid and are not adequate to measure response to volume [63]. These measurements should serve to trigger providers to consider intervention, such as a fluid challenge. In fact, response to a fluid challenge is an optimal method to dynamically assess true intravascular volume status [60].

Goal-directed fluid therapy (GDFT) focuses on optimizing measured stroke volume (SV) via dynamic parameters of volume status, such as stroke volume variation (SVV) and/or pulse pressure variation (PPV), and optimizing these with the appropriate amount, type, and timing of fluid therapy [34]. Patients may be highly responsive to fluid therapy if SVV or PPV is over 13% [60, 64]. Traditional static measures of systemic blood pressure, hemodynamic indices (i.e., central venous pressure, pulmonary capillary wedge pressure), and urine output may not be efficient and reliable measurements to guide appropriate fluid therapy, but again may alert providers to a need for fluid challenge. Stroke volume optimization via GDFT throughout the perioperative period has been shown to significantly decrease morbidity after major surgery in multiple trials [65, 66].

Opiate-Sparing Analgesia

Opioid medications have significant adverse effects that may act to inhibit or prolong return to homeostasis following surgery. In the gastrointestinal tract, opioids act to decrease gastric emptying and increase pyloric sphincter tone, which may result in nausea and vomiting. Blockade of peristalsis activated by luminal distention results in delayed small intestinal transit and paralytic ileus. Moreover, inhibition of ion channels and membrane hyperpolarization impair fluid and ion transport, resulting in further ileus and constipation, as well as abdominal distention.

Optimal pain management strategies within ERAS employ both a multimodal and multidisciplinary approach using an opiate-sparing strategy that begins preoperatively. Nonnarcotic adjunct combinations may be administered preemptively, such as oral pregabalin, gabapentin, NSAIDs (i.e., celecoxib), and acetaminophen. An important component of opiate-sparing approaches includes regional anesthesia techniques, such as neuraxial blocks and field blocks (i.e., transversus abdominus plane [TAP] blocks, quadratus lumborum [QL] blocks, and erector spinae [ES] blocks). The majority of guidelines published by the ERAS Society recommend pre-anesthesia multimodal nonnarcotic analgesia and regional anesthesia techniques to achieve an opiate-sparing pain management approach [13, 67–71].

Postoperative multimodal analgesia approaches are an imperative component of ERAS and pain management, and many types of pain medications may be used in parallel to minimize the need for opioids after surgery. Nonnarcotic adjuncts that may be used include neuromodulators (i.e., pregabalin), nonsteroidal anti-inflammatory drugs (COX-2 inhibitors, ibuprofen, Toradol), and potentially muscle-relaxing medications (methocarbamol). Other medication options exist, and many of these may be started in the preoperative setting. Nonnarcotic adjuncts should be started immediately preoperatively in order to allow for opioid minimization early after surgery. The goal of the team should be to balance narcotic minimization with a tolerable level of pain that allows for full activity and function.

The benefit of regional anesthetic techniques is to augment pain control and, in turn, reduce opioid need in the immediate postoperative period for patients following major surgery. The impact of regional anesthesia on opioid requirements has been demonstrated in multiple studies. For example, as compared to intravenous patient-controlled analgesia (IV-PCA), use of thoracic epidural anesthesia (TEA) is associated with an improved patient experience following major hepatobiliary surgery through improved pain control and less overall opioid use, without increasing length of stay or complications [72]. Moreover, use of TEA is associated with the lowest inpatient opioid use following pancreatectomy [73]. Randomized clinical trials of regional anesthesia techniques and their impact on opioid use following major surgery are ongoing, including the RESQU-Block Trial (NCT03745794), which includes a repeated or "rescue" QL block on the fourth postoperative day following pancreatectomy. Due to the potential for augmentation of patient pain experience and an opiate-sparing approach to pain control, regional anesthesia remains a cornerstone of ERAS.

Perioperative Antimicrobial Prophylaxis and SSI Prevention

The Surgical Care Improvement Project (SCIP) guidelines are part of an initiative by the Centers for Medicare and Medicaid Services (CMS) and the Centers for Disease Control and Prevention (CDC) aimed at reducing postoperative complications [74]. These guidelines are easily incorporated within an ERAS. Antimicrobial prophylaxis should be administered perioperatively to prevent SSI. Guideline-based prophylaxis should be administered less than 1 h prior to surgical incision for most patients and should be re-dosed as indicated during the operation to maintain adequate antimicrobial coverage [34, 75]. For patients undergoing operations that may result in intra-abdominal contamination, coverage for gram-negative and anaerobic organisms should be considered. Unless there is documented concern for confirmed source of infection that would require prolonged antimicrobial treatment, all prophylactic medications should be stopped within 24 h of the index operation.

Skin preparation prior to operative incision is imperative and aimed at reducing the amount of microorganisms residing on the skin that may contribute to SSI. Hair should be clipped, rather than shaved. Solutions commonly employed include povidone-iodine or chlorhexidine always combined with alcohol, which are commercially available.

Venous Thromboembolism Prophylaxis

Venous thromboembolism (VTE) following surgery results in substantial morbidity and mortality, and thus prevention of these adverse events contributes to the success of ERAS. Despite widely disseminated guidelines for prophylaxis against VTE, compliance remains suboptimal and VTE rates following surgery continue to be high [76–80]. Interventions such as graduated compression stockings and intermittent pneumatic compression/sequential compression devices (SCDs) should be placed prior to induction of anesthesia and discontinued once early ambulation occurs [81]. Appropriate anticoagulant VTE prophylaxis may include low-dose unfractionated heparin 5000 units subcutaneously every 8–12 h or low-molecular-weight heparin. For example, following liver surgery at MD Anderson Cancer Center, the first dose of VTE is unfractionated heparin once hemostasis is ensured, followed by conversion to daily subcutaneous enoxaparin for the remainder of the hospitalization. Typically, after oncologic resection, VTE prophylaxis is continued in the outpatient setting for 14–28 days postoperatively [34].

Early Ambulation

Early initiation of ambulation following surgery is a core component of ERAS pathways aimed at rapid return to homeostasis. Early ambulation may have great impact on return of gastrointestinal function and reduction of ileus, improved pulmonary function, and decreasing VTE. Limiting placement or early removal of surgical drains, catheters, IV tubing, and other devices may facilitate early ambulation and encourage patients to return to normal activity faster. For select patients, goals for mobility may be greatly augmented by early involvement of physical and occupational therapists.

Perioperative Opioid Use and Enhanced Recovery Protocols

Opioid Epidemic and Surgery

Opioid abuse has been at epidemic levels in the United States in recent times, with opioid overdose responsible for the majority of injury-related mortalities [82]. This has been largely fueled by a parallel rapid increase in opioid prescriptions over the same time period, which has led to chronic use and diversion [83–85]. Surgery contributes significantly to this crisis, as approximately 6–15% of opioid-naïve patients undergoing surgery will go on to use opioids beyond the perioperative period [86]. Surgeons and care providers managing patients after surgery must be aware of the adverse effects of opioid prescriptions after patients are discharged from the hospital. Perioperative pain management may impact long-term opioid use, thus highlighting the importance of ERAS principles in potentially stemming outpatient opioid need.

The concept of ERAS providing streamlined care and eliminating variation may greatly impact opioid use after surgery. There is wide variation and much provider bias in opioid prescribing in the perioperative setting, and in particular at discharge. This is a primary driver of excess opioids that leave the hospital setting, only to be available in the community, leading to chronic use and diversion. Following common general surgical procedures, Hill and colleagues found a large range in opioids prescribed, with the median number of pills prescribed for patients following the same procedure to have varied by a factor of 3 [87]. Even more shocking is that only 28% of opioid pills prescribed were actually taken, leaving one to understand the community burden of available opioids from postoperative prescriptions. Patient-centered opioid discharge prescribing strategies within ERAS may lead to dramatic decreases in outpatient opioid prescriptions, and thus limit excess medication.

Perioperative Opioids and Discharge Prescriptions

There is mounting evidence implicating inpatient opioid use or exposure as potential predictors of discharge opioid prescriptions and outpatient use. Opiate-sparing analgesia is a core pillar of ERAS, and thus identification of patients at risk for high opioid use may allow for interventions integrated within ERAS. Studies that characterize patterns of opioid use following surgery are imperative to effectively employ opioid-sparing approaches. In an attempt to decipher drivers of opioid use following pancreatectomy, we found that epidural use predicted the lowest opioid use, whereas having a preoperative opioid prescription, longer operative time, and longer LOS predicted the highest opioid use [73]. Studies such as this reveal the great variation in opioid use by our patients after surgery, and that there are relatively few patient factors that drive opioid administration, and highlight the great need for an objective approach to opioid prescription while in the hospital.

A major contributor to the opioid epidemic is overprescription, as the majority of opioids abused in the community were diverted from a friend or relative's prescription [88]. Moreover, overprescription has been shown to occur after surgery, and this is in part related to increased amounts of opioids being prescribed for various surgeries in recent times [87, 89, 90]. Interestingly, despite 36% of patients using zero opioids in the final 24 hours of inpatient stay following surgery, Chen and colleagues found that almost half of these patients received opioids at discharge anyway [91]. We confirmed this following pancreatectomy but to a great degree, with 36% of patients using zero opioids in their final 24 h of hospitalization, but shockingly 91% of these patients received opioids at discharge [92]. Moreover, opioid prescriptions at discharge following pancreatectomy were impacted mostly by which team of providers care for the patient while in the hospital, rather than patient factors [92]. This revealed that discharge opioid prescriptions have been historically based upon provider bias, rather than actual measures of patient need. Implementation of opioid-sparing analgesia approaches as part of an ERAS may have great impact on outpatient opioid use, particularly if discharge prescriptions are objectively based on inpatient use by patients.

ERAS and Outpatient Opioids

In the era of ERAS that has revolutionized the perioperative care of the surgery patient, outcomes have been improved by coordinated and evidence-based approaches. These ERAS principles have led to decreased opioid use by patients postoperatively, by including regional anesthetic techniques and multimodal analgesia. However, the impact that ERAS has on opioid prescriptions at discharge and outpatient use is underreported and is a potential benefit of ERAS that may extend beyond the immediate postoperative period. We believe that to reach maximal potential on the full recovery of the surgical patient, the opioid-sparing pillar of ERAS should continue well beyond inpatient hospitalization.

Despite this, reports on the impact of ERAS on opioid discharge prescriptions have been mixed. Efforts to determine the impact of ERAS on opioid prescriptions at discharge have been reported following hepatobiliary surgery. Strategies to limit excess opioid use following discharge from hepatobiliary surgery are complex, given the magnitude of these operations, their often large open approaches, and need for further adjuvant treatment modalities after surgery [93]. Compared to traditional perioperative management, Lillemoe and colleagues found that patients managed on ERAS pathways following liver surgery were less likely to be discharged with a traditional opioid prescription and were much less likely to require opioids at their initial postoperative clinic visit [93]. Importantly, these patients reported similar pain scores as patients cared for along traditional recovery pathways. However, Brandal and colleagues found no effect of ERAS on opioid prescriptions for patients following colectomy despite decreased opioid need while inpatient [94]. The fact that the great majority of patients in their study who had low inpatient opioid use still received an opioid prescription at discharge highlights the need for objective discharge prescription practices integrated within ERAS. Standardization of discharge prescriptions via evidence-based approaches has been successful on large scales, with recent reports from Englesbe and colleagues from the Michigan Opioid Prescribing Engagement Network and Michigan Surgical Quality Collaborative regarding their successful implementation of statewide opioid prescribing guidelines [95]. After implementation of evidence-based prescribing guidelines, they found a significant decrease in discharge opioid prescriptions without any clinically relevant decrease in pain scores. This highlights the importance of patient-centered, evidence-based practices as part of larger patient care pathways after surgery.

Conclusion

Coordinated, efficient, multidisciplinary perioperative care via ERAS has revolutionized many surgical disciplines. The core principles of ERAS, such as the "four pillars," have resulted in improved safety and efficiency following both routine and complex operations. Moreover, ERAS has continued potential to positively impact patient recovery beyond the immediate postoperative period, such as decreased outpatient opioid use. The systematic approach to perioperative care delineated by ERAS, beginning with preoperative patient education and expectations, continues to improve not only surgical safety and efficiency, but also patient and provider satisfaction.

References

1. Engelman RM, Rousou JA, Flack JE 3rd, Deaton DW, Humphrey CB, Ellison LH, et al. Fast-track recovery of the coronary bypass patient. Ann Thorac Surg. 1994;58(6):1742–6.
2. Kehlet H. Multimodal approach to control postoperative pathophysiology and rehabilitation. Br J Anaesth. 1997;78(5):606–17.
3. Nygren J, Hausel J, Kehlet H, Revhaug A, Lassen K, Dejong C, et al. A comparison in five European Centres of case mix, clinical management and outcomes following either conventional or fast-track perioperative care in colorectal surgery. Clin Nutr. 2005;24(3):455–61.
4. Ljungqvist O, Scott M, Fearon KC. Enhanced recovery after surgery: a review. JAMA Surg. 2017;152(3):292–8.
5. Bokey EL, Chapuis PH, Fung C, Hughes WJ, Koorey SG, Brewer D, et al. Postoperative morbidity and mortality following resection of the colon and rectum for cancer. Dis Colon Rectum. 1995;38(5):480–6; discussion 6–7.
6. Schoetz DJ Jr, Bockler M, Rosenblatt MS, Malhotra S, Roberts PL, Murray JJ, et al. "Ideal" length of stay after colectomy: whose ideal? Dis Colon Rectum. 1997;40(7):806–10.
7. Bradshaw BG, Liu SS, Thirlby RC. Standardized perioperative care protocols and reduced length of stay after colon surgery. J Am Coll Surg. 1998;186(5):501–6.

8. Khoo CK, Vickery CJ, Forsyth N, Vinall NS, Eyre-Brook IA. A prospective randomized controlled trial of multimodal perioperative management protocol in patients undergoing elective colorectal resection for cancer. Ann Surg. 2007;245(6):867–72.
9. Bardram L, Funch-Jensen P, Jensen P, Crawford ME, Kehlet H. Recovery after laparoscopic colonic surgery with epidural analgesia, and early oral nutrition and mobilisation. Lancet. 1995;345(8952):763–4.
10. Fearon KC, Ljungqvist O, Von Meyenfeldt M, Revhaug A, Dejong CH, Lassen K, et al. Enhanced recovery after surgery: a consensus review of clinical care for patients undergoing colonic resection. Clin Nutr. 2005;24(3):466–77.
11. Lassen K, Soop M, Nygren J, Cox PB, Hendry PO, Spies C, et al. Consensus review of optimal perioperative care in colorectal surgery: enhanced recovery after surgery (ERAS) group recommendations. Arch Surg. 2009;144(10):961–9.
12. Lassen K, Coolsen MM, Slim K, Carli F, de Aguilar-Nascimento JE, Schafer M, et al. Guidelines for perioperative care for pancreaticoduodenectomy: enhanced recovery after surgery (ERAS®) society recommendations. Clin Nutr. 2012;31(6):817–30.
13. Melloul E, Hubner M, Scott M, Snowden C, Prentis J, Dejong CH, et al. Guidelines for perioperative care for liver surgery: enhanced recovery after surgery (ERAS) society recommendations. World J Surg. 2016;40(10):2425–40.
14. Thorell A, MacCormick AD, Awad S, Reynolds N, Roulin D, Demartines N, et al. Guidelines for perioperative care in bariatric surgery: enhanced recovery after surgery (ERAS) society recommendations. World J Surg. 2016;40(9):2065–83.
15. Nelson G, Altman AD, Nick A, Meyer LA, Ramirez PT, Achtari C, et al. Guidelines for pre- and intra-operative care in gynecologic/oncology surgery: Enhanced Recovery After Surgery (ERAS®) Society recommendations—Part I. Gynecol Oncol. 2016;140(2):313–22.
16. Mortensen K, Nilsson M, Slim K, Schafer M, Mariette C, Braga M, et al. Consensus guidelines for enhanced recovery after gastrectomy: enhanced recovery after surgery (ERAS®) society recommendations. Br J Surg. 2014;101(10):1209–29.
17. Manso M, Schmelz J, Aloia T. ERAS-anticipated outcomes and realistic goals. J Surg Oncol. 2017;116(5):570–7.
18. Marcus RK, Lillemoe HA, Rice DC, Mena G, Bednarski BK, Speer BB, et al. Determining the safety and efficacy of enhanced recovery protocols in major oncologic surgery: an institutional NSQIP analysis. Ann Surg Oncol. 2019;26(3):782–90.
19. Gustafsson UO, Hausel J, Thorell A, Ljungqvist O, Soop M, Nygren J, et al. Adherence to the enhanced recovery after surgery protocol and outcomes after colorectal cancer surgery. Arch Surg. 2011;146(5):571–7.
20. Varadhan KK, Neal KR, Dejong CH, Fearon KC, Ljungqvist O, Lobo DN. The enhanced recovery after surgery (ERAS) pathway for patients undergoing major elective open colorectal surgery: a meta-analysis of randomized controlled trials. Clin Nutr. 2010;29(4):434–40.
21. Greco M, Capretti G, Beretta L, Gemma M, Pecorelli N, Braga M. Enhanced recovery program in colorectal surgery: a meta-analysis of randomized controlled trials. World J Surg. 2014;38(6):1531–41.
22. Lillemoe HA, Marcus RK, Kim BJ, Narula N, Davis CH, Aloia TA. Detours on the road to recovery: what factors delay readiness to return to intended oncologic therapy (RIOT) after liver resection for malignancy? J Gastrointest Surg. 2019;23(12):2362–71.
23. Kim BJ, Caudle AS, Gottumukkala V, Aloia TA. The impact of postoperative complications on a timely return to intended oncologic therapy (RIOT): the role of enhanced recovery in the cancer journey. Int Anesthesiol Clin. 2016;54(4):e33–46.
24. Aloia TA, Zimmitti G, Conrad C, Gottumukalla V, Kopetz S, Vauthey JN. Return to intended oncologic treatment (RIOT): a novel metric for evaluating the quality of oncosurgical therapy for malignancy. J Surg Oncol. 2014;110(2):107–14.
25. Day RW, Cleeland CS, Wang XS, Fielder S, Calhoun J, Conrad C, et al. Patient-reported outcomes accurately measure the value of an enhanced recovery program in liver surgery. J Am Coll Surg 2015;221(6):1023–30, e1–2.

26. Visioni A, Shah R, Gabriel E, Attwood K, Kukar M, Nurkin S. Enhanced recovery after surgery for noncolorectal surgery?: a systematic review and meta-analysis of major abdominal surgery. Ann Surg. 2018;267(1):57–65.
27. Nelson G, Kiyang LN, Crumley ET, Chuck A, Nguyen T, Faris P, et al. Implementation of enhanced recovery after surgery (ERAS) across a provincial healthcare system: the ERAS Alberta colorectal surgery experience. World J Surg. 2016;40(5):1092–103.
28. Thiele RH, Rea KM, Turrentine FE, Friel CM, Hassinger TE, McMurry TL, et al. Standardization of care: impact of an enhanced recovery protocol on length of stay, complications, and direct costs after colorectal surgery. J Am Coll Surg. 2015;220(4):430–43.
29. Aloia TA, Keller DS, Kowalski RB, Lin H, Luciano MM, Myers JA, et al. Enhanced recovery program implementation: an evidence-based review of the art and the science. Surg Endosc. 2019;33(11):3833–41.
30. Luciano MM, Aloia TA, Brett JF 4 ways to make evidence-based practice the norm in health care. Harvard Bus Rev; 2019. https://hbr.org/2019/08/4-ways-to-make-evidence-based-practice-the-norm-in-health-care
31. Group EC. The impact of enhanced recovery protocol compliance on elective colorectal cancer resection: results from an international registry. Ann Surg. 2015;261(6):1153–9.
32. Day RW, Fielder S, Calhoun J, Kehlet H, Gottumukkala V, Aloia TA. Incomplete reporting of enhanced recovery elements and its impact on achieving quality improvement. Br J Surg. 2015;102(13):1594–602.
33. Ripolles-Melchor J, Ramirez-Rodriguez JM, Casans-Frances R, Aldecoa C, Abad-Motos A, Logrono-Egea M, et al. Association between use of enhanced recovery after surgery protocol and postoperative complications in colorectal surgery: the postoperative outcomes within enhanced recovery after surgery protocol (POWER) study. JAMA Surg. 2019;154(8):725–36.
34. Kim BJ, Aloia TA. What is "enhanced recovery," and how can I do it? J Gastrointest Surg. 2018;22(1):164–71.
35. Kim BJ, Tzeng CD, Cooper AB, Vauthey JN, Aloia TA. Borderline operability in hepatectomy patients is associated with higher rates of failure to rescue after severe complications. J Surg Oncol. 2017;115(3):337–43.
36. Karnofsky DA. Cancer chemotherapeutic agents. CA Cancer J Clin. 1964;14:67–72.
37. Cleeland CS, Mendoza TR, Wang XS, Chou C, Harle MT, Morrissey M, et al. Assessing symptom distress in cancer patients: the M.D. Anderson symptom inventory. Cancer. 2000;89(7):1634–46.
38. Carey EJ, Steidley DE, Aqel BA, Byrne TJ, Mekeel KL, Rakela J, et al. Six-minute walk distance predicts mortality in liver transplant candidates. Liver Transplant. 2010;16(12):1373–8.
39. Hofheinz M, Mibs M. The prognostic validity of the timed up and go test with a dual task for predicting the risk of falls in the elderly. Gerontol Geriatr Med. 2016;2:2333721416637798.
40. Nordin E, Lindelof N, Rosendahl E, Jensen J, Lundin-Olsson L. Prognostic validity of the timed up-and-go test, a modified get-up-and-go test, staff's global judgement and fall history in evaluating fall risk in residential care facilities. Age Ageing. 2008;37(4):442–8.
41. van Rooijen S, Carli F, Dalton S, Thomas G, Bojesen R, Le Guen M, et al. Multimodal prehabilitation in colorectal cancer patients to improve functional capacity and reduce postoperative complications: the first international randomized controlled trial for multimodal prehabilitation. BMC Cancer. 2019;19(1):98.
42. Granziera E, Guglieri I, Del Bianco P, Capovilla E, Dona B, Ciccarese AA, et al. A multidisciplinary approach to improve preoperative understanding and reduce anxiety: a randomised study. Eur J Anaesthesiol. 2013;30(12):734–42.
43. Cavallaro PM, Milch H, Savitt L, Hodin RA, Rattner DW, Berger DL, et al. Addition of a scripted pre-operative patient education module to an existing ERAS pathway further reduces length of stay. Am J Surg. 2018;216(4):652–7.
44. Weimann A, Braga M, Harsanyi L, Laviano A, Ljungqvist O, Soeters P, et al. ESPEN guidelines on enteral nutrition: surgery including organ transplantation. Clin Nutr. 2006;25(2):224–44.
45. Guenter P, Robinson L, DiMaria-Ghalili RA, Lyman B, Steiger E, Winkler MF. Development of sustain: A.S.P.E.N.'s national patient registry for nutrition care. J Parenter Enter Nutr. 2012;36(4):399–406.

46. Djaladat H, Bruins HM, Miranda G, Cai J, Skinner EC, Daneshmand S. The association of preoperative serum albumin level and American Society of Anesthesiologists (ASA) score on early complications and survival of patients undergoing radical cystectomy for urothelial bladder cancer. BJU Int. 2014;113(6):887–93.
47. Lucas DJ, Haider A, Haut E, Dodson R, Wolfgang CL, Ahuja N, et al. Assessing readmission after general, vascular, and thoracic surgery using ACS-NSQIP. Ann Surg. 2013;258(3):430–9.
48. Wagner D, DeMarco MM, Amini N, Buttner S, Segev D, Gani F, et al. Role of frailty and sarcopenia in predicting outcomes among patients undergoing gastrointestinal surgery. World J Gastrointest Surg. 2016;8(1):27–40.
49. Ljungqvist O, Jonathan E. Rhoads lecture 2011: insulin resistance and enhanced recovery after surgery. J Parenter Enter Nutr. 2012;36(4):389–98.
50. Brady M, Kinn S, Stuart P. Preoperative fasting for adults to prevent perioperative complications. Cochrane Database Syst Rev. 2003;(4):CD004423.
51. Gustafsson UO, Scott MJ, Schwenk W, Demartines N, Roulin D, Francis N, et al. Guidelines for perioperative care in elective colonic surgery: enhanced recovery after surgery (ERAS®) society recommendations. World J Surg. 2013;37(2):259–84.
52. Pogatschnik C, Steiger E. Review of preoperative carbohydrate loading. Nutr Clin Pract. 2015;30(5):660–4.
53. Bilku DK, Dennison AR, Hall TC, Metcalfe MS, Garcea G. Role of preoperative carbohydrate loading: a systematic review. Ann R Coll Surg Engl. 2014;96(1):15–22.
54. Nygren J, Thorell A, Ljungqvist O. Preoperative oral carbohydrate nutrition: an update. Curr Opin Clin Nutr Metab Care. 2001;4(4):255–9.
55. Hausel J, Nygren J, Lagerkranser M, Hellstrom PM, Hammarqvist F, Almstrom C, et al. A carbohydrate-rich drink reduces preoperative discomfort in elective surgery patients. Anesth Analg. 2001;93(5):1344–50.
56. Svanfeldt M, Thorell A, Hausel J, Soop M, Rooyackers O, Nygren J, et al. Randomized clinical trial of the effect of preoperative oral carbohydrate treatment on postoperative whole-body protein and glucose kinetics. Br J Surg. 2007;94(11):1342–50.
57. Chestovich PJ, Lin AY, Yoo J. Fast-track pathways in colorectal surgery. Surg Clin North Am. 2013;93(1):21–32.
58. Curran MP, Robins GW, Scott LJ, Perry CM. Alvimopan. Drugs. 2008;68(14):2011–9.
59. Brandstrup B, Tonnesen H, Beier-Holgersen R, Hjortso E, Ording H, Lindorff-Larsen K, et al. Effects of intravenous fluid restriction on postoperative complications: comparison of two perioperative fluid regimens: a randomized assessor-blinded multicenter trial. Ann Surg. 2003;238(5):641–8.
60. Miller TE, Roche AM, Mythen M. Fluid management and goal-directed therapy as an adjunct to enhanced recovery after surgery (ERAS). Can J Anaesth. 2015;62(2):158–68.
61. Chappell D, Jacob M, Hofmann-Kiefer K, Conzen P, Rehm M. A rational approach to perioperative fluid management. Anesthesiology. 2008;109(4):723–40.
62. Lobo DN, Bostock KA, Neal KR, Perkins AC, Rowlands BJ, Allison SP. Effect of salt and water balance on recovery of gastrointestinal function after elective colonic resection: a randomised controlled trial. Lancet. 2002;359(9320):1812–8.
63. Bundgaard-Nielsen M, Holte K, Secher NH, Kehlet H. Monitoring of peri-operative fluid administration by individualized goal-directed therapy. Acta Anaesthesiol Scand. 2007;51(3):331–40.
64. Marik PE, Cavallazzi R, Vasu T, Hirani A. Dynamic changes in arterial waveform derived variables and fluid responsiveness in mechanically ventilated patients: a systematic review of the literature. Crit Care Med. 2009;37(9):2642–7.
65. Roche AM, Miller TE, Gan TJ. Goal-directed fluid management with trans-oesophageal Doppler. Best Pract Res Clin Anaesthesiol. 2009;23(3):327–34.
66. Miller TE, Roche AM, Gan TJ. Poor adoption of hemodynamic optimization during major surgery: are we practicing substandard care? Anesth Analg. 2011;112(6):1274–6.
67. Gustafsson UO, Scott MJ, Hubner M, Nygren J, Demartines N, Francis N, et al. Guidelines for perioperative care in elective colorectal surgery: Enhanced Recovery After Surgery (ERAS®) Society recommendations: 2018. World J Surg. 2019;43(3):659–95.

68. Engelman DT, Ben Ali W, Williams JB, Perrault LP, Reddy VS, Arora RC, et al. Guidelines for perioperative care in cardiac surgery: enhanced recovery after surgery society recommendations. JAMA Surg. 2019;154(8):755–66.
69. Batchelor TJP, Rasburn NJ, Abdelnour-Berchtold E, Brunelli A, Cerfolio RJ, Gonzalez M, et al. Guidelines for enhanced recovery after lung surgery: recommendations of the Enhanced Recovery After Surgery (ERAS®) Society and the European Society of Thoracic Surgeons (ESTS). Eur J Cardiothorac Surg. 2019;55(1):91–115.
70. Temple-Oberle C, Shea-Budgell MA, Tan M, Semple JL, Schrag C, Barreto M, et al. Consensus review of optimal perioperative care in breast reconstruction: Enhanced Recovery after Surgery (ERAS) Society recommendations. Plast Reconstr Surg. 2017;139(5):1056e–71e.
71. Nelson G, Bakkum-Gamez J, Kalogera E, Glaser G, Altman A, Meyer LA, et al. Guidelines for perioperative care in gynecologic/oncology: Enhanced Recovery After Surgery (ERAS) Society recommendations-2019 update. Int J Gynecol Cancer. 2019;29(4):651–68.
72. Aloia TA, Kim BJ, Segraves-Chun YS, Cata JP, Truty MJ, Shi Q, et al. A randomized controlled trial of postoperative thoracic epidural analgesia versus intravenous patient-controlled analgesia after major hepatopancreatobiliary surgery. Ann Surg. 2017;266(3):545–54.
73. Newhook TE, Dewhurst WL, Vreeland TJ, Wang X, Soliz J, Speer BB, et al. Inpatient opioid use after pancreatectomy: opportunities for reducing initial opioid exposure in cancer surgery patients. Ann Surg Oncol. 2019;26:3428.
74. Jones RS, Brown C, Opelka F. Surgeon compensation: "pay for performance," the American College of Surgeons National Surgical Quality Improvement Program, the Surgical Care Improvement Program, and other considerations. Surgery. 2005;138(5):829–36.
75. Bratzler DW, Houck PM. Surgical infection prevention guideline writers W. antimicrobial prophylaxis for surgery: an advisory statement from the National Surgical Infection Prevention Project. Am J Surg. 2005;189(4):395–404.
76. Aloia TA, Geerts WH, Clary BM, Day RW, Hemming AW, D'Albuquerque LC, et al. Venous thromboembolism prophylaxis in liver surgery. J Gastrointest Surg. 2016;20(1):221–9.
77. Bergqvist D, Agnelli G, Cohen AT, Eldor A, Nilsson PE, Le Moigne-Amrani A, et al. Duration of prophylaxis against venous thromboembolism with enoxaparin after surgery for cancer. N Engl J Med. 2002;346(13):975–80.
78. Gould MK, Garcia DA, Wren SM, Karanicolas PJ, Arcelus JI, Heit JA, et al. Prevention of VTE in nonorthopedic surgical patients: antithrombotic therapy and prevention of thrombosis, 9th ed: American College of Chest Physicians evidence-based clinical practice guidelines. Chest. 2012;141(2 Suppl):e227S–e77S.
79. Tzeng CW, Curley SA, Vauthey JN, Aloia TA. Distinct predictors of pre- versus post-discharge venous thromboembolism after hepatectomy: analysis of 7621 NSQIP patients. HPB (Oxford). 2013;15(10):773–80.
80. Bellini G, Teng A, Kotecha N, Sutton E, Yang CK, Passeri M, et al. The identification of risk factors for venous thromboembolism in gastrointestinal oncologic surgery. J Surg Res. 2016;205(2):279–85.
81. Ho KM, Tan JA. Stratified meta-analysis of intermittent pneumatic compression of the lower limbs to prevent venous thromboembolism in hospitalized patients. Circulation. 2013;128(9):1003–20.
82. Chen LH, Hedegaard H, Warner M. Drug-poisoning deaths involving opioid analgesics: United States, 1999–2011. NCHS Data Brief. 2014;166:1–8.
83. Bicket MC, Long JJ, Pronovost PJ, Alexander GC, Wu CL. Prescription opioid analgesics commonly unused after surgery: a systematic review. JAMA Surg. 2017;152(11):1066–71.
84. Feinberg AE, Chesney TR, Srikandarajah S, Acuna SA, McLeod RS, Best Practice in Surgery G. Opioid use after discharge in postoperative patients: a systematic review. Ann Surg. 2018;267(6):1056–62.
85. Dart RC, Severtson SG, Bucher-Bartelson B. Trends in opioid analgesic abuse and mortality in the United States. N Engl J Med. 2015;372(16):1573–4.

86. Clarke H, Soneji N, Ko DT, Yun L, Wijeysundera DN. Rates and risk factors for prolonged opioid use after major surgery: population based cohort study. BMJ. 2014;348:g1251.
87. Hill MV, McMahon ML, Stucke RS, Barth RJ Jr. Wide variation and excessive dosage of opioid prescriptions for common general surgical procedures. Ann Surg. 2017;265(4):709–14.
88. Jones CM, Paulozzi LJ, Mack KA. Sources of prescription opioid pain relievers by frequency of past-year nonmedical use United States, 2008-2011. JAMA Intern Med. 2014;174(5):802–3.
89. Bates C, Laciak R, Southwick A, Bishoff J. Overprescription of postoperative narcotics: a look at postoperative pain medication delivery, consumption and disposal in urological practice. J Urol. 2011;185(2):551–5.
90. Wunsch H, Wijeysundera DN, Passarella MA, Neuman MD. Opioids prescribed after low-risk surgical procedures in the United States, 2004-2012. JAMA. 2016;315(15):1654–7.
91. Chen EY, Marcantonio A, Tornetta P 3rd. Correlation between 24-hour predischarge opioid use and amount of opioids prescribed at hospital discharge. JAMA Surg. 2018;153(2):e174859.
92. Newhook TE, Vreeland TJ, Dewhurst WL, Wang X, Prakash L, Feng C, et al. Clinical factors associated with practice variation in discharge opioid prescriptions after pancreatectomy. Ann Surg. 2020;272(1):163–9.
93. Lillemoe HA, Marcus RK, Day RW, Kim BJ, Narula N, Davis CH, et al. Enhanced recovery in liver surgery decreases postoperative outpatient use of opioids. Surgery. 2019;166(1):22–7.
94. Brandal D, Keller MS, Lee C, Grogan T, Fujimoto Y, Gricourt Y, et al. Impact of enhanced recovery after surgery and opioid-free anesthesia on opioid prescriptions at discharge from the hospital: a historical-prospective study. Anesth Analg. 2017;125(5):1784–92.
95. Vu JV, Howard RA, Gunaseelan V, Brummett CM, Waljee JF, Englesbe MJ. Statewide implementation of postoperative opioid prescribing guidelines. N Engl J Med. 2019;381(7):680–2.

"I Can't Ventilate!" Intraoperative Anesthesia Safety Events and Airway Management

18

Marwan Sarkis Rizk, Sarada Eleswarpu,
and Chakib Maurice Ayoub

Introduction

Airway catastrophes and hypoxia have been identified as the leading causes of neurological injury and death during anesthesia or resuscitation. In the American Society of Anesthesiology Closed Claims Analysis, failure to oxygenate patients with respiratory failure was associated with major morbidity and mortality [1]. Difficult airway management (DAM) is important and critical.

For its latest practice guidelines, the American Society of Anesthesiologists defines a difficult airway as "a clinical situation in which a conventionally trained anesthesiologist experiences difficulty with face mask ventilation of the upper airway, difficulty with tracheal intubation, or both" [2]. Planning and preparedness in these situations can save lives, and there is advocacy for an algorithm-based strategy. Many international bodies such as the American Society of Anesthesiologists, European Resuscitation Council, and Difficult Airway Society have developed recommendations and algorithms that facilitate a basic pathway for the management of difficult airway.

It is crucial that all stakeholders involved in patient airway management be familiar with the techniques and tools needed to provide adequate oxygenation [3]. The literature provides insights into the various types of protocols, advanced airway devices [4, 5], and availability of such equipment in different countries [6, 7]. The important role of simulators to acquire and maintain skills in difficult airway management is also widely established [8]. This chapter focuses on the organization of resource and staff during catastrophic airway situations.

M. S. Rizk (✉)
Department of Anesthesiology, American University of Beirut, Beirut, Lebanon
e-mail: mr04@aub.edu.lb

S. Eleswarpu · C. M. Ayoub
Department of Anesthesiology, Duke University school of Medicine, Durham, NC, USA

J. J. Hoballah et al. (eds.), *Principles of Perioperative Safety and Efficiency*,
https://doi.org/10.1007/978-3-031-41089-5_18

Difficult Airway Management (DAM): Key Factors

Current clinical practices based on established guidelines emphasize airway evaluation, basic preparation, and algorithm-based strategies for intubation. Respiratory failure can be caused by many reasons, and it is important that non-patient factors are also acknowledged. If not addressed, these factors can present a risk that could complicate airway management and threaten patient safety [9, 10].

"Complexity factors"—a term that is commonly used to describe factors contributing to the complexity of a procedure and includes experience, time pressure, available equipment, position, location, and human factors—should be identified and considered [11]. In the context of difficult airway, complexity factors encompass one or more of the following adverse outcomes: failures in technique and equipment; wrong head position; side effects of certain drugs; and pathological airway obstruction.

The possibility of difficult airway occurring is a risk if underlying causes that are contributing factors are not addressed. For example, obstructive sleep apnea patients constitute a recurring risk unless the pharyngeal pathology is corrected [12]. The depth of anesthesia can also play a significant role in precipitating a difficult airway scenario or securing a safe airway; laryngeal spasm due to light anesthesia may result in difficult mask ventilation (DMV), while adequate anesthesia depth will likely result in easy mask ventilation (MV) [13]. "Composite failure" of airway management is another prominent observation from previous studies: a phenomenon in which if one airway management technique is difficult or fails, the chance of alternative techniques being difficult or failing is significantly higher [14].

Emergency Conditions

Airway management is sensitive to both context and time; it is influenced by the clinical condition of the patient, physician expertise, urgency of the situation, and the environment in which the procedure takes place [15].

Intubating conditions fluctuate with changes in the clinical picture as well as environmental context. For example, a patient who is known to be an easy intubation may become "difficult" when presenting in septic shock with a low oxygen saturation to a remote hospital that has limited resources. If this same patient was in an intensive care unit in a busy metropolitan hospital, the availability of more resources and experienced providers would influence the approach to this patient's airway management. While preparing for a challenging intubation, the most experienced provider should be performing the intubation to minimize adverse events. The clinical picture can also evolve, often due to factors including time delay, worsening of the disease pathology, or tiring out after a period of increased work of breathing. For example, a patient with an epiglottitis may be able to protect the native airway upon initial presentation to a hospital; over time, the patient may become tired due to a period of increased work of breathing and may require immediate establishment of a secured airway. It is the responsibility of the anesthesiologist to continuously monitor patients and readjust the strategy accordingly.

A pitfall to avoid during a challenging difficult airway situation is "plan continuation error," which is a validated detrimental factor in aviation crashes [16]. The initial airway management plan, seemingly clear and rock solid in the beginning, could prove inapplicable as the circumstances change. For example, if a tumor starts bleeding during intubation, the view of a video laryngoscope or fiber-optic bronchoscope will be obscured and the physician may have to use another device that does not rely on a camera for securing the airway. It is crucial that the physician does not ignore the warning signs and adapts his or her strategy to the changing dynamics of the situation to avoid adverse events. Experience and training raise awareness of plan continuation error and avert any potential hazards.

Operator Conditions

Mask ventilation (MV) is a basic technique for providing oxygenation before intubation. Prompt diagnosis of difficult mask ventilation (DMV) could maximize risk management strategy and avoid catastrophic complications. Most operators rely on their subjective assessments such as thoracic movement and resistance of the anesthetic bag. In the literature, DMV is interpreted as inadequate mask seal, increased airway resistance, and decreased respiratory compliance. Clinical skills can be taught to address difficulties in each of these categories [17].

Elling et al. showed that more than 50% of emergency medical technicians were not able to ventilate a mannequin, and De Regge et al. showed that around 84% of emergency room nurses were not able to adequately perform mask ventilation [18, 19]. The dexterity of face mask ventilation is acquired through proper training and maintained subsequently by daily practice. Learning curves are more rapidly acquired and less variable for mask ventilation than for tracheal intubation. Komatsu et al. showed that novice interns reached a 20% failure rate or better after a median of 25 procedures [20]. Davidovic et al. showed that trainee participants in a pediatric context demonstrated improved tidal volumes and inspiratory pressures when practicing two-person compared to one-person MV [21]. Cocucci et al. showed that training accurate respiratory rates during pediatric MV can be improved with the use of a metronome [22].

Simple maneuvers might be used to achieve a tight seal in patients with distorted anatomy. Examples include inverting the face mask over a cast nose or keeping the dentures in edentulous patients [23]. In obese patients with relatively large facial structures, it is recommended to use both hands; as with only one hand, it is practically difficult to appropriately perform airway maneuvers including mouth opening. After failed intubation during rapid-sequence intubation, inadequately applied cricoid pressure may induce airway obstruction and result in DAM [24].

Equipment Conditions

During an emergency airway situation, time is of major importance whether the patient is difficult to intubate or is difficult to ventilate. The location and storage of equipment in operating rooms are important for easy and quick accessibility. Storing all the necessary equipment in a designated "difficult airway cart" (DAC) will save time and effort when an emergency occurs. It is recommended that the DAC should include a jet ventilator, fiber-optic bronchoscope, intubating stylet, video laryngoscope, intubating laryngeal mask airway, Combitube, various laryngoscope blades (i.e., Miller and Macintosh), an articulating laryngoscope, and different sizes of oropharyngeal and nasopharyngeal airways (OPAs and NPAs).

The DAC drives efficiency in all the units where intubations are frequently performed, i.e., emergency room (ER), intensive care unit (ICU), and operating room (OR). It is also very effective in areas outside the general operating room where advanced airway equipment may not be readily available for surgical use.

The availability of a DAC with many new alternative airway devices, adoption of the ASA difficult airway algorithm, and better monitoring techniques have resulted in safer airway management practices and reduced the incidence of these serious complications [25, 26].

Patient Conditions

Head Position

Suboptimal head and neck positioning may lead to DAM [27]. The sniffing position increases the pharyngeal space, which may render MV more efficient [28, 29]. Neck flexion, head extension, chin lift, and jaw thrust (the triple maneuver) are important simple techniques to increase pharyngeal patency.

Obesity

Obesity is recognized as one of the risk factors for difficult and challenging MV [30]. Lung volume, pharyngeal collapse, and increased chest wall rigidity impact difficult MV, particularly in patients with sleep-disordered breathing (SDB) and obesity. Obesity negatively impacts SDB by increasing pharyngeal airway collapsibility through structural mechanisms such as excessive soft tissue for the craniofacial size and reduced lung volume. Preoperative screening for obesity, lingual tonsils, and patients with a history of SDB is crucial in an effort to prevent difficult MV [31–33].

In their study comparing mask ventilation in normal patients and patients with multiple risk factors for SDB, Sato et al. found that expiratory flow limitation (EFL) and obesity independently account for reduction of mask ventilation efficiency. The study indicated that the use of two hands can effectively, though not perfectly, compensate for the structural abnormalities resulting in acceptable MV even in severe

SDB patients. The tidal volume during one-handed MV increased by more than 70% during the first minute [31]. This has been attributed to the deepening of anesthesia and onset of neuromuscular blockade.

Safar et al. recommended the use of oral or nasal airways to prevent the EFL at the soft palate and further improve the MV [16]. Also, the right positioning may improve conditions for effective mask ventilation, such as adopting anti-Trendelenburg or Fowler positions to reduce abdominal pressure on the diaphragm [34].

Trauma

Trauma patients should be managed as having difficult airway. Special strategies are required for airway management in trauma patients. When dealing with a trauma patient, one has to take into account several predisposing factors for difficult airway such as cervical spine injury, full stomach, hemodynamic instability, and lack of cooperation. Choices for airway management may be limited due to lack of patient cooperation and time pressure. The option of waking a trauma patient after failure to secure a patent airway might not be possible. The gold standard is an awake fiber-optic intubation, which might turn out to be impractical or impossible in massive face trauma bleeding. Thus, in certain cases, it might be safer to proceed with a surgical front-of-neck access.

Other Patient Considerations

Opioid Induced

High doses of opioids may cause DMV by decreasing ventilatory compliance. This phenomenon was first described by Hamilton and Cullen in 1953. The chest and abdominal wall rigidity induced by opioids was always thought to be the main reason for DMV [35]. In 1983, Scamman showed that patients with tracheostomies experienced only a slight decrease in pulmonary compliance after high doses of fentanyl induction [35]. Later, Abrams et al. published similar findings in intubated preinduction patients who received high-dose opioid [36]. Bennet et al. went further in demonstrating closure of the glottis and supraglottic structures as the proximate cause of difficult ventilation after induction with 3 microg/kg sufentanil by using a fiber-optic bronchoscope to examine the vocal cords before and after narcotics. Vocal cord closure occurred in 28 of 30 patients after sufentanil administration and improved only after muscle relaxant administration. They concluded that vocal cord closure is the main mechanism of opioid-induced DMV [37]. Animal studies show that the underlying mechanism of vocal cord spasm and muscle rigidity is central stimulation of microreceptors through efferent motor traffic, particularly to the laryngeal muscles [38].

Succinylcholine-Induced Masseter Spasm

The masseter muscle responds to the initial depolarization by a contracture. Usually, this response is transient, and masseter spasm resolves when fasciculation stops. Moreover, succinylcholine is known to cause significant masseter spasm in children when used in conjunction with volatile anesthetics such as halothane. Sometimes in adults, it can result in clinically significant jaw rigidity (jaw of steel), impeding ventilation and intubation attempts [39]. Masseter spasm can be a benign phenomenon, but it may also be an early sign of malignant hyperthermia [40].

Non-depolarizing Muscle Relaxation (NDMR) and Light Anesthesia

The effect of administration of NDMR on the ease of mask ventilation is controversial. Immediately after anesthesia induction, there may be some difficulty with MV. However, with the onset of muscle relaxation, this phenomenon gradually eases, and adequate MV is eventually established. Full neuromuscular blockade might facilitate mask ventilation by increasing chest wall compliance or by reducing upper airway tone; alternatively, it could make mask ventilation more difficult by inducing upper airway collapse [41, 42]. Therefore, it was concluded that muscle tone was the factor behind the initial resistance to MV.

In accordance with Ikeda et al., our data showed that MV was not significantly affected with the use of NDMR [43]. We observed only a minimal and nonsignificant increase in the percentage of patients with Cormack and Lehane (C&L) grade I who were easy to ventilate before (93% of patients) and after (98% of patients) administration of NDMR. Furthermore, patients with C&L grades II and III exhibited a statistically nonsignificant trend toward a change in the quality of MV before (68% easy, 32% difficult) and after (60% easy, 40% difficult) administration of NDMR. The nonsignificant increase in the percentage of difficult MV in patients with C&L grades II and III before (32%) and after (40%) NDMR could be attributed to the relaxation of the oropharyngeal muscles and subsequent obstruction of the submandibular tissues, in a group of patients already predisposed (i.e., C&L II and III) to difficult MV [44]. It is worth mentioning that impossible MV was not encountered in our patient population before and after administration of NDMR, similar to previous studies [42, 45, 46].

On the other hand, light anesthesia may induce coughing, increased chest wall muscle tone, and paradoxical vocal cord movement and may be complicated by tracheobronchial spasm. This phenomenon may cause DMV by reducing compliance and, consequently, decreasing chest wall expansion [47]. This critical situation can be resolved by deepening of the anesthesia or by using muscle relaxants.

Upper Airway Obstruction

The most common causes of upper airway obstruction include pharyngeal wall collapse in morbidly obese and sleep apnea patients; this is mostly attributed to either a proportionally large tongue in relation to the pharyngeal space, tonsillar hyperplasia, or redundant tissues [48]. Upper airway obstruction can also occur after induction of general anesthesia with posterior displacements of the soft palate, base of tongue, and epiglottis. Attempts at inspiration during anesthesia were found to cause major secondary collapse of the pharynx with multiple sites of obstruction, similar to that found in obstructive sleep apnea [49]. In patients with a slight increased BMI with no apparent signs of airway abnormalities, a difficult airway may not be anticipated, leading to a more difficult airway management, whereas there is a low threshold for awake intubation in morbidly obese patients [50].

Other causes such as pharyngeal and neck tumors may obstruct the upper airway [51]. Facial and maxillary tumors may cause face deformity, leading to impingement on the upper airway and DAM [52]. Other tumors affecting the thyroid or the larynx can all produce different levels of upper airway obstruction leading to DAM [53]. Trauma to the upper airway, including iatrogenic trauma induced by repeated attempts at tracheal intubation, can lead to bleeding, swelling, and edema of the pharyngeal and laryngeal structures [54]. Carotid pseudo-aneurysms may bulge into the pharynx, causing partial obstruction [55].

Distal Airway Obstruction

It is recommended that patients with distal airway obstruction, mostly tracheomalacia and mediastinal masses, should be intubated while awake. In these cases, induction with muscle relaxant will cause relaxation of the parasternal muscles leading to extrinsic airway compression. Subsequently, this will lead to decreased expiratory flow and elimination of diaphragmatic movement leading to impossible ventilation.

DMV might also be caused by severe bronchospasm, stiff lungs, bronchopleural fistula, pneumothorax, foreign body aspiration, bronchial tumors, severe kyphoscoliosis, and chest wall deformity, all of which impede lung expansion and reduce compliance [56]. In these situations, the practice of testing the possibility of MV prior to the administration of neuromuscular blockers is no longer supported [40].

When facing a DAM, it is imperative to go through this list of differential diagnoses to try to correct the reversible causes, or consider alternative interventions if initial measures fail.

Evaluation of Difficult Airway Management

Expertise in airway management is a critical clinical skill for anesthesiologists. Major morbidities due to complicated airway management can be the most life-threatening. MV is a core skill in airway management, as it proves to be a lifesaving technique when all others fail. The Difficult Airway Society in 2015 shared guidelines for the management of unanticipated difficult intubation (DI) in adults. It states MV as the third step after the failure of tracheal intubation and supraglottic airway insertion [57].

Even though MV can be a critical solution in difficult airway management, it can also be difficult, challenging, or a source of complication. Aspiration is a common complication of MV, which can be prevented. The patient should observe fasting guidelines whenever possible. Draining the gastric content before proceeding to airway management is another option. Application of cricoid pressure during MV might help to reduce gastric distension, keeping in mind that cricoid pressure might sometimes impede the ease of MV. Most of the time, a DMV can be improved by some maneuvers such as administering neuromuscular blockade, head-up positioning, jaw thrust, two-handed mask ventilation, and use of oropharyngeal and nasopharyngeal airways [40]. Successful MV requires good technique and regular practice. Poor MV performance can have adverse physiological complications, particularly during emergency airway management when the operator starts to hyperventilate forcefully. This hyperventilation leads to decreased PaCO2, vasoconstriction, and gastric insufflation. Ventilating with small tidal volumes (6–7 mL/kg) and short inflation duration of 1 s are recommended; also avoid rapid or forceful breaths [37].

Several algorithms for difficult airway management have been developed; the most common component is the preoperative assessment to predict the difficult airway [4, 5]. Prediction is mainly based on factors focusing on difficult tracheal intubation. Yet the most critical situation is the case in which intubation is impossible and mask ventilation is, or becomes, inadequate. The prediction of difficult mask ventilation (DMV) is therefore of vital importance. Unfortunately, the factors to predict DMV remain unknown and have not been defined in practice guidelines for the management of difficult airway [4, 5]. Many authors have tried to predict DMV. Asai et al. failed to anticipate DMV in 57% of the patients who were ultimately difficult to ventilate before anesthesia induction [58].

Expected Difficult Tracheal Intubation (DTI)

Before the procedure, patient airway evaluation is crucial. Patient's history, oral and maxillofacial anatomy, pharyngeal and laryngeal structures, and cervical spine mobility must be assessed for signs that predispose to airway difficulty. Both the Mallampati score and the thyromental distance require special attention. A view of the oral cavity can show the size of the tongue, adequacy of mouth opening, and condition of the teeth and uvula. The less the uvula is visualized behind the tongue and the closer the chin is to the chest wall with the head in mid-position, the more difficult the intubation is expected to be. Moreover, obesity, wide neck circumference, and a drastic overbite promote difficulty in airway management.

If a difficult airway is anticipated, awake fiber-optic intubation is recommended to be performed in cooperative patients. Physicians who do not routinely perform fiber-optic intubations should not attempt a difficult airway, except in an emergency setting. Failed intubation attempts may lead to trauma and increase in bleeding, secretions, and edema in the periglottic structures. This will further complicate subsequent intubation attempts and may render intubation impossible by completely obstructing the airway, leaving an urgent surgical airway the only resort [1].

An ASA closed claims analysis of difficult airway management cases indicated that when DTI was expected, almost 70% of anesthetists still decided to proceed with routine general anesthesia and paralysis. Of those cases, more than 60% evolved to CICV (cannot intubate, cannot ventilate) and poor outcomes were significantly more common than in cases intubated differently. Very similar results were found in other surveys in other countries for more than 20 years [59, 60].

However, even with a careful assessment of these findings, occasionally patients will be surprisingly difficult. If one encounters a difficult airway case, one needs to make an informed decision about how to proceed based on the availability of equipment, preferably before the onset of desaturation. The options for difficult airway tools include the intubating laryngeal mask airway, fiber-optic bronchoscope, intubating stylet, articulating laryngoscope, video laryngoscope (VL), and cricothyrotomy [3].

As for any procedure, the patient should be prepared adequately. The first step is to have the patient positioned ideally on the bed. The body should be located just at the head of the bed so that the occiput is supported on the edge. The head is placed in neutral alignment with the vertebral axis and, if the cervical spine is stable, the head is slightly extended to achieve the so-called sniffing position. The bed is then raised or lowered to the proper height required by the person doing the procedure [61–63]. All required equipment should be immediately available at the bedside, and all necessary medications should be drawn up in syringes. A reliable intravenous access should be confirmed first and foremost.

If the patient is breathing on his or her own, it would be prudent to hold off the administration of neuromuscular blocking drugs. Often, in traumatic airways, the only way to identify the tracheal opening is to watch the subglottic area for spontaneous respiration.

In elective intubations, the patient with a history of difficult intubation can be intubated awake. The airway is prepped with nebulized viscous lidocaine 4% 5 cc to 10 cc for 15 minutes to achieve topicalization of the buccal, subglottic structures and trachea. A fiber-optic bronchoscope with a preloaded endotracheal tube is introduced through the nares, which leads to a less acute angle on approaching the vocal cords. The vocal cords are identified, and the scope is passed through the true cords. After visualization of the tracheal rings, an endotracheal tube is passed over the bronchoscope, and position is confirmed through direct visualization. The bronchoscope is removed, and the patient is sedated and ventilated after reconfirmation of the right position of the endotracheal tube by capnography. Fiber-optic bronchoscopy has the disadvantages of being operator dependent; therefore, considerable experience is a prerequisite. It can also be difficult to visualize laryngeal structures when the airway is bloody or full of secretions, since the aspiration port on the scope is small, and it can be difficult to suction large volumes or thick mucus.

Expected DMV

Most of the studies confirm the opinion of Langeron that increased BMI, advanced age, history of snoring, and presence of a beard are independent predictors of DMV [30]. The presence of a beard is the only reversible risk factor for DMV, which is why it is preferable that the patient shaves prior to the operation if he has associated other risk factors for DMV. The mandibular protrusion test is a key predictor for DMV. Takenaka et al. suggested that abnormalities in mandibular protrusion may be a common indicator of both DI and DMV [64].

Most of the patients labeled as difficult to ventilate also have signs of a potential DI and are candidates for awake fiber-optic intubation [65]. On the other hand, some patients with risk factors for DMV may have indicators of easy intubation (Mallampati, thyromental distance, etc.) or a previous history of "easy" tracheal intubation. In this category of patients, it is recommended to address preoperatively the reversible factors of DMV [40].

When anesthesia induction is planned, the team should be prepared for any possible scenario [66]. Preparation should include the readiness of the difficult airway cart and jet ventilation in the room, availability of an experienced assistant in case help is needed, and rapid reversal (sugammadex) of neuromuscular blockade in the need to resume spontaneous breathing. Some anesthesiologists may elect to induce with a short-acting neuromuscular blocking agent like succinylcholine. Adequate preoxygenation with 100% oxygen before loss of consciousness is crucial. Apneic oxygenation affords the anesthesiologist several minutes to manage the airway before oxygen desaturation [67].

Unexpected DTI

If problems in intubating the trachea are encountered, bag-mask ventilation can provide a bridge to the patient while equipment is being prepared or more skilled hands arrive for intubation. A quick decision, whether to awaken the patient or to proceed with alternative intubation techniques, should be made (e.g., different laryngoscope blades, flexible fiber-optic scope or other fiber-optic techniques, lighted wand, retrograde intubation, or surgical airway). In the potentially life-threatening "cannot intubate, cannot ventilate" situation, either transtracheal jet ventilation, laryngeal mask airway, esophageal-tracheal Combitube, or a surgical airway must be performed/inserted immediately. Anesthesiologists should train under routine conditions on these alternative techniques in order to be comfortable with these critical situations [1].

Denitrogenation of the lungs should be performed routinely before anesthesia induction. This is accomplished with giving the patient 100% oxygen via a face mask for 5 min before administration of any induction dose of apneic drug. This will oxygenate the patient by diffusion, allowing some apneic time during a potentially prolonged intubation attempt. Patients who are obtunded should be mask ventilated with 100% oxygen before any intubation attempt to achieve the same denitrogenation. In the obtunded patient, the mouth and posterior pharynx should be explored and suctioned before mask ventilation, as aspiration events and inability to protect the airway are likely in altered mental states.

When intubation is difficult, publications showed that anesthetists may tend to repeat the same technique at intubation several times, most of the time followed by another anesthetist doing the same. This was shown by the fourth National Audit Project of the Royal College of Anaesthetists and Difficult Airway Society (NAP4) to increase the risk of progression to CICV leading to an increase in death and brain damage [59]. According to Mort, there is a dramatic increase in airway complications when more than two direct laryngoscopies were attempted [68]. All national unanticipated DTI guidelines stress that alternative techniques should be attempted when direct laryngoscopy fails, and to limit the number of trials [69, 70]. Further trials of laryngoscopy have a close to 80% failure rate, but alternative techniques (SAD, indirect laryngoscopy) might be more successful. In a UK study of failed obstetric intubation, 50% of failures were followed by management that deviated from known recommendations [60].

Unexpected DMV

According to the ASA algorithm, once DMV is encountered, the patient's head position should be optimized. In most situations, it is advisable to avoid the development of the difficulty, e.g., by applying continuous positive airway pressure (CPAP) ventilation to stent the airway open, as it may collapse after loss of consciousness. Partial obstruction may result in negative pressure efforts that lead to further collapse and complete airway obstruction, creating a vicious cycle that is difficult to break [33].

DMV and DTI

In some instances, unanticipated difficult laryngeal visualization may be faced after an "easy" MV. When MV is difficult in some cases, a grade 1 view may be obtained with direct laryngoscopy [30]. Difficulty in one of these techniques does not necessarily mean that the other will also be difficult. Studies have shown that a relationship exists between DMV and incidence of DI. Langeron et al. demonstrated that patients with DMV have a higher incidence of DI than those with easy MV. They found the incidence of DI to be 8% in easy-to-ventilate patients, and 30% in those who had DMV, a fourfold increase [50]. Also, the incidence of impossible intubation increased 12-fold (0.5% vs. 6%) in patients who had DMV. Although the average of DI is probably around 8%, most of those patients should be suspected to have DMV. Kheterpal et al. identified many factors that predispose to DMV and also to DI [30]. Obstructive sleep apnea, history of snoring, obese neck anatomy, limited mandibular protrusion, and BMI of 30 kg/m^2 or more are shared predictors for both DMV and DI. However, despite this association, a large percentage of patients who experienced DMV in that study eventually had successful tracheal intubation. On the other hand, minimal data were found in the literature about the relationship between invasive mechanical ventilation (IMV) and DI. Of 37 patients (0.16%) who experienced IMV, 26 were easily intubated, 10 had DI but were eventually intubated, and only 1 patient required emergency cricothyrotomy [30]. Although this is the largest reported group of patients with IMV, the number is still too small to draw any conclusions.

Distinguishing difficult intubation from difficult ventilation is important. If the patient is difficult to intubate, adequacy of bag-mask ventilation becomes paramount, especially if the patient is already paralyzed or not breathing on their own. The incidence of difficult and impossible MV determined by the four-point grading scale is reported to be 1.4–5% and 0.15%, respectively [30, 50, 71]. DMV combined with DI occurs in 0.14% of adult patients undergoing general anesthesia [72].

Following initially unsuccessful attempts at intubation, no single subsequent technique is superior to others in all circumstances. For example, in one series of 698 patients with both difficult mask ventilation and difficult laryngoscopy, intubation was eventually successful with direct laryngoscopy in 177, direct laryngoscopy with bougie introducer in 284, VL in 163, and other techniques in 73; one patient required emergent cricothyrotomy [72]. After failed intubation in the AIMS study, 1 in 7 patients also exhibited DMV, and in an obstetric failed intubation setting, DMV occurred in 30% and IMV in 10% of cases [73, 74].

The ASA practice guideline on difficult airway management urges anesthetists to routinely examine patients to identify predictors of airway technique failure [70]. When such features are elicited, we should optimize our intubation option, knowing that the best shot is the first attempt. If it fails, the feasibility of rescue techniques should be planned ahead of time.

Regarding laryngeal masks, failure of laryngeal mask airway (LMA) placement was associated with a threefold increase in the likelihood of DMV from 1.9 to 5.6% [75]. In the ASACCP dataset, it was suggested that "LMA rescue ability may be hindered by effects of multiple preceding intubation attempts" [59]. Finally, as emphasized previously, multiple attempts at direct laryngoscopy are associated with the development of both DMV and CICV [30].

Based on the review of large datasets, expert groups have recommended that VL should be the first rescue technique when direct laryngoscopy and/or mask or SGA ventilation have failed, because of its high success rates. In a large, multicenter retrospective study of failed DL utilizing the Multicenter Perioperative Outcomes Database, in 1619 rescue attempts, VL resulted in the highest success rate (92%), compared with FSI (78%), use of an SGA as a conduit for intubation (78%), or use of a lighted stylet (77%) [76].

Management of Difficult Airway

After induction of anesthesia, management of DMV is a dynamic process in which close observation of the efficacy of oxygenation should be accompanied simultaneously by adjustments of the maneuvers, use of adjuncts, and call for help as soon as difficulty is encountered. The most commonly used maneuvers to open the airway are head tilt, chin lift, and jaw thrust. The placement of an oropharyngeal or nasopharyngeal airway can also facilitate ventilation. Operator change or two-person MV technique might be successful.

Figure 18.1 shows the failure progression of DMV and the management steps that can be followed to establish adequate ventilation. The figure is based on the ASA difficult airway algorithm and other evidence from the literature [40, 66, 70, 77–82].

If MV is still impossible, the anesthesiologist should seriously consider discontinuing the anesthetic and awaken the patient. When recovery from anesthesia induction is possible and spontaneous breathing is resumed, the case can be rescheduled, or an awake tracheal intubation technique performed. Recovery time is critical, and waiting for the patient to spontaneously breathe is not always a safe option and might lead to fatal outcome. Reversal of neuromuscular blockade can consume time. Bisschops et al. observed that the total time to prepare and administer sugammadex turned out to be 8.9 min [83]. Makris et al. pointed out that a readily available syringe preloaded with sugammadex placed in the difficult airway trolley would reduce this time [84]. Naquib et al. showed that recovery of neuromuscular function only took 4.5 min with 1.2 mg kg^{-1} rocuronium at induction of anesthesia, followed 3 min later by 16 mg kg^{-1} sugammadex [85]. Despite these results, the

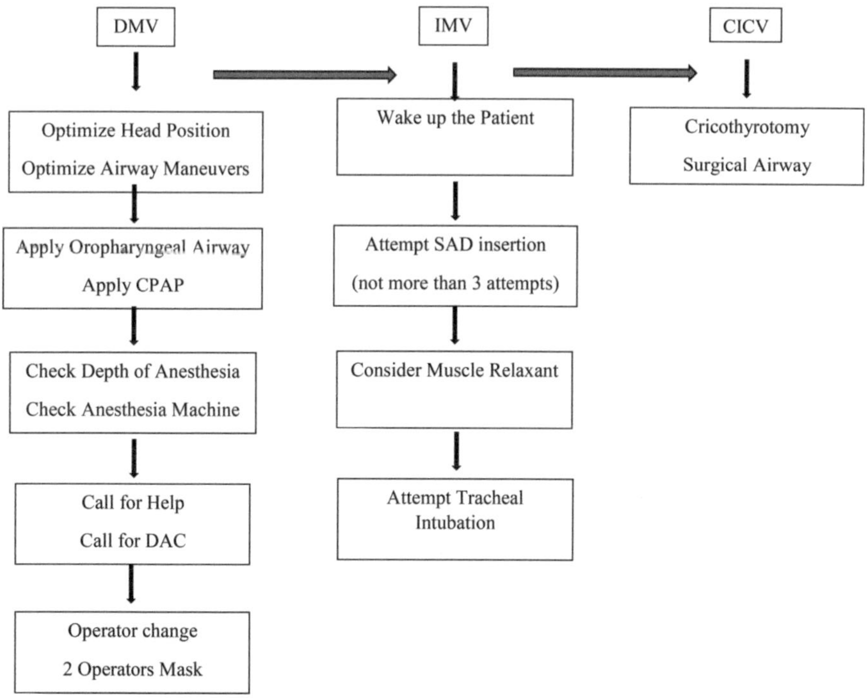

Fig. 18.1 Failure progression of DMV, and steps to take to establish ventilation

duration of apnea after sugammadex reversal may last as long as 15 min, mainly in obese patients. During this rescue, if ventilation is unsuccessful, oxygen desaturation will occur despite full reversal of neuromuscular blockade. Therefore, in a CICV scenario, the clinical maneuvers such as restoration of a patent airway and oxygenation are vital and should come before any pharmacological tools [86].

Meanwhile, the operator may either proceed with tracheal intubation or use an alternative ventilatory device. Crosby et al. [77] considered an attempt at tracheal intubation a prudent first intervention in cases of IMV. As previously noted, Kheterpal et al. [30] reported successful tracheal intubation in 36 of 37 patients who had IMV, and only 1 patient required cricothyrotomy. Based on these results (because this was the largest group of IMV patients studied), limited trials of direct laryngoscopy and tracheal intubation should be considered.

The decision to proceed with either technique will be dictated by its availability, urgency to establish ventilation, and the patient's oxygen saturation. The laryngeal mask airway (LMA) is considered by many to be the first-choice rescue ventilation device [59]. Because of its success rate, ease of insertion, and increased familiarity with its use, the LMA was included in the ASA difficult airway algorithm as an early option to be considered whenever it is difficult or impossible to ventilate [70]. Success with supraglottic airway ventilation relies on the clinician's skill and experience with specific devices. The Combitube or other supraglottic airway devices may be tried if both face mask and LMA fail to establish adequate ventilation [70, 79, 80]. Two relatively new supraglottic devices deserve mention because of the reported success in their use to rescue ventilation. These are the laryngeal tube (LT) and the LMA CTrach. The LT (King Systems, Noblesville, IN) is a silicone tube with a proximal (pharyngeal) cuff and a distal (esophageal) cuff and ventilatory apertures in between [87]. This device is easily inserted even by inexperienced personnel [88]. Its ventilatory efficiency has been demonstrated with both controlled and spontaneous ventilation [89, 90]. There are many reports of the LT used as a rescue ventilation device in difficult airway situations [80, 91]. Placement, however, may sometimes be difficult or impossible in patients with upper airway masses. The LT cannot prevent or treat airway obstruction at or beyond the glottis [92]. The LMA CTrach (LMA North America, San Diego, CA) is another device that was successfully used in patients with difficult airways [93]. It is a modification of the intubating LMA that incorporates a built-in fiber-optic system to transmit images to a small screen. The device can be used to rescue ventilation while simultaneously performing tracheal intubation under visualization [94]. More time is required, however, for its accurate placement [95]. More clinical trials are currently needed on the use of these two promising devices and their role in difficult airway management.

Several other devices have also been introduced. The choice of the proper device should be based on the etiology of the problem, limitations of the device, experienced clinical judgment, and familiarity with its use, which can be crucial to its successful application.

If all previously described techniques fail, the patient could not be ventilated or intubated—an emergency surgical airway (ESA) is needed. As soon as the airway is labeled as potentially difficult, a surgeon should be consulted. Transtracheal jet ventilation may be considered when supraglottic ventilation devices fail, but the operator must be familiar with its use [81]. If all other measures fail to establish ventilation, cricothyrotomy may be the only lifesaving alternative [70, 82]. There are also kits available using a Seldinger technique, with a needle inserted through the cricothyroid membrane. On successful aspiration of air, a wire is passed into the trachea, and the needle removed. A small incision is made in the skin, and a dilator is passed over the wire. This should produce a large air leak on positive ventilation, confirming the placement. Then, a cricothyrotomy tube is passed through the opening and the patient ventilated. Proper placement of an airway device should always be confirmed with an end-tidal carbon dioxide (CO_2) device immediately and radiographically later to document the placement of the tube tip proximal to the carina.

ESA is a rescue technique and is performed in 1 in 50,000 general anesthesia cases where CICV occurs and increases 15-fold the risk of a poor outcome. However, failure of ESA puts the patient at a significant risk of death, and it accounts for more than 25% of all anesthesia-related deaths [60, 71, 72].

The rarity, invasiveness, and emergency nature of ESA make its study difficult, and much of the evidence is derived from models and simulations whose fidelity is uncertain. NAP4 included a cohort of 80 cases of ESA (43% of all reports), perhaps the largest in-hospital series. Thirteen of these patients died (16%), and seven suffered permanent harm (25% permanent harm or death). Despite high rates of failure of ESA in this series, most patients made a full recovery. Failed initial ESA was rescued variously by intubation, supraglottic airway device (SAD) placement, patient awakening, or an alternative ESA technique.

CICV and attempted ESA occurred in several cases where NMBA was intentionally avoided and an airway rescue by a SGA was not attempted [60]. The NAP4 report recommended the use of NMBA and SGA whenever CICV is encountered and before it progresses to ESA. The ASA closed claim reported that the use of narrow-bore cricothyroidotomy in CICV cases was associated with high rates of failed ventilation and of barotrauma [59]. It was also reported in NAP4 that needle cricothyroidotomy performed by anesthetists had a high failure rate (63%) compared to surgical tracheostomy/cricothyroidotomy with 100% success rate. However, it is worth mentioning that the former procedure was performed by an anesthesiologist in extreme emergency situations, but the open technique was performed by a surgeon on a relatively stabilized patient where the anesthesiologist was maintaining his oxygenation. Consequently, no conclusion could be drawn on which technique is safer.

Evidence from a large series of various ESA techniques in sheep in a "wet lab" suggests that well-trained anesthetists have a high success rate with needle cricothyroidotomy in lifelike situations [96].

Delay in performance of ESA is as important as equipment choice. In the ASACCP analysis of difficult airway management, 79 (42%) cases progressed from intubation difficulty to CICV, and in two-thirds, a surgical airway was performed, but too late to prevent an adverse outcome [59]. ESA was often performed when the patient was either moribund or in fact dead. Similarly, in NAP4, there was clear evidence of delay in performing ESA and even cases where ESA was not performed at all despite clear need [72]. There is a natural reluctance to perform such techniques, but the evidence is clear: when ESA is required, it is not the procedure that kills patients, but delaying or not doing it that causes harm [97]. Training programs could usefully emphasize behavioral aspects of cricothyroidotomy as equally important as technical training.

When CICV occurs after general anesthesia, it is important to remember that the primary task is to oxygenate the patient, and not to intubate the trachea: the patient may need to be awakened, surgical airway obtained, or cardiopulmonary bypass established. To make a right decision, it is necessary to know the advantages and disadvantages of each option, as well as of each airway device, and to be acquainted with these devices during routine anesthesia.

Conclusion

In summary, many airway devices exist to assist in the successful management of the difficult airway. Proper identification is paramount to avoiding an airway disaster and the feared "cannot intubate, cannot ventilate" scenario. Any difficult airway should be left to the best trained personnel available. When a difficult airway is encountered, healthcare workers should refrain from repeating the same attempts at intubation. Each practitioner should have a number of intubation techniques and tools with which they are most comfortable and should know when to call for help.

References

1. Krafft P, Frass M. The difficult airway. Wien Klin Wochenschr. 2000;112(6):260–70.
2. Apfelbaum JL, Hagberg CA, Caplan RA, Blitt CD, Connis RT, Nickinovich DG, et al. Practice guidelines for management of the difficult airway: an updated report by the American Society of Anesthesiologists Task Force on Management of the Difficult Airway. Anesthesiology. 2013;118:251–70.
3. Kollmeier BR, Boyette LC, Beecham GB, Khetarpal S. Difficult airway. Treasure Island, FL: StatPearls Publishing; 2020.
4. Caplan RA, Benumof JL, Berry FA, Blitt CD, Bode RH, Cheney FW, et al. Practice guidelines for management of the difficult airway: a report by the ASA Task Force on Management of the Difficult Airway. Anesthesiology. 1993;78:597–602.
5. Boisson-Bertrand D, Bourgain JL, Camboulives J, Crinquette V, Cros AM, Dubreuil M, et al. Difficult intubation. French Society of Anesthesia and Intensive Care. A collective expertise. Ann Fr Anesth Réanim. 1996;15:207–14. [Article in French].
6. Ovassapian A. The difficult airway, fiberoptic endoscopy and the difficult airway. 2nd ed. Philadelphia: Lippincott-Raven; 1996. p. 185–99.
7. Horton WA, Fahy L, Charters P. Defining a standard intubating position using "angle finder". Br J Anaesth. 1989;62:6–12.
8. Hanley JA, Mc Neil BJ. The meaning and use of the area under a receiver operating characteristic (ROC) curve. Radiology. 1982;143:29–36.
9. Flin R, Fioratou E, Frerk C, Trotter C, Cook TM. Human factors in the development of complications of airway management: preliminary evaluation of an interview tool. Anaesthesia. 2013;68:817–25.

10. Endsley M. Toward a theory of situation awareness in dynamic systems. Hum Factors. 1995;37:32–64.
11. Azim SW. Understanding and managing project complexity. PhD Thesis, The University of Manchester; 2010. https://www.escholar.manchester.ac.uk/api/datastream?publicationPid=uk-ac-manscw:121030&datastreamId=FULL-TEXT.PDF. Accessed 23 Nov 2019.
12. Chung SA, Yuan H, Chung FC. A systemic review of obstructive sleep apnea and its implications for anesthesiologists. Anesth Analg. 2008;107:1543–63.
13. Landsman IS. Mechanisms and treatment of laryngospasm. Int Anesthesiol Clin. 1997;35:67–73.
14. Rocke DA, Murray WB, Rout CC, Gouws EB. Relative risk analysis of factors associated with difficult intubation in obstetric anesthesia. Anesthesiology. 1992;77:67–73.
15. Hung O, Murphy O. Context sensitive airway management. Anesth Analg. 2010;110:982–3.
16. McCoy CE, Mickunas A. The role of context and progressive commitment in plan continuation error. Proceed Hum Factors Ergonom Soc Ann Meet. 2000;44:26–9.
17. Saddawi-Konefka D, Hung SL, Kacmarek RM, et al. Optimizing mask ventilation: literature review and development of a conceptual framework. Respir Care. 2015;60(12):1834–40.
18. Elling R, Politis J. An evaluation of emergency medical technicians' ability to use manual ventilation devices. Ann Emerg Med. 1983;12:765–8.
19. De Regge M, Vogels C, Monsieurs KG, Calle PA. Retention of ventilation skills of emergency nurses after training with the SMART BAG compared to a standard BAG-valve-mask. Resuscitation. 2006;68:379–84.
20. Komatsu R, Kasuya Y, Yogo H, Sessler DI, Mascha E, Yang D, et al. Learning curves for bag-and-mask ventilation and orotracheal intubation: an application of the cumulative sum method. Anesthesiology. 2010;112(6):1525–31.
21. Davidovic L, LaCovey D, Pitetti RD. Comparison of 1- versus 2-person bag valve-mask techniques for manikin ventilation of infants and children. Ann Emerg Med. 2005;46(1):37–42.
22. Cocucci C, Madorno M, Aguilar A, Acha L, Szyld E, Musante G. A metronome for pacing manual ventilation in a neonatal resuscitation simulation. Arch Dis Child Fetal Neonatal Ed. 2015;100(1):F47–9.
23. Conlon NP, Sullivan RP, Herbison PG, Zacharias M, Buggy DJ. The effect of leaving dentures in place on bag-mask ventilation at induction of general anesthesia. Anesth Analg. 2007;105:370–3.
24. Ho AM, Wong W, Ling E, Chung DC, Tay BA. Airway difficulties caused by improperly applied cricoid pressure. J Emerg Med. 2001;20:29–31.
25. Chung YT, Wu HS, Lin YH, Hsieh AY, Chen CL. Frequent use of alternative airway techniques makes difficult intubation less and easier. Acta Anaesthesiol Taiwanica. 2004;42:141–5.
26. Ezri T, Szmuk P, Warters RD, Katz J, Hagberg CA. Difficult airway management practice patterns among anesthesiologists practicing in the United States: have we made any progress? J Clin Anesth. 2003;15:418–22.
27. Greenberg RS. Facemask, nasal and oral airway devices. Anesthesiol Clin N Am. 2002;20:833–61.
28. Isono S, Tanaka A, Ishikawa T, Tagaito Y, Nishino T. Sniffing position improves pharyngeal airway patency in anesthetized patients with obstructive sleep apnea. Anesthesiology. 2005;103:489–94.
29. El-Orbany M. The optimal head position for mask ventilation. Anaesthesia. 2007;62:855.
30. Kheterpal S, Han R, Tremper KK, Shanks A, Tait AR, O'Reilly M, et al. Incidence and predictors of difficult and impossible mask ventilation. Anesthesiology. 2006;105:885–91.
31. Sato S, Hasegawa M, Okuyama M, Okazaki J, Kitamura Y, Sato Y, et al. Mask ventilation during induction of general anesthesia: influences of obstructive sleep apnea. Anesthesiology. 2017;126(1):28–38.
32. Ovassapian A, Glassenberg R, Randel GI, Klock A, Mesnick PS, Klafta JM. The unexpected difficult airway and lingual tonsil hyperplasia: a case series and a review of the literature. Anesthesiology. 2002;97(1):124–32.

33. Hillman DR, Platt PR, Eastwood PR. The upper airway during anaesthesia. Br J Anaesth. 2003;91(1):31–9.
34. Baker P. Mask ventilation. F1000 Faculty Rev. 2018;7:1683. https://doi.org/10.12688/f1000research.15742.1. eCollection 2018.
35. Comstock M, Scamman F, Moyers J, Stevens W. Rigidity and hypercarbia associated with high dose fentanyl induction of anesthesia. Anesth Analg. 1981;60:362–3.
36. Abrams JT, Horrow JC, Bennet JA, Van Riper DF, Storella RJ. Upper airway closure: a primary source of difficult ventilation with sufentanil induction of anesthesia. Anesth Analg. 1996;83:629–32.
37. Bennett JA, Abrams JT, Van Riper DF, Horrow JC. Difficult or impossible ventilation after sufentanil-induced anesthesia is caused primarily by vocal cord closure. Anesthesiology. 1997;87:1070–4.
38. Vancova ME, Weinger MB, Chen DY, Bronson JB, Motis V, Koop GF. Role of central Mu, delta-1 and kappa-1 opioid receptors in opioid-induced muscle rigidity in the rat. Anesthesiology. 1996;85:574–83.
39. Bauer SJ, Orio K, Adams BD. Succinylcholine induced masseter spasm during rapid sequence intubation may require a surgical airway: case report. Emerg Med J. 2005;22:456–8.
40. El-Orbany M, Woehlck HJ. Difficult mask ventilation, review article. Anesth Analg. 2009;109:1870–80.
41. Odeh M, Schnall R, Gavriely N, Oliven A. Effect of upper air-way muscle contraction on supraglottic resistance and stability. Respir Physiol. 1993;92:139–50.
42. Van Lunteren E, Strohl KP. The muscles of the upper airways. Clin Chest Med. 1986;7:171–88.
43. Ikeda A, Isono S, Sato Y, Yogo H, Sato J, Ishikawa T, et al. Effects of muscle relaxants on mask ventilation in anesthetized persons with normal upper airway anatomy. Anesthesiology. 2012;117:487–93.
44. Rizk MS, Zeineldine SM, El-Khatib MF, Yazbeck-Karam VG, Ayoub SD, Bou-Khalil PK, et al. Nondepolarizing muscle relaxant improves direct laryngoscopy view with no effect on face mask ventilation. Rev Bras Anestesiol. 2017;67(4):383–7. [Article in Portuguese].
45. Pandit JJ. Checking the ability to mask ventilate before administering long-acting neuromuscular blocking drugs. Anaesthesia. 2011;66:520–2.
46. Warters RD, Szabo TA, Spinale FG, DeSantis SM, Reves JG. The effect of neuromuscular blockade on mask ventilation. Anaesthesia. 2011;66:163–7.
47. Fletcher ME, Stack C, Ewart M, Davies CJ, Ridley S, Hatch DJ, Stocks JJ. Respiratory compliance during sedation, anesthesia, and paralysis in infants and young children. J Appl Physiol. 1991;70:1977–82.
48. Partinen M, Guilleminault C, Quera-Salva MA, Jamieson A. Obstructive sleep apnea and cephalometric roentgenograms: the role of anatomic upper airway abnormalities in the definition of abnormal breathing during sleep. Chest. 1988;93:1199–205.
49. Nandi PR, Charlesworth CH, Taylor SJ, Nunn JF, Dore´ CJ. Effect of general anaesthesia on the pharynx. Br J Anaesth. 1991;66:157–62.
50. Langeron O, Masso E, Huraux C, Guggiari M, Bianchi A, Coriat P, Riou B. Prediction of difficult mask ventilation. Anesthesiology. 2000;92:1229–36.
51. Sofferman RA, Johnson DL, Spencer RF. Lost airway during anesthesia induction: alternatives for management. Laryngoscope. 1997;107:1476–82.
52. Asai T, Matsumoto H, Shingo K. Awake tracheal intubation through the intubating laryngeal mask. Can J Anaesth. 1999;46:182–4.
53. Keon TP. Anesthesia for airway surgery. Int Anesthesiol Clin. 1985;23:87–116.
54. Davies JM, Weeks S, Crone LA, Pavlin E. Difficult intubation in the parturient. Can J Anaesth. 1989;36:668–74.
55. White JA, MacRae D. Airway obstruction secondary to extracranial carotid-artery pseudoaneurysm. J Otolaryngol. 1999;28:105–7.
56. Gabbott DA, Baskett PJ. Management of the airway and ventilation during resuscitation. Br J Anaesth. 1997;79:159–71.

57. Frerk C, Mitchell VS, McNarry AF, et al. Difficult Airway Society 2015 guidelines for management of unanticipated difficult intubation in adults. Br J Anaesth. 2015;115(6):827–48.
58. Asai T, Koga K, Vaughan RS. Respiratory complications associated with tracheal intubation and extubation. Br J Anaesth. 1998;80:767–75.
59. Peterson GN, Domino KB, Caplan RA, Posner KL, Lee LA, Cheney FW. Management of the difficult airway: a closed claims analysis. Anesthesiology. 2005;103:33–9.
60. Cook TM, MacDougall-Davis SR. Complications and failure of airway management. Br J Anaesth. 2012;109(S1):68–85.
61. Krebs M, Müller-Lobeck L, Francis RCE. Management of pediatric airway in anesthesia. Anasthesiol Intensivmed Notfallmed Schmerzther. 2018;53(11–12):754–65. [Article in German].
62. Tsao M, Vargas AA, Hajduk J, Singh R, Jagannathan N. Pediatric airway management devices: an update on recent advances and future directions. Expert Rev Med Devices. 2018;15(12):911–27.
63. Glasheen J, Hooper J, Donohue A, Murray-Smith B, Finn E. Endotracheal intubation for traumatic cardiac arrest by an Australian air medical service. Air Med J. 2018;37(6):371–3.
64. Takenaka I, Aoyama K, Kadoya T. Mandibular protrusion test for prediction of difficult mask ventilation. Anesthesiology. 2001;94:935.
65. Benumof JL. Management of the difficult adult airway. With special emphasis on awake tracheal intubation. Anesthesiology. 1991;75:1087–110.
66. Practice guidelines for management of the difficult airway: A report by the American Society of Anesthesiologists' task force on management of the difficult airway. Anesthesiology. 1993;78:597–602.
67. Benumof JL. Preoxygenation: best method for both efficacy and efficiency. Anesthesiology. 1999;91:603–5.
68. Mort TC. Emergency tracheal intubation: complications associated with repeated laryngoscopic attempts. Anesth Analg. 2004;99:607–13.
69. Henderson JJ, Popat MT, Latto IP, Pearce AC, Difficult Airway Society. Difficult airway society guidelines for management of the unanticipated difficult intubation. Anaesthesia. 2004;59:675–94.
70. American Society of Anesthesiologists Task Force on Management of the Difficult Airway. Practice guidelines for management of the difficult airway: an updated report by the American Society of Anesthesiologists Task Force on Management of the Difficult Airway. Anesthesiology. 2003;98:1269–77.
71. Kheterpal S, Martin L, Shanks AM, Tremper KK. Prediction and outcomes of impossible mask ventilation: a review of 50,000 anesthetics. Anesthesiology. 2009;110:891–7.
72. Kheterpal S, Healy D, Aziz MF, Shanks AM, Freundlich RE, Linton F, et al. Multicenter Perioperative Outcomes Group (MPOG) Perioperative Clinical Research Committee. Incidence, predictors, and outcome of difficult mask ventilation combined with difficult laryngoscopy: a report from the multicenter perioperative outcomes group. Anesthesiology. 2013;119:1360–9.
73. Williamson JA, Webb RK, Szekely S, Gillies ER, Dreosti AV. The Australian Incident Monitoring Study. Difficult intubation: an analysis of 2000 incident reports. Anaesth Intensive Care. 1993(21):602–7.
74. Hawthorne L, Wilson R, Lyons G, Dresner M. Failed intubation revisited: 17-yr experience in a teaching maternity unit. Br J Anaesth. 1996;76:680–4.
75. Ramachandran SK, Mathis MR, Tremper KK, Shanks AM, Kheterpal S. Predictors and clinical outcomes from failed Laryngeal Mask Airway Unique™: a study of 15,795 patients. Anesthesiology. 2012;116:1217–26.
76. Aziz MF, Brambrink AM, Healy DW, Willett AW, Shanks A, Tremper T, et al. Success of intubation rescue techniques after failed direct laryngoscopy in adults: a retrospective comparative analysis from the Multicenter Perioperative Outcomes Group. Anesthesiology. 2016;125:656.
77. Crosby ET, Cooper RM, Douglas MJ, Doyle DJ, Hung OR, Labrecque P, et al. The unanticipated difficult airway with recommendations for management. Can J Anaesth. 1998;45:757–76.

78. Bogetz MS. Using the laryngeal mask airway to manage the difficult airway. Anesthesiol Clin N Am. 2002;20:863–70.
79. Krafft P, Schebesta K. Alternative management techniques for the difficult airway: esophageal-tracheal Combitube. Curr Opin Anaesthesiol. 2004;17:499–504.
80. Winterhalter M, Kirchoff K, Groschel W, Lullwitz E, Heermann R, Hoy L, et al. The laryngeal tube for difficult airway management: a prospective investigation in patients with pharyngeal and laryngeal tumours. Eur J Anaesthesiol. 2005;22:678–82.
81. Mchugh R, Kumar M, Sprung J, Bourke D. Transtracheal jet ventilation in management of the difficult airway. Anaesth Intensive Care. 2007;35:406–8.
82. Scrase I, Woollard M. Needle vs surgical cricothyroidotomy: a short cut to effective ventilation. Anaesthesia. 2006;61:962–74.
83. Bisschops MMA, Holleman C, Huitink JM. Can sugammadex save a patient in a simulated 'cannot intubate, cannot ventilate' situation? Anaesthesia. 2010;65:936–41.
84. Makris N. Sugammadex following rocuronium rapid sequence induction. Anaesthesia. 2011;66:224.
85. Naguib M, Brewer L, LaPierre C, Kopman AF, Johnson KB. The myth of rescue reversal in "can't intubate, can't ventilate" scenarios. Anesth Analg. 2016;123:82–92.
86. Bailey C. Sugammadex: when should we be giving it? Anaesthesia. 2017;72(10):1170–5.
87. Dorges V, Ocker H, Wenzel V, Schmucker P. The laryngeal tube: a new simple airway device. Anesth Analg. 2000;90:1220–2.
88. Asai T, Hidaka I, Kawachi S. Efficacy of LT by inexperienced personnel. Resuscitation. 2002;55:171–5.
89. Cook TM, McCormick B, Asai T. Randomized comparison of laryngeal tube with classical laryngeal mask airway for anaesthesia with controlled ventilation. Br J Anaesth. 2003;91:373–8.
90. Hagberg C, Bogomolny Y, Gilmore C, Gibson V, Kaitner M, Khurana S. An evaluation of insertion and function of a new supraglottic airway device, the King LTTM, during spontaneous ventilation. Anesth Analg. 2006;102:621–5.
91. Matioc AA, Olson J. Use of the laryngeal tube in two unexpected difficult airway situations: lingual tonsillar hyperplasia and morbid obesity. Can J Anaesth. 2004;51:1018–21.
92. Cook TM, Hommers C. New airways for resuscitation? Resuscitation. 2006;69:371–87.
93. Goldman AJ, Rosenblatt WH. The LMA CTrach in airway resuscitation: six case reports. Anaesthesia. 2006;61:975–7.
94. Liu EH, Goy RW, Chen FG. The LMA CTrach, a new laryngeal mask airway for endotracheal intubation under vision: evaluation in 100 patients. Br J Anaesth. 2006;96:396–400.
95. Liu EH, Goy RW, Lim Y, Chen FG. Success of tracheal intubation with intubating laryngeal mask airways: a randomized trial of the LMA Fastrach and LMA CTrach. Anesthesiology. 2008;108:621–6.
96. Heard AM, Green RJ, Eakins P. The formulation and introduction of a 'can't intubate, can't ventilate' algorithm into clinical practice. Anaesthesia. 2009;64:601–8.
97. Greenland KB, Acott C, Segal R, Goulding G, Riley R, Merry AF. Emergency surgical airway in life-threatening acute airway emergencies-why are we so reluctant to do it. Anaesth Intensive Care. 2011;39:578–84.

"Don't Yell at Me!" Disruptive Behavior in the OR

19

Julia R. Coleman and Richard Schulick

Introduction

Surgical team dynamics, operating room environment, and surgical culture are paramount to perioperative safety, and all of these are adversely affected by disruptive behavior in the operating room (OR). The American Medical Association has defined disruptive physician behavior as "conduct, whether verbal or physical, that negatively affects or that potentially may negatively affect patient care" [1]. Disruptive conduct has also been described as a behavior that is interpersonal (directed toward others or in the presence of others), results in perceived threats to victim and/or witnesses, and violates a reasonable person's standard of respectful behavior [2]. Unfortunately, disruptive behavior from physicians is particularly prevalent, with an American College of Physician executive survey reporting that 30% of the 16,000 physician executive respondents experience disruptive behavior at least monthly with physicians in their work environment [3]. This is even more pronounced among surgeons, with over double the rate of complaints about disruptive conduct as compared to their nonsurgical physician peers [4]. Given the prevalence and potential consequences of disruptive behavior in the OR, it is important to consider its effects on surgeon and staff, the learner (whether a resident or medical student), and ultimately the patient and perioperative safety. In this chapter,

J. R. Coleman (✉)
Department of Surgery, University of Colorado–Denver, Aurora, CO, USA
e-mail: julia.coleman@cuanschutz.edu

R. Schulick
University of Colorado Department of Surgery, Aurora, CO, USA

University of Colorado Cancer Center, Aurora, CO, USA

University of Colorado Anschutz Medical Campus, Aurora, CO, USA

J. J. Hoballah et al. (eds.), *Principles of Perioperative Safety and Efficiency*,
https://doi.org/10.1007/978-3-031-41089-5_19

definitions and causes of disruptive behavior will be explored, as well as its downstream effects on perioperative safety. Strategies for addressing and discouraging disruptive behavior in the OR at an individual, team, and systems level will also be discussed.

Disruptive Behavior in the Operating Room: Causes and Manifestations

Disruptive behavior in the operating room from surgeons can manifest in a myriad of overt to more subtle demonstrations, from aggressive verbal outbursts or throwing of items to more subtle, passive behavior including avoidance and failure to communicate (Table 19.1), all of which affect the anxiety level, performance, and safety in the operating room [5]. In a qualitative study of interviews with perioperative staff (residents, anesthesiologists, scrub technicians, and perioperative nurses) focused on types and causes of disruptive surgeon behavior in the perioperative environment, Cochran and colleagues report the four themes of disruptive behavior by surgeons: unprofessional behavior, situational stressors, cultural conditions, and personality traits, all of which dynamically interact and contextualize operating room staff behavior and disruptive behavior of surgeons [6]. Categories of unprofessional behavior range from "yelling," "swearing," "threatening," and "disparaging remarks" to hitting or throwing equipment. Situational stressors may include physical environment and patient-specific factors, such as unexpected outcomes in operating course, more difficult technical demands, and issues with equipment malfunctioning. Cultural conditions can create complacency and power differentials, which result in perpetuation disruptive behavior. And lastly, personality traits of surgeons may also be linked to more disruptive behavior and are generally linked to a lack of teamwork attitude. All of these individual- and systems-related variables—from workplace logistics, intrapersonal aspects, and broader cultural environment to workplace relationships—dynamically interact and lead to disruptive behavior on the part of the surgeon [7]. It is essential to understand not just the upstream factors affecting disruptive behavior in the operating room, but also the downstream effects, on the surgeon, the learners and team, and the patient (Fig. 19.1).

Table 19.1 Categories and examples of disruptive surgeon behaviors

Category	Example
Verbal outbursts	Yelling, derogatory comments, profanity, threats, inappropriate anger
Physical aggression	Throwing objects, hitting equipment, striking others
Intrapersonal	Irritability, hyperactive, complaining
Interpersonal	Dismissive comments, bullying, condescending conduct, argumentative, blaming
Passive aggressive	Ignoring, avoiding, refusal to perform tasks or work with others, reluctance to answer questions, ineffective use of team, uncooperative attitude

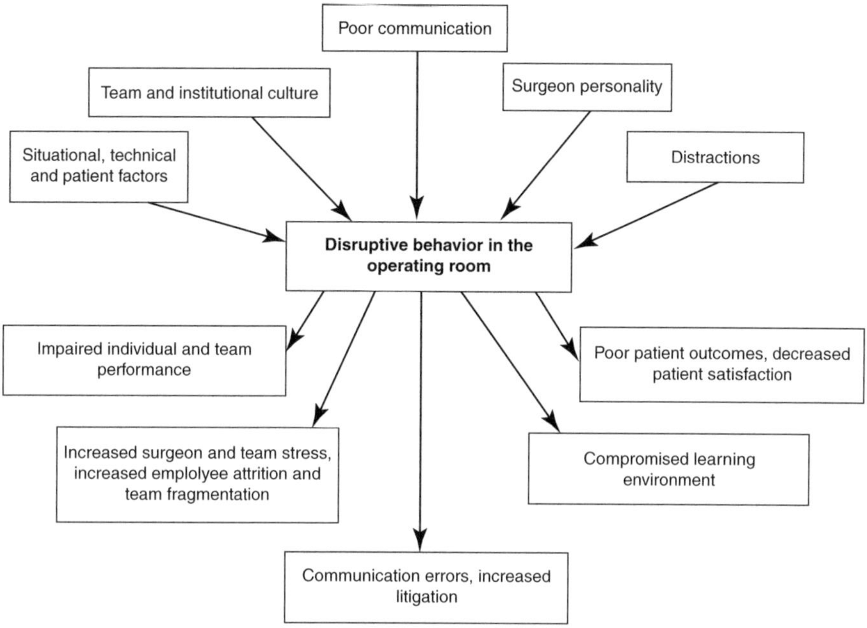

Fig. 19.1 Upstream and downstream effects of disruptive behavior in the operating room

Consequences of Disruptive Behavior: Effect on Surgeon and Staff

Disruptive behavior in the operating room (OR) is commonly associated with the surgeon as the source; however, it is imperative to understand the stress that causes disruptive behavior in the first place and how it affects the surgeon, staff rapport and performance, and safety in the OR. While surgery commands undivided attention for both the simple and complex operative tasks, there are on average 20 distracting events and/or interruptions during a single operation [8]. Stress is commonly reported in the operating room by surgeons [9], and high levels of stress strongly negatively correlate with surgeon performance [7, 10, 11]. These distractions can vary from conversations unrelated to the task at hand to people entering and leaving the OR to equipment issues, all of which translate to increased workload, decreased communication, and poor coordination on the part of the surgical team [12]. These distracting events that compromise communication and teamwork can ultimately lead to and/or be catalyzed by disruptive behavior by the surgeon, including verbal outbursts, unprofessional treatment of operating room staff, and passive aggression. The downstream effect is compromised team performance deviation, with inconsistent completion of tasks in the operating room, deviation from protocols, lower completion of patient checklists with the surgeons and nurses intraoperatively, and compromised perioperative safety [13]. A prospective observational study of complex general surgery cases in an academic hospital found that problems in communication and information flow, in addition to workload and competing tasks, had a measurable negative impact on team performance [14]. Another prospective observational study of 48 surgical procedures and 90 h of surgical teams at work identified that one-third of communication errors, including disruptive verbal communication, resulted in "visible effects on the system processes" including inefficiency, team tension, resource waste, delay, and procedural error [15].

The effects of disruptive behavior and interruptions on the surgeon and team highlight the importance of teamwork for perioperative safety. Davies and colleagues describe the six components of effective teamwork in the operating room (situational awareness, problem identification, decision-making, workload distribution, time management, and conflict resolution). Several of the components involve minimizing, addressing, and/or managing disruptive behavior in the OR [16].

Disruptive behavior in the OR not only alters the team dynamics of providers, but also burdens the surgeon and staff individually. One study of focus groups with OR nurses and surgeons at five different hospitals revealed that disruptive behavior and harsh language cause conflict in OR teams and negative culture, which ultimately can lead to termination of effective, working relationships [17]. Bullying of staff registered nurses in the workplace, from other nurses and surgeons, in the form of public humiliation, isolation, and/or excessive criticism often results in staff leaving the workplace [18, 19]. This rate of turnover in staff can perpetuate fragmentation of teams, which hampers team cohesion and communication, both essential for perioperative safety. Further, disruptive behavior in the operating room can also affect the wellness of individual surgeons, with higher levels of burnout [20] and depression and decreased self-esteem [21] in those with higher occupational stress. From physical performance to mental health and wellness, disruptive behavior has distinct effects on operating surgeons and staff, which has implications for their learners and patients.

Consequences of Disruptive Behavior: Effect on Learner

It is paramount to consider the effects of disruptive behavior in the operating room on the learners, in particular medical students and residents who are instrumental in perpetuating a culture of safety in patient care. In a survey of more than 400 trainees (medical students, interns, residents, and fellows), the majority reported experiencing mistreatment during their education, in the form of verbal abuse, specialty-choice discrimination, noneducational tasks, withholding learning opportunities, neglect, and gender/racial insensitivity [22]. This mistreatment is particularly prevalent within surgery, with surveyed medical students reporting the highest rate perception of mistreatment within surgery specifically [23, 24]. Disruptive behavior in the operating room or among surgical teams directed at the learner is not limited to medical students, with an EAST Multicenter Trial published in 2019 reporting that surveyed surgical residents commonly report discrimination and harassment [25]. Due to the hierarchal structure of surgical teams, residents and medical students often not only are the brunt of demeaning and disrespectful behavior, but also feel disempowered to address such unprofessional behavior. This has implications for perioperative safety, in that learners feel further disempowered by the culture created from disruptive behavior to address concerns about perioperative safety when they arise [26]. This is significant, given that students' speaking up about safety concerns is linked to improved patient safety [27].

The power differential between attending surgeons and learners in the setting of disruptive surgeon behavior can ultimately cause undue stress in the operating room, which ultimately permeates into the learner's didactic experience. Surgeons and surgical trainees report a culture against complaining about stress because "stress is seen as a failing" [28]. In a series of group and individual surgical residents and surgeons, Musselman and colleagues found that despite surgery residents reporting intimidation and harassment in the operating room, they rationalized dysfunctional, disruptive behavior in the operating room as functional educational tools necessary for advancement [29]. Stress related to disruptive behavior in the operating room can ultimately hamper a culture conducive to learning. Medical students and residents may not perform as well [30] or feel as comfortable asking questions [31] in a tense environment caused and propagated by disruptive behavior. In a study of 24 medical students and residents, ability to perform laparoscopic skills in the setting of increased stress was compromised such that negative stress-coping strategies correlated with longer time to complete tasks, more apt for errors, and less economy of motion [11]. An effective learning environment mandates a culture of professionalism and respect, with a zero-tolerance policy for disrespectful, disruptive behavior [32].

Not only does an environment free of disruptive behavior aimed at medical students and/or residents optimize the learning experience, but also contributes to a new culture in the rising generation of surgeons, which discourages disruptive behavior in the OR and promotes perioperative safety. The "hidden curriculum" of medical school and residency training is often thought of as learning the behavioral norms and values of the surgical culture [33]. When a learner (whether medical student or resident) witnesses disruptive behavior on the part of the attending surgeon, it can normalize and perpetuate such behavior patterns [7]. Further, medical students who are exposed to disruptive attending behavior and/or perceived mistreatment are less likely to have an interest in and respect for surgical specialties [6, 34]. Beyond influencing career choice, the high levels of stress from disruptive interactions can also negatively impact resident wellness, contributing to burnout and depression [35].

Consequences of Disruptive Behavior: Effect on Perioperative Safety and Patient

While disruptive behavior in the OR creates anxiety and compromised intraoperative team communication, the most important downstream effect is on the performance of the team and consequent perioperative safety and patient outcomes [36]. Compromised performance can be in the form of communication problems or technical errors on the part of the surgeon, with the ultimate end consequence of compromised perioperative safety. In a retrospective cohort study using the American College of Surgeons National Surgical Quality Improvement Program database of more than 10,000 surgical procedures performed by general and vascular surgeons, there was a direct link between number of complaints about a surgeon and adverse surgical outcomes [37].

Since the "To Err is Human" report was published in 1999, there has been a renewed focus in the medical community and lay community at large in understanding, preventing, and managing medical error [38]. Of malpractice claims filed against surgeons, nearly 80% are related to an error in the intraoperative phase of care [39]. While there have been few studies to perform root-cause analyses of error in the operating room, surveys from attending and resident surgeons suggest that errors can result from being distracting from communication problems and interpersonal conflict in the operating room. In an observational study of surgical teams in the operating room, Catchpole and colleagues report that surgeons with high levels of leadership and management skills and situational awareness fostered teamwork and had fewer surgical errors [40]. This correlation has been described in other observational studies of surgical teams, one of which identified increased odds of complications and patient death when surgical teams do not demonstrate teamwork and open communication, including speaking up during critical moments, along with disruptive interactions [41]. Other studies have also described near misses and compromised patient safety due to a lack of leadership and/or communication errors in the operating room [14]. A surgeon review of 444 surgical malpractice claims from four liability insurers identified 60 cases involving communication breakdown resulting in harm to patients, the majority of which involved an attending surgeon (and occasionally a resident) [42]. Not only can communication errors occur with disruptive behavior in the OR, but disruptive behavior can also affect clinical decision-making among clinicians, translating into poor patient outcomes [2, 43]. This highlights the fact that the greatest victim of disruptive behavior in the OR is not the surgeon, staff, or learner, but the patient.

The most concerning aspect of disruptive surgeon behavior on patient care is that the environment created by disruptive behavior may prevent or discourage OR team members from speaking up about discomfort with operative or postoperative course events and decision-making, similar to the hesitancy reported by residents [6]. In a cross-sectional study of 244 surgeons and surgical nurses, disruptive behavior was reported by the majority of respondents (83%), and reported to be perpetuated because of lack of consequences and hesitance to report or address disruptive behavior due to fear of retaliation, lack of change, lack of security, and culture [44]. Other surveys of perioperative staff that work with surgeons report difficulty voicing opinions about disagreement or perceived problems in patient care [45, 46]. While situational stressors unique to a patient case may arise, disruptive behavior may be perpetuated by cultural factors; staff in the OR may not feel that there is "social infrastructure" to voice concerns about disruptive behavior and communication problems in the operating room, ultimately posing higher risk of medical and surgical errors [47].

Strategies for Preventing, Addressing, and Managing Disruptive Behavior in the OR

While the factors that influence disruptive behavior in the operating room are complex and interactive, so must the solutions be to create an environment in which disruptive behavior can be prevented, managed, and/or addressed effectively.

Individual Level

While a shift in culture and "top-down" approaches from leadership are ultimately required to prevent and address disruptive behavior in the OR, programming at the individual level is crucial. This should be done at every level of participant in the surgical team and should start early. Despite the pervasiveness of self-reported mistreatment by medical students in the operating room, there is no systematic, institutional strategy for helping medical students dealing with stress and promoting a culture of safety [28]. Trainees are not instructed on how to manage intraoperative stressors, how to cope through observing similar scenarios, or how to speak up about concerns related to perioperative safety. Crisis or stress management interventions, consisting of didactics, simulation exercises, and individualized specific feedback, have yet to be widely adopted into medical student and resident training, despite their established effectiveness [28]. One academic program described medical students as feeling more comfortable addressing disruptive behavior in the operating room after a "mistreatment course" incorporating into their surgery clerkship didactics, which included lectures and hands-on role-playing scenarios [48]. Other programs have incorporated a year-long curriculum into third- or fourth-year curriculum, which focuses on tenants of professionalism and discourages disruptive behavior in the OR on the part of the individual, but also as an observer of disruptive behavior [49]. In the era of increasing incorporation of simulation into didactics for medical students and residents, there is also great opportunity to utilize simulation labs for learning communication and working within a teamwork-focused environment with the ability to prevent and/or address disruptive behavior and downstream safety in the OR [50–52]. Gettman and colleagues describe a simulation lab didactics in which urology residents are faced with two clinical scenarios (insufflator failure or carbon dioxide embolism): one before-and-after simulation didactics that focused on teamwork improved residents' consequent adherence to best safe practice and maintenance of positive rapport among team members [53].

Training should be implemented not only at the resident level to optimize teamwork and communication skills, but also at the level of the attending surgeons. Surgeons, as leaders in the operating room, should be cognizant of their internal and external stressors, which may affect their performance levels and behavior in an undisrupted environment. This type of self-awareness can come from leadership and professional development in conjunction with development in surgical skills, in which stress management, conflict resolution, and teamwork are emphasized. Stress management education, not dissimilar to what is taught in the aviation and military field, focused on self-awareness, focus, relaxation, positive self-talk, visualization, and team building and has been shown to optimize surgical performance [54].

Team Level

Preventing, minimizing, and addressing disruptive behavior in the OR require a team culture and team approach. Team training programs focused on dealing with intraoperative stressors, and fostering an environment of respectful, open communication is key to creating the cultural shift required to prevent disruptive behaviors in the OR. These programs should include training for situations in which disruptive behaviors occur, along with effective strategies such as discussing situations with involved individuals and articulating problems and possible solutions [5] and/or coaching programs to staff about addressing and preventing disruptive behavior [55]. One such program is TeamSTEPPS, a federally sponsored evidence-based team training program for health care professionals [56]. The program involves a top-down approach with initial leadership training for Chairs and OR Directors, followed by training of all staff and appointment of team "champions," which focuses on teamwork in the OR, minimizing disruptive behavior in the OR, and addressing it when it arises. Self-rated communication and teamwork among residents and attending surgeons, as well as other OR staff, increase significantly after implementation of the nine-month TeamSTEPPS training [56]. Similar to TeamSTEPPS, Medical Team Training (MTT) is a one-day intensive training for OR staff aimed at improving teamwork, minimizing disruption in the OR, and optimizing patient safety through didactic modules, videos, and role-playing. Such a program has been shown to increase subjective sense of teamwork and patient safety among OR staff, as well as improved efficiency in case turnover [57]. There are other descriptions of individual institution's assessment of their own hospital and surgery staff team needs, and creation of a unified stance on professionalism and communication in the operating room, followed by training with the whole OR staff with focus on addressing disruptive behavior [58]. The program implementation improved conflict resolution and teamwork with the operative staff after 6 months, highlighting that investment in teams can have a lasting effect on the surgical culture of an institution.

Systems Level

Despite the pervasively reported high levels of disruptive behavior from surgeons, only 3–4% of physicians are referred for remediation for unprofessional, disruptive behavior [59]. This discordance highlights a potential area of systemic intervention. Not only should a culture of reporting and proactively addressing disruptive behavior be encouraged in the spirit of patient safety, but also when it is, appropriate mechanisms should be in place for remediating surgeons. This can be fostered by professional standards that shift the culture toward a no-tolerance policy against disruptive behavior in the OR. In 2008, the Joint Commission on Accreditation of Healthcare Organizations (JCAHO) announced that disruptive behaviors would be considered "sentinel events" and included any "intimidation and disruptive acts that might foster errors, contribute to poor patient care, increase costs, and discourage teamwork" [5]. JCAHO also recommends that "disruptive" physicians be non-punitively educated and rehabilitated. This announcement has catalyzed professional societies, including the American College of Surgeons, to update and publish professional standards and competencies, including interpersonal and communication skills and professionalism [60]. The result of these recommendations from leadership is a call to hospitals to teach operative staff about how to identify and be accountable for addressing disruptive behavior, as well as create accessible, nonpunitive processes for reporting disruptive behavior. After reports have been investigated, the institution should be obligated to have a transparent, consistent system in place for dealing with and addressing these behaviors from surgeons. This can be done with an intentional, organized OR and team structure, with clear expectations of behavior and roles, multidisciplinary process improvement teams, bilateral active feedback of team members, team-building initiatives, informal leaders, and rapidly and consistently addressing disruptive behavior [61]. Villafranca and colleagues, who have researched disruptive behavior and its effects on surgeons, surgical staff, and patients, report that the key to mitigating disruptive behavior is prevention by setting behavioral standards, helping clinicians to meet those standards, and selectively recruiting and hiring employees who are less likely to act disruptively [2]. This can be in the form of macro-level (institutional, cultural) solutions like monitoring compliance and enforcing standards, to microlevel solutions (individual, team based) that support witnesses and those affected by disruptive behavior with support to respond appropriately.

Conclusion: Call to Leadership for Surgeons

Disruptive behavior in the operating room can manifest in many forms and is the product of individual, team, and cultural environment. The downstream effects of disruptive behavior have implications for surgeons, teams, learners, surgical culture at large, perioperative safety, and patient outcomes. As leaders of the operating team, it is essential that surgeons do not contribute to disruptive behavior, either in individual conduct or in perpetuation of a complicit culture. Understanding how to recognize, address, manage, and ultimately prevent disruptive behavior in the operating room is of great importance, given that disruptive behavior has negative effects on the surgeon, surgical teams, learners, and most importantly patients.

Preventing and addressing disruptive behavior in the operating room mandate a multitiered approach. With a combination of systemic, institutional changes and team-based approaches to promote a culture of open communication and teamwork, a cultural shift can be instigated and perpetuated. Ultimately, interventions to effectively prevent and manage operating room conflicts are successful when the focus remains on improved patient care and outcomes [62]. As champions of patients and team leaders, surgeons must have an integral role in leading a culture of respect and safety, void of disruptive behavior both in the operating room and within surgical teams.

References

1. American Medical Association. Report of the Council on Ethical and Judicial Affairs: physicians with disruptive behavior. https://www.ama-assn.org/delivering-care/ethics/physicians-disruptive-behavior. Accessed 6 June 2019.
2. Villafranca A, Hamlin C, Enns S, Jacobsohn E. Disruptive behaviour in the perioperative setting: a contemporary review. Can J Anaesth. 2017;64(2):128–40.
3. Weber DO. Poll results: doctors' disruptive behavior disturbs physician leaders. Physician Exec. 2004;30(5):6–14.
4. Tibble HM, Broughton NS, Studdert DM, Spittal MJ, Hill N, Morris JM, et al. Why do surgeons receive more complaints than their physician peers? ANZ J Surg. 2018;88(4):269–73.
5. Halverson AL, Neumayer L, Dagi TF. Leadership skills in the OR: part II: recognizing disruptive behavior. Bull Am Coll Surg. 2012;97(6):17–23.
6. Cochran A, Elder WB. Effects of disruptive surgeon behavior in the operating room. Am J Surg. 2015;209(1):65–70.
7. Villafranca A, Fast I, Jacobsohn E. Disruptive behavior in the operating room: prevalence, consequences, prevention, and management. Curr Opin Anaesthesiol. 2018;31(3):366–74.
8. Healey AN, Primus CP, Koutantji M. Quantifying distraction and interruption in urological surgery. Qual Saf Health Care. 2007;16(2):135–9.
9. Arora S, Hull L, Sevdalis N, Tierney T, Nestel D, Woloshynowych M, et al. Factors compromising safety in surgery: stressful events in the operating room. Am J Surg. 2010;199(1):60–5.
10. Berguer R, Smith WD, Chung YH. Performing laparoscopic surgery is significantly more stressful for the surgeon than open surgery. Surg Endosc. 2001;15(10):1204–7.
11. Hassan I, Weyers P, Maschuw K, Dick B, Gerdes B, Rothmund M, et al. Negative stress-coping strategies among novices in surgery correlate with poor virtual laparoscopic performance. Br J Surg. 2006;93(12):1554–9.
12. Weber J, Catchpole K, Becker AJ, Schlenker B, Weigl M. Effects of flow disruptions on mental workload and surgical performance in robotic-assisted surgery. World J Surg. 2018;42(11):3599–607.
13. Sevdalis N, Undre S, McDermott J, Giddie J, Diner L, Smith G. Impact of intraoperative distractions on patient safety: a prospective descriptive study using validated instruments. World J Surg. 2014;38(4):751–8.
14. Christian CK, Gustafson ML, Roth EM, Sheridan TB, Gandhi TK, Dwyer K, et al. A prospective study of patient safety in the operating room. Surgery. 2006;139(2):159–73.
15. Lingard L, Espin S, Whyte S, Regehr G, Baker GR, Reznick R, et al. Communication failures in the operating room: an observational classification of recurrent types and effects. Qual Saf Health Care. 2004;13(5):330–4.
16. Davies JM. Team communication in the operating room. Acta Anaesthesiol Scand. 2005;49(7):898–901.
17. Rogers D, Lingard L, Boehler ML, Espin S, Klingensmith M, Mellinger JD, et al. Teaching operating room conflict management to surgeons: clarifying the optimal approach. Med Educ. 2011;45(9):939–45.
18. Vessey JA, Demarco RF, Gaffney DA, Budin WC. Bullying of staff registered nurses in the workplace: a preliminary study for developing personal and organizational strategies for the transformation of hostile to healthy workplace environments. J Prof Nurs. 2009;25(5):299–306.
19. Walinder R, Runeson-Broberg R, Arakelian E, Nordqvist T, Runeson A, Rask-Andersen A. A supportive climate and low strain promote Well-being and sustainable working life in the operation theatre. Ups J Med Sci. 2018;123(3):183–90.

20. Laschinger HK, Grau AL, Finegan J, Wilk P. New graduate nurses' experiences of bullying and burnout in hospital settings. J Adv Nurs. 2010;66(12):2732–42.
21. Pfifferling JH. The disruptive physician. A quality of professional life factor. Physician Exec. 1999;25(2):56–61.
22. Kulaylat AN, Qin D, Sun SX, Hollenbeak CS, Schubart JR, Aboud AJ, et al. Perceptions of mistreatment among trainees vary at different stages of clinical training. BMC Med Educ. 2017;17(1):14.
23. Richardson DA, Becker M, Frank RR, Sokol RJ. Assessing medical students' perceptions of mistreatment in their second and third years. Acad Med. 1997;72(8):728–30.
24. Lebenthal A, Kaiserman I, Lernau O. Student abuse in medical school: a comparison of students' and faculty's perceptions. Isr J Med Sci. 1996;32(3–4):229–38.
25. Fitzgerald CA, Smith RN, Luo-Owen X, Turay D, Ferrada P, Han J, et al. Screening for harassment, abuse, and discrimination among surgery residents: an EAST multicenter trial. Am Surg. 2019;85(5):456–61.
26. Fagan A, Parker V, Jackson D. A concept analysis of undergraduate nursing students speaking up for patient safety in the patient care environment. J Adv Nurs. 2016;72(10):2346–57.
27. Dwyer J, Faber-Langendoen K. Speaking up: an ethical action exercise. Acad Med. 2018;93(4):602–5.
28. Arora S, Sevdalis N, Nestel D, Tierney T, Woloshynowych M, Kneebone R. Managing intraoperative stress: what do surgeons want from a crisis training program? Am J Surg. 2009;197(4):537–43.
29. Musselman LJ, MacRae HM, Reznick RK, Lingard LA. 'You learn better under the gun': intimidation and harassment in surgical education. Med Educ. 2005;39(9):926–34.
30. Moawad GN, Tyan P, Kumar D, Krapf J, Marfori C, Abi Khalil ED, et al. Determining the effect of external stressors on laparoscopic skills and performance between obstetrics and gynecology residents. J Surg Educ. 2017;74(5):862–6.
31. Coats RD, Burd RS. Intraoperative communication of residents with faculty: perception versus reality. J Surg Res. 2002;104(1):40–5.
32. Spruce L. Back to basics: speak up. AORN J. 2014;99(3):407–12; quiz 13–5.
33. Ludwig B, Turk B, Seitz T, Klaus I, Loffler-Stastka H. The search for attitude—a hidden curriculum assessment from a central European perspective. Wien Klin Wochenschr. 2018;130(3–4):134–40.
34. Stratton TD, McLaughlin MA, Witte FM, Fosson SE, Nora LM. Does students' exposure to gender discrimination and sexual harassment in medical school affect specialty choice and residency program selection? Acad Med. 2005;80(4):400–8.
35. Lebares CC, Guvva EV, Ascher NL, O'Sullivan PS, Harris HW, Epel ES. Burnout and stress among US surgery residents: psychological distress and resilience. J Am Coll Surg. 2018;226(1):80–90.
36. Schiff L, Tsafrir Z, Aoun J, Taylor A, Theoharis E, Eisenstein D. Quality of communication in robotic surgery and surgical outcomes. JSLS. 2016;20(3):e2016.00026.
37. Catron TF, Guillamondegui OD, Karrass J, Cooper WO, Martin BJ, Dmochowski RR, et al. Patient complaints and adverse surgical outcomes. Am J Med Qual. 2016;31(5):415–22.
38. Bates DW, Singh H. Two decades since To Err Is Human: an assessment of progress and emerging priorities in patient safety. Health Aff (Millwood). 2018;37(11):1736–43.
39. Rogers SO Jr, Gawande AA, Kwaan M, Puopolo AL, Yoon C, Brennan TA, et al. Analysis of surgical errors in closed malpractice claims at 4 liability insurers. Surgery. 2006;140(1):25–33.
40. Catchpole K, Mishra A, Handa A, McCulloch P. Teamwork and error in the operating room: analysis of skills and roles. Ann Surg. 2008;247(4):699–706.
41. Mazzocco K, Petitti DB, Fong KT, Bonacum D, Brookey J, Graham S, et al. Surgical team behaviors and patient outcomes. Am J Surg. 2009;197(5):678–85.
42. Greenberg CC, Regenbogen SE, Studdert DM, Lipsitz SR, Rogers SO, Zinner MJ, et al. Patterns of communication breakdowns resulting in injury to surgical patients. J Am Coll Surg. 2007;204(4):533–40.

43. Rosenstein AH, O'Daniel M. Invited article: managing disruptive physician behavior: impact on staff relationships and patient care. Neurology. 2008;70(17):1564–70.
44. Maddineshat M, Hashemi M, Tabatabaeichehr M. Evaluation of the disruptive behaviors among treatment teams and its reflection on the therapy process of patients in the operating room: the impact of personal conflicts. J Educ Health Promot. 2017;6:69.
45. Minhas MS, Muzzammil M, Effendi J. Assessment of safety levels in operation rooms at two major tertiary care public hospitals of Karachi. Safe surgery saves life. J Ayub Med Coll Abbottabad. 2017;29(4):580–6.
46. Smetzer JL, Cohen MR. Intimidation: practitioners speak up about this unresolved problem. Jt Comm J Qual Patient Saf. 2005;31(10):594–9.
47. Rydenfalt C, Johansson G, Larsson PA, Akerman K, Odenrick P. Social structures in the operating theatre: how contradicting rationalities and trust affect work. J Adv Nurs. 2012;68(4):783–95.
48. Hasty BN, Miller SE, Bereknyei Merrell S, Lin DT, Shipper ES, Lau JN. Medical student perceptions of a mistreatment program during the surgery clerkship. Am J Surg. 2018;215(4):761–6.
49. Hultman CS, Connolly A, Halvorson EG, Rowland P, Meyers MO, Mayer DC, et al. Get on your boots: preparing fourth-year medical students for a career in surgery, using a focused curriculum to teach the competency of professionalism. J Surg Res. 2012;177(2):217–23.
50. Graafland M, Bemelman WA, Schijven MP. Appraisal of face and content validity of a serious game improving situational awareness in surgical training. J Laparoendosc Adv Surg Tech. 2015;25(1):43–9.
51. Naguib S, Meyr AJ. Reliability, surgeon preferences, and eye-tracking assessment of the stress examination of the tarsometatarsal (Lisfranc) joint complex. J Foot Ankle Surg. 2019;58(1):93–6.
52. Anton NE, Beane J, Yurco AM, Howley LD, Bean E, Myers EM, et al. Mental skills training effectively minimizes operative performance deterioration under stressful conditions: results of a randomized controlled study. Am J Surg. 2018;215(2):214–21.
53. Gettman MT, Pereira CW, Lipsky K, Wilson T, Arnold JJ, Leibovich BC, et al. Use of high fidelity operating room simulation to assess and teach communication, teamwork and laparoscopic skills: initial experience. J Urol. 2009;181(3):1289–96.
54. Goldberg MB, Mazzei M, Maher Z, Fish JH, Milner R, Yu D, et al. Optimizing performance through stress training—an educational strategy for surgical residents. Am J Surg. 2018;216(3):618–23.
55. Kleiner C, Link T, Maynard MT, Halverson CK. Coaching to improve the quality of communication during briefings and debriefings. AORN J. 2014;100(4):358–68.
56. Armour Forse R, Bramble JD, McQuillan R. Team training can improve operating room performance. Surgery. 2011;150(4):771–8.
57. Wolf FA, Way LW, Stewart L. The efficacy of medical team training: improved team performance and decreased operating room delays: a detailed analysis of 4863 cases. Ann Surg. 2010;252(3):477–83.
58. Larson BA, Martinson DJ. Words can hurt. Dealing with verbal abuse in the operating room. AORN J. 1990;52(6):1238–41.
59. Hickson GB, Pichert JW, Webb LE, Gabbe SG. A complementary approach to promoting professionalism: identifying, measuring, and addressing unprofessional behaviors. Acad Med. 2007;82(11):1040–8.
60. American College of Surgeons. Statements on principles; 2016. https://www.facs.org/about-acs/statements/stonprin#anchor1256362016. Accessed 6 June 2019.
61. Sax HC. Building high-performance teams in the operating room. Surg Clin N Am. 2012;92(1):15–9.
62. Rogers DA, Lingard L, Boehler ML, Espin S, Schindler N, Klingensmith M, et al. Foundations for teaching surgeons to address the contributions of systems to operating room team conflict. Am J Surg. 2013;206(3):428–32.

"Code Red!" Preventing and Managing Fire and Smoke Hazards in the OR

20

Wilton C. Levine and Yasmine Tameze

Introduction

An estimated 550–650 surgical fires occur in the United States per year, leading to devastating repercussions to patients, in addition to significant legal and economic consequences for the surgical team and the facility involved [1, 2]. Together with retained sponges and wrong-site surgery, patient safety groups consider surgical fires as "never events"—events that can be avoided entirely with organizational checks and balances [3]. Fire risk can be minimized when the operating room team understands fire hazards presented by each side of the fire triangle, and appropriate steps are taken to minimize these risks. This chapter describes the risks, prevention, response, and impact of fires in the operating room and procedural areas.

The Risks: The Fire Triad

A fire requires three components: (1) an oxidizer, (2) an ignition source, and (3) a fuel. This is also known as the "fire triangle" (Fig. 20.1).

W. C. Levine (✉) · Y. Tameze
Department of Anesthesia, Critical Care and Pain Medicine, Massachusetts General Hospital, Boston, MA, USA
e-mail: wlevine@mgh.harvard.edu

J. J. Hoballah et al. (eds.), *Principles of Perioperative Safety and Efficiency*,
https://doi.org/10.1007/978-3-031-41089-5_20

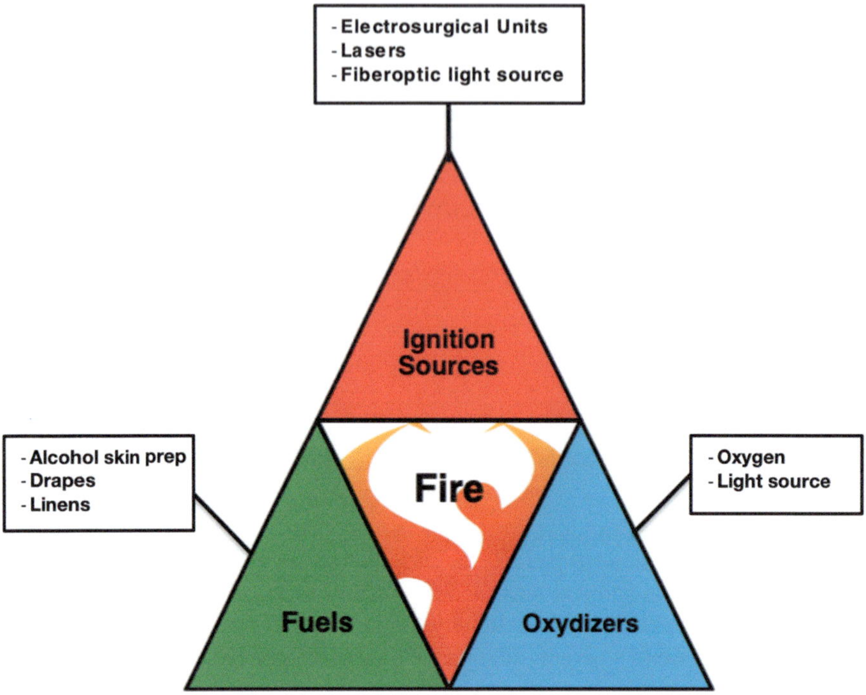

Fig. 20.1 The classic "fire triangle" and examples of components found in the operating room. Used with permission from Anesthesia Patient Safety Foundation; www.apsf.org

Oxidizers

In surgical fires, oxidizers typically include oxygen and/or nitrous oxide. In the OR, oxygen is provided to the patient via tracheal tubes, laryngeal mask airways, face masks, or nasal cannulas. These are especially hazardous when contributing to an oxidizer-enriched atmosphere (i.e., any oxygen concentration of more than 21%, or the presence of any concentration of nitrous oxide). Such environments are also created when the configuration of draping and oxygen sources promote the trapping or pooling of an oxidizer-rich atmosphere [4]. Redraping such that no "tent" covers the field helps decrease the possibility of an oxygen-rich environment [5]. It is recommended that an open draping technique (where the face is partially covered or not covered at all) be used to reduce the risk of accumulated oxygen under the drape when surgery is required in proximity to the oxygen source [6]. These oxidizer-enriched environments increase the likelihood and intensity of combustion in the surgical field.

Ignition Sources

In OR fires, the ignition source may encompass any source of energy in the operating room that can start a fire in the presence of fuel and oxidizer. These include, but are not limited to, electrocautery (ECU) or electrosurgery (ESU) units, lasers, fiber-optic light cords, and cable connections. Of the reported surgical fires, between 70% and 90% had ESU equipment as their ignition source, 10% were caused by lasers, and the rest were caused by a variety of other ignition sources [2, 7]. One of these other ignition sources worth mentioning is the fiber-optic light cord. As the frequency of cases done robotically and laparoscopically increases, the fiber-optic light is emerging as an important ignition source, as it can burn quickly through the drapes and cause thermal injury to patients. In appropriate settings, these lights can ignite an operating room fire; therefore, it is important that they are on "standby" mode when not in use [8].

Fuels

Fuels include any flammable sources including alcohol preps, surgical drapes, linens, sponges, towels, surgical drapes, and the patient (see Fig. 20.1). When using alcohol-based surgical prep solutions, it is critical to use the smallest possible solution preparation and to follow the manufacturer's instructions for use (IFU). Typically, alcohol-based surgical prep is required to dry for a minimum of 3 min before placing the surgical drapes. This is to allow drying and evaporation of any remaining liquid prep.

The Risks: Assessing the Preoperative Surgical Fire Risk

A key element to fire prevention in the OR is the communication amongst each of the OR team members regarding fire risk assessment and the plan to minimize the risk [5, 7]. Ideally, this should be done at the beginning of the case and included in the surgical "time-out" [3, 4]. Several professional organizations have highlighted the importance of a surgical time-out at the beginning of the case that includes the fire risk assessment [9]. One tool to assess fire safety risk is the Silverstein Fire Risk Assessment [10], where each case is given a score from 0 to 3 (Table 20.1). The

Table 20.1 Silverstein Fire Risk Assessment Tool

Risk factor	Yes	No
Surgery above the xiphoid	1	0
Open oxygen source	1	0
Available ignition source	1	0
Total score	–	–

From Scoring fire risk for surgical patients. OR Manager. 2006;22(1):19–20. Used with permission from Access Intelligence scoring is based on the surgical location, oxygen source, and presence of a source of ignition. Based on the score, the surgery is considered high risk (3 points), intermediate risk (2 points), or low risk (0–1 point) [2, 10]. The plan for surgical fire prevention will be based on the level of risk. As the patient's fire risk score increases, the OR team should follow the guidelines listed for the patient's highest score along with the standard fire safety precautions of the lower scores [9]. For example, if a patient has a fire risk score of 3 (high fire risk), the OR team should implement all of the recommended guidelines listed under "high risk" along with the standard fire safety recommendations.

Prevention Measures Based on Risk Assessment

For all procedures (score 0–3), the following standard prevention measures should be taken [4]:

- Surgical drapes should minimize the accumulation of oxidizer under the drapes.
- Before placing the surgical drapes, flammable skin solutions must be allowed to dry for at least 3 min or according to the package insert, before draping.
- Gauze and sponges should be moistened before use in proximity to ignition source.
- Protect heat sources (i.e., keep the active electrode tip in holster when not in use).

For intermediate-risk procedures (2 points):

These procedures have the potential to convert to being high risk. The OR staff should follow the prevention measures described above, but be prepared to initiate high-risk precautions if necessary.

For high-risk procedures (3 points) such as procedures above xyphoid requiring the use of an open oxygen source in the presence of an ignition source (i.e., ENT surgery, dermatology/plastic procedures), the key to prevention is altering one or more of these components to avoid combustion. This implies (a) minimizing or avoiding an oxidizer-rich atmosphere near the surgical site, (b) safely managing ignition sources, and (c) safely managing fuels [2].

Minimizing or Avoiding an Oxidizer-Rich Atmosphere Near the Surgical Site

The open delivery of oxygen from a direct source, such as through nasal cannula or face mask, is the predominant oxidizer cause in OR fires, accounting for about 85% of operating room fires reviewed by a closed claim analysis [7]. In fact, many materials that will not burn or sustain a flame in ambient air do burn in an oxygen-rich environment: for example, polyvinyl chloride (PVC) plastic, a component of endotracheal tubes, requires 26% oxygen to maintain burning [2].

For high-risk procedures:

- Delivery of supplemental oxygen (i.e., via nasal cannula or face mask) should be avoided.
- If not able to maintain adequate delivery with oxygen concentration of ≤30% with an open source, secure the airway with an endotracheal tube or a supraglottic device

Airway Surgery

- Patients are usually intubated; therefore, monitoring both the fraction of inspired oxygen concentration (FiO_2) and fraction of expired oxygen (FeO_2) is possible. Both FiO_2 and FeO_2 should be ≤30% before activation of any ignition source.
- If using laser in the airway, the airway should be secured using a cuffed laser-resistant endotracheal tube, and the cuff should be filled with saline and colored with an indicator dye. The dye serves as a marker, to rapidly demonstrate inadvertent cuff perforation by the laser.

Exceptional cases exist when procedures above the xyphoid require conscious sedation, and oxygen delivery via nasal cannula or mask is necessary to maintain adequate oxygen saturation. These include (awake) carotid artery surgery, awake craniotomies, and some pacemaker implantations. In such high-risk procedures, where eliminating the use of an open oxygen source by securing the airway is not an option, the recommendations are as follows [2, 4]:

- Use an oxygen blender or adaptor to use the lowest concentration of oxygen required to maintain adequate hemoglobin saturations as monitored via pulse oximetry (≥92%). If an oxygen blender or common gas outlet is not available, oxygen concentration adjustment can be made using a standard wye breathing circuit [5].
- The surgeon must communicate with the anesthetist or sedation nurse when about to use an ignition source to allow for further reduction of fraction of inspired oxygen concentration (≤30%) or discontinue nitrous oxide. There should be a delay of 3–5 min before using an ignition source to allow for dissipation of oxygen on the surgical field. To further minimize the oxygen buildup, the anesthetist or sedation nurse can "flush" with high-flow medical air or scavenge the operating field with suction.

Safely Managing Ignition Sources

Electrosurgical units (ESUs) are the most common ignition source in surgical fires [7]. It is recommended to avoid using any ESU devices in high-risk procedures. If an ESU is necessary, avoiding the use of monopolar ESU and instead using a bipolar tip or harmonic scalpel at the lowest effective energy setting are the best way to reduce any chances of combustion. Bipolar ESU uses low power across the forceps tips and little to no sparking, which might be the reason why there has not been as many reported cases of OR fires with bipolar ESU [2, 11].

Surgical lasers are the second most frequent cause of ignition in surgical fires [2]. While less common than the fires caused by ESUs, their fires are more serious, as they deliver power as high as 120 W focused in a small area. Laser energy can penetrate drapes and ignite towels and linens that may burn for some time before being noticed. As mentioned earlier, it is essential that the surgeon communicates clearly to the team prior to the use of ignition to make sure that there is enough time for the nitrous oxide and oxygen to have dissipated from the surgical field. The recommendations to minimize ignition source risk include the following [2]:

- Place the electrosurgical active electrode in a holster when not in active use.
- The surgeon should activate the unit or laser only when the active electrode tip is in direct view.
- If open oxygen sources are employed, use bipolar ESU, a scalpel, or harmonic scalpel whenever possible. If not replaceable, use ESU with extreme caution.
- During a tracheostomy, do not use ESU or ECU to cut into the trachea; use a scalpel instead.
- Give the anesthetist or sedation nurse adequate notice of 3–5 min before activating the ESU, to allow enough time for oxygen concentration $\leq 30\%$ and NO_2 discontinued, and the anesthetist or sedation nurse and surgeon should together confirm the current oxygen concentration before use of the ESU.
- Use the lowest effective setting once ESU is activated.

Safely Managing Fuels

The nurses and OR staff typically handle the fuels, which include most of the materials that come in contact with the patient (including the patient), such as alcohol-based skin preparation solutions, sponges, drapes, and towels. Alcohol fires can be difficult to detect because they are able to burn in room air, and their flames are hard to visualize with the naked eye. The recommendations to minimize fuel risks include the following [2]:

Prep Solution

1. Avoid pooling or spilling of flammable liquid preps and apply alcohol-based prep solutions using an appropriately sized applicator.
2. Avoid re-prepping any area. Re-prepping the area may lead to pooling of the alcohol-based prep and a fuel reservoir.

3. Allow flammable liquids to dry fully before draping: Most solutions have a minimum drying time of 3 min for hairless skin, but this time increases when the solution is applied to unclipped skin. Prep dry time must be monitored and adhered to, and follow the manufacturer's IFU.

Drape Management

1. Remove any solution-soaked materials from the operating room prior to draping or use of the ignition source [12].
2. Draping should be done to avoid accumulation of oxidizers under the drape. If available, use an adherent incise drape to isolate the head, face, and neck incisions from oxidizer-enriched atmosphere.
3. Coat head and facial hair within the surgical field with water-soluble surgical lubricating jelly [9].

A large part of reducing the fire risk in the OR relies on minimizing the interaction between each side of the fire triangle. Assessing the risk of the procedure at the beginning of the procedure allows each member of the OR team to understand and communicate fire risks [9].

Prevention of Operating Room Fires: Education

In addition to safely managing oxidizers, ignition sources, and fuel, an effective response to OR fire includes education and practice. Every member of the OR team should receive training on OR fire prevention and management and should be familiar with their institutional fire safety protocols [4]. Another tool to enhance the OR team response to OR fires is OR fire drills and team simulation, which have been shown to improve staff response to a fire [4]. These OR drills allow each member of the OR to be familiar with their pre-assigned role in managing a fire and enhance communication amongst OR team members and with the local authorities [9]. In high-risk cases, having a brief discussion during surgical time-out might be useful to review/assign roles in the case of a fire. Finally, it is useful to understand the different types of fire extinguishers and uses during OR fires. Fire extinguishers should not be the first choice during surgical fires but might be needed in cases where the fire engulfs a patient, has migrated off the patient, involves material that continues to burn after being removed from the patient, or involves equipment in the OR [2]. Fire extinguishers are classified according to the agent used (Table 20.2).

The ECRI and APSF recommend CO_2 extinguishers as they are nontoxic, readily dissipate, and are not likely to result in thermal injury.

Table 20.2 Fire extinguisher chart.

Extinguisher		Type of Fire			
Color	Type	Solid (Paper)	Flammable Liquids	Flammable Gas	Electrical Equipment
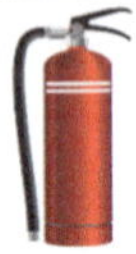	Water	✓	✗	✗	✗
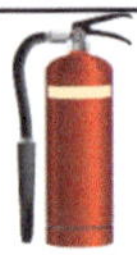	Foam	✓	✓	✗	✗
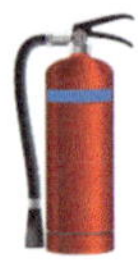	Dry Powder	✓	✓	✓	✓
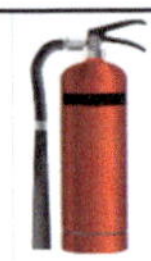		✗	✓	✗	✓
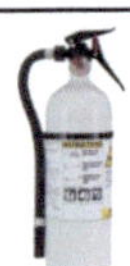	MRI Compatible	✓	✓	✗	✓
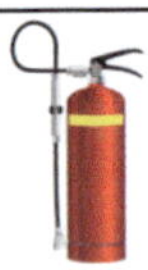	Wet Chemical	✓	✗	✗	✗

Management of Operating Room Fires

In nonoperating room fires, the RACE acronym (rescue, alarm, confine, and extinguish) is commonly used. In the operating room, this sequence may not be appropriate, depending on the type of fire. Operating room fires can be divided into fires occurring on the patients, in the patient (i.e., airway fires), and in the operating room environment.

Fires Occurring on the Patient

About 44% of the fires occurring on the patient occur on the head, neck, or upper chest [2]. Managing the fires that happen on the patient needs a team effort, with each performing their pre-assigned fire management tasks, which include [4]:

1. Calling for help.
2. Stopping the procedure.
3. Stopping the flow of all airway gases: removing the oxidizer can allow for the fire to subside.
4. Removing all drapes and burning material from the patient—even if the fire appears to be extinguished—to assess for lingering flames or fire elements hidden underneath the flames.
5. Extinguishing all burning materials in, on, and surrounding the patient with saline or water, or smothering with wet towels or sponges.

If the fire is not extinguished by these measures:

1. Use a carbon dioxide fire extinguisher, if no success.
2. Initiate the RACE fire protocol:
   (a) Rescue: move the patient from the burning source to a safe location.
   (b) Activate the fire alarm system.
   (c) Confine: close the door to the room after evacuation and turn off medical gas supply to the room. The medical gas zone valves should be shut off to prevent piped gas and vacuum systems from sustaining the fire damage or prevent potential explosion.
   (d) Extinguish: if possible, use a fire extinguisher as you retreat from the area. Do not pour saline or water on an electric fire.

Fires Occurring in the Patient: Airway Fires

About 21% of the fires occurring in the patient are airway fires (Fig. 20.2) [2]. As soon as an airway fire is suspected:

1. Remove the tracheal tube at the same time as disconnecting the breathing circuit from the tracheal tube (Fig. 20.3).

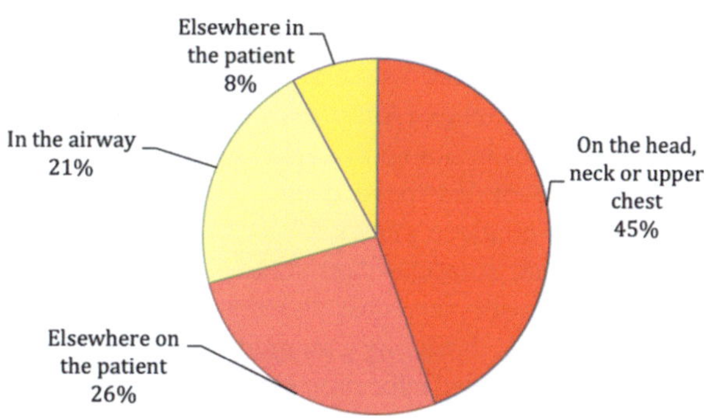

Fig. 20.2 Location of surgical fires (yellow: fires in patient; red: fire on the patient)From Health Devices. 2009;38(10):314–32. Used with permission from ECRI Institute; www.ecri.org

Fig. 20.3 Tracheal tube with oxygen flowing through it. Note the fire coming out of the tube as well as the fire progressing inside the tube against the flow of oxygen. Used with permission from Anesthesia Patient Safety Foundation; www.apsf.org

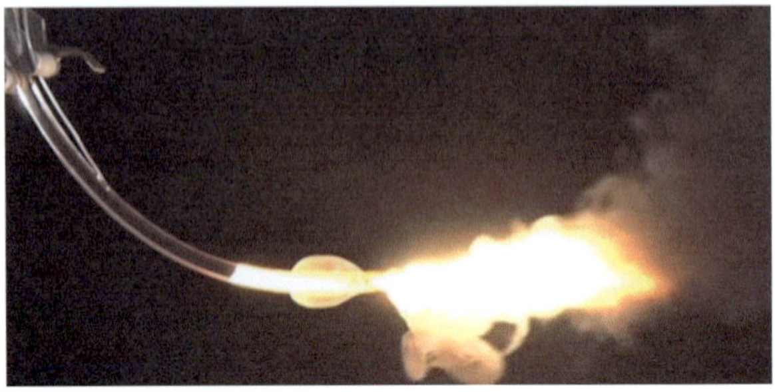

2. Stop the flow of all airway gases.
3. Remove all flammable and burning materials from the airway. Pour saline into the patient's airway.

Once the fire is extinguished:

1. Reestablish ventilation by mask, avoiding supplemental oxygen and nitrous oxide.
2. Examine the endotracheal tube to assess if fragments were left in the airway—consider rigid bronchoscopy to further evaluate the airway.
3. Consider referral to burn center, based on the extent of the injury.
4. Assess for smoke inhalation injury in non-intubated patients, including OR team members.

Fires in the Operating Room, But Not on or in the Patient

In fires that occur in the operating room but do not involve the patient, electrical equipment is often involved. The equipment at fault should be unplugged safely and removed from the OR. If not possible, the same steps followed in fires on the patient (but not the airway) should be followed, and a fire extinguisher might be needed to extinguish the device in the room. The entire operating suite should be evacuated, as the possibility of fireball explosions from bottled alcohol or gas cylinders still exists [13].

Conclusion

Operating room fires are rare but can have tragic consequences for both the injured patient and healthcare workers. In recent years, there has been an initiative from professional societies (Anesthesia Patient Safety Foundation (APSF), American Society of Anesthesiologists (ASA) ECRI, and Joint Commission), to raise awareness and prevent this "never event." This effort has been echoed by hospital-based initiatives to heighten clinicians' awareness of surgical fires by including surgical fire assessment scores to their surgical time-out, in addition to conducting yearly OR fire drills with mandatory attendance by surgeons, anesthesia providers, nurses, and technicians. Fostering communications between surgical team members, in addition to continued education about the three basic elements of surgical fires and management of OR fires, is key in reducing the incidence of this "never event."

References

1. Smith LP, Roy S. Operating room fires in otolaryngology: risk factors and prevention. Am J Otolaryngol. 2011;32(2):109–14.
2. Emergency Care Research Institute. New clinical guide to surgical fire prevention. Patients can catch fire—here's how to keep them safer. Health Devices. 2009;38(10):314–32.
3. Clarifications and expectations. Preventing surgical fires. Making fire safety a top priority in the OR. Jt Comm Perspect. 2013;33(4):8–9, 11, 12.
4. Apfelbaum JL, Caplan RA, Barker SJ, Connis RT, Cowles C, Ehrenwerth J, et al. Practice advisory for the prevention and management of operating room fires: an updated report by the American Society of Anesthesiologists Task Force on Operating Room Fires. Anesthesiology. 2013;118(2):271–90.
5. Anesthesia Patient Safety Foundation. Prevention and management of operating room fires; 2010. https://www.apsf.org/videos/or-fire-safety-video/. Accessed 31 May 2019.
6. Rinder CS. Fire safety in the operating room. Curr Opin Anaesthesiol. 2008;21(6):790–5.
7. Mehta SP, Bhananker SM, Posner KL, Domino KB. Operating room fires: a closed claims analysis. Anesthesiology. 2013;118(5):1133–9.
8. Jones TS, Black IH, Robinson TN, Jones EL. Operating room fires. Anesthesiology. 2019;130(3):492–501.
9. Association of Perioperative Registered Nurses. Fire risk safety tool kit; 2019. https://test.aorn.org/guidelines/clinical-resources/tool-kits/fire-safety-tool-kit.
10. Mathias JM. Scoring fire risk for surgical patients. OR Manager. 2006;22(1):19–20.
11. Akhtar N, Ansar F, Baig MS, Abbas A. Airway fires during surgery: management and prevention. J Anaesthesiol Clin Pharmacol. 2016;32(1):109–11.
12. NFPA 99: health care facilities code. Quincy, MA: National Fire Protection Association; 2015.
13. A clinician's guide to surgical fires. How they occur, how to prevent them, how to put them out. Health Devices. 2003;32(1):5–24.

"I Got Stuck!" Blood Exposure in the OR: Prevention and Management of Sharp Injuries and Infectious Disease Exposure

21

Tala Ballouz, Carine Sakr, and Nesrine A. Rizk

Background

The first report of occupational exposure to human immunodeficiency virus (HIV) through a needlestick prick was reported in 1984 in the United Kingdom [1]. Since then, several strategies, such as the Occupational Safety and Health Administration (OSHA) Bloodborne Pathogens Standard [2], have been implemented to provide guidance for the prevention of such incidents. Yet, needlesticks and other types of injuries continue to occur in healthcare settings. It is estimated that 600,000–800,000 needlestick and other percutaneous injuries occur among healthcare workers (HCWs) in the United States annually [3]. Elseviers et al. calculated a rate of 3.7 sharp injures per 100 healthcare workers per year, based on data from Australia, Europe, Africa, and North America [4]. Surgical personnel carry an increased risk because of potential injuries caused by sharp surgical instruments [5]. In a recent study, Makary et al. reported that 83% of surgery residents reported a needlestick injury during their training [6]. These injuries are typically associated with substantial financial costs related to the testing, prophylaxis, and counseling needed, as well

T. Ballouz · N. A. Rizk (✉)
Department of Internal Medicine, Division of Infectious Diseases, American University of Beirut, Beirut, Lebanon
e-mail: nr00@aub.edu.lb

C. Sakr
Department of Employee Health, American University of Beirut Medical Center, Beirut, Lebanon

J. J. Hoballah et al. (eds.), *Principles of Perioperative Safety and Efficiency*,
https://doi.org/10.1007/978-3-031-41089-5_21

as lost productivity [7, 8]. In addition, most HCWs experience psychological distress after such injuries, affecting their productivity and work time and thus leading to more economic costs [8–11].

In this chapter, we will discuss the risks and management of occupational exposure to the three most commonly reported blood-borne pathogens (BBPs): hepatitis B virus (HBV), hepatitis C virus (HCV), and HIV. We will also mention the standards of prevention of exposure including the standard issued by OSHA. Throughout the chapter, as our focus is exposure to blood-borne pathogens in the healthcare setting, we will follow the Centers for Disease Control and Prevention (CDC) nomenclature and use the term "source" to refer to the source patient (SP) [12]. We will refer to the exposed healthcare worker as "exposed employee" (EE).

Definitions

According to OSHA, **blood-borne pathogens** are "*pathogenic microorganisms that are present in human blood and can cause disease in humans*" [3]. They are transmitted through contact with contaminated blood and result in an infection in the exposed individual. The most frequently described pathogens are HBV, HCV, and HIV. Other less frequently reported pathogens include *Brucella*, syphilis, varicella zoster virus, Ebola virus, and malaria [13].

The most significant means of transmission in healthcare settings is intravenous exposure to contaminated blood. According to OSHA, blood is defined as human blood and any blood components or products made from human blood. Other potentially infectious products include (1) human body fluids, including, but not limited to, semen, vaginal secretions, and cerebrospinal, pleural, or pericardial fluids; (2) any unfixed tissue or organ from a living or dead human; and (3) HIV-containing cell or tissue or organ cultures, HIV- or hepatitis virus-containing culture medium, or blood, organs, or other tissues from experimental animals infected with HIV, HBV, or HCV. Fluids that do not transmit HIV unless they contain blood include tears, nasal secretions, saliva, sputum, gastric secretions, feces, and urine [3, 12].

When a mucous membrane (including eye, mouth, nose) or non-intact skin comes in contact with blood, bloody fluids contaminated with blood, or any of the previously mentioned infectious material, it is known as an **exposure incident**. When this exposure occurs in the setting of a person's work duties, it is known as an **occupational exposure** [3]. The main mode of exposure in healthcare personnel is percutaneous injury through a contaminated sharp object such as a hollow-bore needle, suture needle, scalpel, or glass. However, other modes of exposure have been reported and include mucous membrane exposure, non-intact skin exposure, and bites. Potential exposures to blood and body fluids could also occur through large-volume spills.

In the healthcare setting, most significant exposures occur within the context of surgery and surgical procedures, as those are usually associated with exposure to a large volume of blood and deep injuries.

Table 21.1 Risk of acquisition of blood-borne pathogens by mode of exposure

Mode of exposure	HBV	HCV	HIV
Percutaneous	6–30%	1.8%	0.3%
Mucous membrane	Unknown	Unknown	0.09%
Non-intact skin	Unknown	Unknown	<0.1%, incomplete
Bite	Unknown	Unknown	Unknown

HBV Hepatitis B virus, *HCV* Hepatitis, *HIV* Human immunodeficiency virus

Risk of Acquisition After Occupational Exposure to HBV, HCV, or HIV

The risk of transmission of HBV, HCV, and HIV depends on several factors and varies across settings. These factors include the baseline prevalence of these pathogens within both the general and healthcare facility populations, the type of injury (deep or shallow), the nature of the body fluid involved (with blood being the most infectious), the concentration of the virus in the fluid, and the availability of postexposure prophylaxis [12, 14]. Table 21.1 summarizes the risk of acquisition of bloodborne pathogens by mode of exposure in the healthcare setting.

Risk of Transmission of HBV

The highest titers of hepatitis B have been found to be in blood, blood products, and serous exudates [12]. It is present in moderate titers in saliva, semen, and vaginal secretions [15, 16]. The lowest titers can be found in urine, tears, and feces [15, 17, 18]. Outside of the body, HBV is relatively stable and can survive up to 7 days on surfaces at room temperature [19]. HBV transmission depends on the hepatitis B status of the source and the immunity of the exposed individual. The hepatitis B surface antigen (HBsAg) and hepatitis B e antigen (HBeAg) of the source determine infectivity. In a nonimmune healthcare worker, the risk of transmission after a needlestick prick ranges from 30% to 62% if the source is HBsAg and HBeAg positive, and 6% to 30% if the source is HBsAg positive and HBeAg negative. The risk of infection is tremendously reduced in the immune EE [12, 20].

Risk of Transmission of HCV

Similar to HBV, HCV circulates at the highest titers in blood. In addition, studies have shown that HCV can be detected in different human body fluids including saliva, semen, urine, sweat, and tears [21–24]. However, only serum has been proven infectious in human and experimental models. HCV can also survive for long periods of time on surfaces and inside needles, with one study recovering viable HCV for up to 6 weeks from dried spots of blood [25]. The most common way of occupational HCV acquisition is through percutaneous exposure through sharp and needlestick injuries. Studies estimate the average incidence of anti-HCV seroconversion from percutaneous injuries from a known HCV-positive source to be 1.8% (range: 0–7%) [12]. The risk of infection with other modes of exposure is less well defined, with two case reports describing HCV transmission after blood splash to the conjunctiva [26, 27].

Risk of Transmission of HIV

HIV is the most reported and studied blood-borne pathogen. Studies have estimated the average risk of HIV acquisition in HCWs after percutaneous injury with inoculation of blood from an HIV-positive source to be around 0.3% (95% confidence interval: 0.2–0.5%). This risk is lower after a mucous membrane exposure to HIV-infected blood and is almost 0.09% (95% confidence interval: 0.006–0.5%) [28]. The risk of transmission of HIV through intact skin is not well quantified, with most experts reporting the risk to be less than that of mucous membrane exposure. Risk factors that increase occupational HIV acquisition are well described in epidemiological studies. Some of those factors relate to the type of equipment, with the highest risk occurring after deep-wound injuries, as well as percutaneous injuries with hollow-bore blood-filled needles, blood-contaminated devices, and devices or needles recently used in an artery or vein [29]. A high viral burden in the source is another important determinant of infectivity, with a greater risk associated with a source patient with terminal acquired immunodeficiency syndrome (AIDS), or with a detectable high HIV viral load.

Management: Initial and Specific

Although prevention remains the best strategy for protecting healthcare workers from blood-borne pathogens, there is still a risk that exposure might occur during invasive procedures and surgical interventions. In such cases, institutions should have a clear system in place that guides incident reporting, evaluation, initial management, counseling, and follow-up of exposed cases, while ensuring confidentiality and privacy of the source and exposed individuals. Additionally, healthcare personnel should be adequately educated and trained in the prevention of occupational exposure. It is crucial that clinicians who provide postexposure care be accessible at all times of the day and night. Similarly, postexposure prophylaxis (PEP), hepatitis B immunoglobulin (HBIG), and hepatitis B vaccine should always be available.

Appropriate management of blood exposure in the healthcare setting, including the operating room, includes some key elements. These include initial management of the wound, exposure reporting and assessment, and providing postexposure prophylaxis and appropriate counseling.

Those exposures cause stress and result in disruption of the workflow and interruption of a procedure and lead to emotional distress and fear. This may disrupt daily life and incur in several ways, especially if pharmacologic interventions are recommended, in addition to the cost to the healthcare system (for testing and retesting, treatment, and appropriate medical follow-up).

The Initial Management of the Wound and Exposed Surface

If a healthcare worker has been exposed to blood or a bloody body fluid, the first step in the management is cleaning of the exposed wound or punctured skin with soap and water. There is no solid evidence behind this practice; however, it is recommended by OSHA, CDC, and WHO [2, 30–32]. Additionally, for exposures involving mucous membranes (eyes, nose, mouth, or skin), the recommendation is to vigorously flush the surface with water. The use of topical antiseptics (e.g., 2–4% chlorhexidine) has not been shown to be beneficial, although their use is not contraindicated. Similarly, squeezing or rubbing the injury site has been shown to be nonbeneficial. The use of caustic agents such as iodine, bleach, and others should be avoided. After the wound has been cleaned, a thorough assessment of the exposure needs to be done by a trained practitioner to assess the risk of infection and appropriately manage the situation [12, 30, 32].

The Reporting of the Incident

When an exposure occurs, prompt and confidential reporting is essential. The Health Insurance Portability and Accountability Act (HIPAA) privacy rules guarantee the respect of the medical information of the source as well as the exposed personnel. The incident is usually reported immediately to a senior practitioner or a supervisor. It is important to document all the following details:

- Details on exposure
  - Date and time
  - Location
- Type of procedure
  - The type of devices involved
  - Description of the injury (depth of wound, type of body fluid, duration and volume of exposure, condition of skin)
- Details on the source of exposure
  - Serologic status for HIV, HBV, or HCV (history of antiviral treatment, viral load if applicable)
  - History of HBV vaccination
- Details on the exposed HCW
  - Serologic status for HIV, HCV, HIV
  - HBV vaccination history
  - Medical history
  - Pregnancy or lactation

Finally, the report should mention what the management steps are and what follow-up will be recommended. This report not only serves as documentation for a particular incident, but also aims at identifying effective preventive strategies and any future risks or hazards. To ensure that this report is being correctly and promptly done, education of healthcare workers on blood-borne exposure risks and importance of reporting incidents as soon as they occur is essential. Several institutions use a comprehensive template for the report, to guarantee adequate documentation and standardization in the reporting and subsequent follow-up. It may be useful to include some guidance to the reporter to expedite the management and ensure compliance.

Assessment of the Exposure Risk

An important part of the evaluation of the exposure is assessing the risk of infection. As detailed above, the risk of transmission is dependent on several factors. These factors may increase or decrease the risk of transmission of blood-borne pathogens. These include the type and extent of exposure/injury, the type and volume of body fluid involved, the status of the source of exposure, and the susceptibility of the exposed HCW. As an example, exposure to a blood-filled hollow needle or visibly bloody device poses a greater risk for HIV or HCV than a needle used for injection. A thorough examination of both the source and the exposed person is needed for the assessment of the transmission risks. In the event that the status of the source is unknown, serological testing for HIV, HBV, and HCV should be performed only after obtaining the necessary consent for such testing. Confidentiality needs to be maintained throughout the process. Any results ought to be communicated to the exposure source, who will be referred accordingly for counseling and treatment.

General Approach to Risk Assessment and Management

Exposure source (source patient): Initial steps include clinical assessment of any evidence or signs of HIV, HBV, or HCV. Additionally, available laboratory results or medical history can help in determining whether the patient already has a blood-borne infection or not.

All source patients should be tested for HIV serology, hepatitis B surface antigen (HBsAg), and hepatitis C virus (anti-HCV), unless they are known to be infected. Some sources do not recommend testing the source for HBV infection if the EE has completed three doses of hepatitis B vaccine with documentation of adequate vaccination response. In that case, only HCV and HIV testing needs to be done. If a patient is known to be infected with HIV, additional information regarding the most recent HIV viral load and antiretroviral treatment history, including any drug resistance information, will be gathered. The same applies to the treatment of hepatitis C infection and any hepatitis B treatment.

Exposed employee (healthcare worker): For any EE, information regarding their immunization status (tetanus and hepatitis B); post-immunization titers; previous HIV, HBV, and HCV testing; and any underlying medical conditions and medications needs to be obtained from their medical/occupational health records.

Specific Approaches to Risk Assessment and Management

Occupational HBV Exposure

Risk Assessment and Management

Postexposure management of any healthcare worker with a possible exposure to HBV depends on two elements: the immune status of the EE and the HBsAg status of the SP.

The medical/occupational health records of all EEs should have evidence of their HBV status (HBsAg, hepatitis B surface antibodies [anti-HBs]). However, if that is not available, prompt baseline testing of the healthcare worker is needed before determining the next steps in postexposure management. The EE and thus postexposure management might fall into several categories (Table 21.2) [32].

Table 21.2 HBV postexposure management

EE status	SP HBsAg status	EE anti-HBs status	Postexposure management	Follow-up
Previous infection	No action needed	No action needed	No action needed	No action needed
Vaccinated, vaccine responder	No action needed	No action needed	No action needed	No action needed
Vaccinated, vaccine nonresponder	Positive or unknown	<10 milli-IU/mL	HBIG *2 separated by 1 month	No action needed
	Negative	<10 milli-IU/mL	No action needed	No action needed
Vaccinated, response unknown	Positive or unknown	<10 milli-IU/mL	HBIG * 1 and revaccinate	Anti-HBs 1–2 months after last vaccine dose
	Negative	<10 milli-IU/mL	Revaccinate	Anti-HBs 1–2 months after last vaccine dose
	Any result	≥10 milli-IU/mL	No action needed	No action needed
Non-vaccinated	Positive		HBIG*1 and HB vaccination series	Anti-HBs 1–2 months after last vaccine dose
	Unknown		HB vaccination series	Anti-HBs 1–2 months after last vaccine dose
	Negative		HB vaccination series	Anti-HBs 1–2 months after last vaccine dose

EE Exposed employee, *SP* Source patient, *HBsAg* Hepatitis B surface antigen, *anti-HBs* Hepatitis B surface antibodies, *HBIG* Hepatitis B immunoglobulin, *IU* International unit, *mL* Milliliter

1. **Evidence of a previous infection** of the EE (anti-HBs and hepatitis B core antibodies [anti-HBc] are positive): in this case, the HCW is deemed to be protected and no postexposure prophylaxis is needed.
2. **Immunized healthcare worker and is a known vaccine responder** (anti-HBs ≥10 milli-international unit [IU/milliliter[mL]]): no baseline testing is required and no postexposure prophylaxis is needed.
3. **Immunized healthcare worker but is a vaccine nonresponder** (anti-HBs <10 milli-IU/mL after receiving 2 full doses of hepatitis B vaccine, i.e., 6 injections): in such case, the status of the source patient needs to be determined. If the source patient has a positive HBsAg or if it is unknown, the healthcare worker should receive two doses of the hepatitis B immunoglobulin (HBIG), separated by 1 month.
4. **Immunized healthcare worker with unknown vaccine status**: immediate testing of the source patient (SP) for HBsAg and of the EE for anti-HBs. If EE's anti-HBs is ≥10 milli-IU/mL, then no additional testing or management is required.

   If the anti-HBs are <10 milli-IU/mL, postexposure management depends on the source patient's status. If HBsAg of the SP is positive, the EE should receive one dose of HBIG and one dose of the hepatitis B vaccine. Afterwards, the EE should receive two more doses of the vaccine to complete the immunization series. Anti-HB testing should be done 1–2 months after the last dose of the hepatitis B vaccine to determine the EE's immunity status. Management is similar if the status of the source patient cannot be determined, where the EE should be managed as if the source is HBsAg positive.

   If the source patient SP has a negative HBsAg, the EE should be immunized for hepatitis B and checked for anti-HBs 1–2 months after completing the last dose.
5. **Healthcare workers who have not received or completed hepatitis B vaccination:** The source patient should be tested for HBsAg. If found positive or cannot be determined, the EE should immediately receive one dose of HBIG and one dose of the hepatitis B vaccine. Afterwards, the EE will receive the additional doses of hepatitis B vaccine to complete the immunization series with anti-HB testing to assess vaccination response. If the source patient is negative for HBsAg, the EE should receive the complete hepatitis B vaccination series followed by anti-HB testing.

Postexposure Prophylaxis with Hepatitis B Immunoglobulin

The role of antivirals in postexposure prophylaxis of hepatitis B has not been established. Guidelines recommend administering HBIG as soon as possible after the exposure (preferably within 24 hours). However, if that is not possible, it can be given up to 7 days after exposure. Studies have shown that if the first dose was initiated within the first week, multiple doses of HBIG are 70–75% effective in preventing HBV infection. Benefit beyond 7 days is unknown [12, 32].

Postexposure Prophylaxis (PEP) with Hepatitis B Vaccine

Similarly, hepatitis B vaccine alone is 70–75% effective in preventing HBV infection [12, 32]. Ideally, HBV vaccine should be given within 24 h of exposure. The mostly highly effective postexposure management is a combination of HBIG and hepatitis B vaccination, where effectiveness reaches 85–95% in HBV infection prevention [32–34].

Follow-Up Counseling and Testing

In cases where the EE has no evidence of HBV immunity at the time of immunity, follow-up testing with anti-HBc and HBsAg needs to done 6 months after exposure to determine HBV transmission. In those that have received hepatitis B vaccinations and HBIG, anti-HB testing should be performed 1–2 months after the last vaccine dose and at least 6 months after the last HBIG dose.

The EE should be counseled to refrain from donating blood, plasma, semen, or organs. However, there is no need to modify sexual practices or breastfeeding. In addition, there is no need to modify any of the patient care responsibilities of the EE. Counseling should include immediate reporting of any illness, symptoms of fever, chills, nausea, vomiting, jaundice, and/or change in color of urine and stools.

If acute hepatitis B infection is documented, evaluation and referral should be performed according to published guidelines and recommendations.

Occupational HCV Exposure

Risk Assessment and Management

To this day, there has been no effective postexposure prophylaxis for individuals exposed to HCV. Despite the availability of highly effective HCV direct-acting antiviral drugs, there is not enough evidence for the use of these drugs in postexposure prophylaxis, and they are not FDA approved in such contexts [35]. Similarly, the use of immunoglobulins as postexposure prophylaxis for hepatitis C has not been recommended due to the lack of data on its effectiveness in preventing such infections [36]. Therefore, in the cases of possible HCV exposure, management lies in the early detection and treatment of HCV.

Based on CDC guidelines for the follow-up of occupational HCV exposures (Table 21.3) [12]:

Table 21.3 Postexposure HCV testing

	Baseline testing			Follow-up		
	Anti-HCV	HCV RNA	ALT	HCV RNA	Anti-HCV	ALT
SP	Yes	If anti-HCV is positive	–	–	–	–
EE	Yes	If anti-HCV is positive	Yes	At 4–6 weeks if earlier diagnosis is desired	At 4–6 months	At 4–6 months

HCV Hepatitis C virus, *ALT* Alanine transaminase, *SP* Source person, *EE* Exposed employee

(a) The SP should be tested for anti-HCV at baseline.
(b) The EE should be tested at baseline, preferably within 48 h, for anti-HCV and alanine transaminase (ALT). Follow-up testing with ALT and anti-HCV is usually performed at 4–6 months; however, if earlier diagnosis is desired, HCV RNA can be done at 4–6 weeks.
(c) If anti-HCV for SP or EE returns positive, a confirmatory test with another anti-HCV testing is needed.

Follow-Up Counseling

At any point, if the EE has evidence of acquiring HCV infection, they should be referred to a specialist for appropriate management. Signs and symptoms of acute hepatitis C infection may be subtle most of the time; however, in certain instances, there may be evidence of constitutional symptoms, jaundice, abdominal pain, etc. Similar to HBV, EEs with possible exposure to HCV do not need to abstain from sexual practices, breastfeeding, or pregnancy during the follow-up period. However, they need to refrain from donating blood, plasma, semen, or organs. Patient care responsibilities do not need to be modified solely on the basis of possible exposure to HCV-infected blood or tissue [12].

Occupational HIV Exposure

Risk Assessment and Management

Healthcare workers who are potentially exposed to HIV should receive immediate evaluation and care. This prompt management critically reduces the likelihood of HIV transmission. Generally, the approach to assessing the risk of HIV exposure includes determining the status of the source patient and EE, assessing the type of body fluid and the nature of the exposure, and finally the timing of the exposure [30].

Testing

1. **Determine the status of the source patient.** If unknown, the HIV status of the source needs to be immediately determined, preferably using a fourth-generation antibody-antigen test [30]. If HIV serology in a source patient is negative, no further testing is normally required. If the testing is going to be delayed, PEP should be initiated right away while awaiting the test results. If the source is later found to be HIV negative, PEP can be discontinued. If HIV serology is negative but there is clinical suspicion of acute HIV infection, PEP should be initiated and the HIV viral load performed.
2. **HIV testing in exposed HCWs.** All EEs need to have a baseline HIV serology testing immediately after exposure. Since seroconversion occurs usually within the first 3 months, it is important to perform follow-up HIV tests. Timing of follow-up testing depends on the test used. Ideally, a fourth-generation combination antibody-antigen test is preferred, since it detects seroconversion earlier, where follow-up testing can be done at six weeks and 4 months after exposure.

However, if an antibody test is used, follow-up should be done at 6 weeks, 3 months, and 6 months postexposure. A longer follow-up is recommended in those with impaired humoral immunity and in those exposed to a source with HIV-HCV co-infection.

In determining statuses of SP or exposed EE, it is important to start with a serology test rather than with HIV RNA, since there is a high likelihood of a false-positive test.

Postexposure Prophylaxis (PEP) for HIV

When a person is exposed to HIV, the virus first replicates in the dendritic cells of the skin and mucous membrane before disseminating. It takes HIV up to 72 h, 5 days, and 8 days to be detected in regional lymph nodes, blood, and cerebrospinal fluid, respectively. This "window of opportunity" allows PEP to prevent HIV acquisition after exposure, if started early enough [37]. A landmark case-control study published in 1997 provides the best available evidence on the effectiveness of PEP in preventing HIV acquisition in healthcare workers. This study included 33 cases (HCW who became infected with HIV) and 665 controls (HCW who did not become infected with HIV). Multivariate analyses revealed that after controlling for other risk factors, the odds of HIV transmission after exposure in those who received zidovudine were reduced by 81% (95% CI 48–94%) [29]. This study, along with other smaller human (mainly on prevention of perinatal transmission) and animal studies (on PEP efficacy), has supported the use of PEP [38].

Indication

PEP is given to EEs on a case-by-case basis, taking into consideration the risk of HIV transmission, weighing it against individual preference, inconvenience, and toxicity of PEP. However, generally PEP is recommended when there is percutaneous mucous membrane or non-intact skin exposure to blood or bloody body fluids from a patient known or suspected to be HIV positive. If the status of the source patient is unknown, PEP is continued until the results of the HIV testing are available. If the source patient cannot be identified, PEP is recommended in settings with a high likelihood of HIV infection, such as in the case of a prick from a needle in a sharps disposal container [30].

Timing and Duration

PEP should be initiated as soon as possible after exposure, preferably within 1–2 h. Animal studies have highlighted the importance of starting PEP soon after an exposure, with a reduced effectiveness if started more than 36–72 h after exposure [39–41]. Unless there is a very-high-risk exposure (such as needle injury that was in an artery or vein of an HIV-infected patient), recommendations state that PEP should not be offered if it has been more than 72 h after the exposure. In the cases of very-high-risk exposures, PEP might be initiated up to 1 week following the exposure (Table 21.4) [30].

Table 21.4 Postexposure HIV follow-up testing and monitoring

	Baseline (within 24 h)	Two weeks	Four weeks	Six weeks	Three months	Four months	Six months
HIV test							
– Fourth-generation	x	–	–	x	–	x	–
– Antibody test	x	–	–	–	x	x	x
Complete blood count, renal and hepatic function, and pregnancy test	x	x	x	–	–	–	–

HIV Human immunodeficiency virus

The optimal duration of PEP is unknown; however, it is generally given for 4 weeks, based on studies assessing zidovudine protectiveness against HIV transmission [29, 39, 40].

Antiretroviral Therapy Regimens

Three-drug regimens are the preferred regimens for occupational PEP. The recommendations for regimens to use in PEP are based on studies evaluating the safety, tolerability, and effectiveness of such regimens in patients with HIV infections, since studies assessing the effectiveness of these regimens as PEP are lacking.

The recommended regimens are:

1. Tenofovir disoproxil fumarate-emtricitabine (300/200 mg once daily) plus dolutegravir (50 mg once daily)
2. Tenofovir disoproxil fumarate-emtricitabine (300/200 mg once daily) plus raltegravir (400 mg twice daily)

   The dolutegravir-based regimen is preferred, due to its once-daily dosing and higher genetic barrier to resistance. The use of dolutegravir in females who are pregnant or of childbearing potential should be carefully discussed with the EE due to some reports of potential serious threat of neural tube defects associated with this drug. The data is still evolving in this field, and up to the time of writing of this chapter, the WHO continues to recommend dolutegravir as the first-line therapy for the treatment of HIV-infected women. The use of dolutegravir for prophylaxis has not been studied in this group.
3. Other regimens include tenofovir disoproxil fumarate-emtricitabine plus a boosted protease inhibitor (such as ritonavir-boosted darunavir or ritonavir-boosted atazanavir) or tenofovir disoproxil fumarate-emtricitabine plus cobicistat-boosted elvitegravir. The latter is not a preferred agent due to potential drug–drug interactions and the restrictions for use that require dosage at the same time daily and with a fatty meal.

Certain regimens should be avoided when selecting PEP, such as nevirapine, due to the potential risk of fatal hepatotoxicity and Stevens-Johnson syndrome. Likewise, abacavir should not be used without appropriate consultation and HLA-B*5701 testing, due to the risk of developing a fatal hypersensitivity reaction. The use of Atripla is not favored due to the potential for viral resistance to the constituent agents and the associated side effects [42].

The National Clinician's Post-Exposure Prophylaxis Hotline (PEPline) provides guidance for choosing a regimen.

PEP in Certain Populations

1. *Known or suspected drug resistance:* Rare cases of PEP failure have occurred due to the transmission of resistant strains from an HIV-infected source. Therefore, if the source is known to be HIV infected, it is important to gather information on their history of antiretroviral treatment and any possible genetic resistance. This allows the tailoring of the PEP regimen. In any suspected or known case, expert consultation is recommended. However, unavailability of an expert or needed information should not delay PEP, and if resistance is suspected, dolutegravir-based or boosted darunavir regimens are preferred until resistance testing is available.
2. *If pregnant or of childbearing potential:* Choosing a PEP regimen in pregnant people is complex. Antiretrovirals may exacerbate physiologic changes in pregnancy, and some drugs are contraindicated and some may have short- or long-term effects on the fetus or newborn. In May 2018, the FDA released a warning on the use of dolutegravir in pregnant or of childbearing females due to a preliminary report suggesting an increased risk of neural tube defects in four infants born to 426 women in Botswana who were on dolutegravir at the time of conception [43, 44]. Following the warning, the HHS Antiretroviral Guideline Panels issued recommendations guiding the use of dolutegravir in such populations. Alternative regimens include tenofovir disoproxil fumarate-emtricitabine plus raltegravir or tenofovir disoproxil fumarate-emtricitabine plus a boosted protease inhibitor [45].

Patient Follow-up and Monitoring

HCWs who have been started on PEP need to be followed up within 72 h of exposure and PEP initiation to assess baseline tolerance of PEP and to provide any needed psychological counseling if needed. Baseline labs should also be performed, and these include complete blood count and renal and hepatic function. In addition the following should be performed:

1. **Follow-up with laboratory testing.** As mentioned previously, exposed EEs need to have repeat HIV testing to detect seroconversion. If a fourth-generation combination antibody-antigen test is used, then follow-up can be done at 6 weeks and 4 months after exposure. However, if an antibody test is used, follow-up should be done at 6 weeks, 3 months, and 6 months postexposure. Repeat laboratory testing includes complete blood count and renal and hepatic function at 2 and 4 weeks. Further laboratory testing might be required if drug toxicity is suspected or ordered according to the medications included in the regimen, such as monitoring of hypoglycemia in those on protease inhibitors.

2. **Extended follow-up.** Several case reports have described delayed cases of seroconversion in healthcare workers who had been exposed to sources that had HIV-HCV co-infection. Therefore, in cases with exposure to such a source, or if the EE has been found to have acquired HCV, a longer follow-up, up to 12 months, is recommended.

Counseling and Education

Counseling and educating EEs on HIV risk acquisition and PEP are very important. This guides them in making educated choices on PEP and helps in reducing stress and anxiety associated with the exposure incident. Additionally, EEs should be advised to use preventative measures 6–12 weeks after exposure, such as barrier contraception, and avoiding breastfeeding and pregnancy, to avoid secondary transmission of HIV.

Psychological Counseling and Stress Management

Exposure incidents are distressing to the EEs, their co-workers, and their families. These events may trigger various psychological reactions including stress, anxiety, and depression and could even lead to post-traumatic stress disorder (PTSD) [11, 46, 47]. Evidence has shown that the lack of social and psychological support may affect the development of PTSD. Therefore, it is essential to provide EEs with psychological counseling to avoid any potential psychological harms [30]. Even though no guidelines outline psychological management of exposure incidents, approaches could include the integration of psychosocial components and education into institutions' postexposure management systems [46].

Prevention

In the United States, OSHA issued the OSHA Bloodborne Pathogens Standard in 1992 because of the significant health risk associated with exposure to viruses and microorganisms that cause blood-borne diseases [2]. The standard applies to all occupational exposures to blood or other potentially infectious materials. The standard requires that the employer must implement an exposure control plan for the worksite. The plan must include industrial hygiene measures designed to decrease the potential for exposure. Such measures include the following:

- **Engineering controls:** use of safer medical devices, such as needleless devices, shielded needle devices, and plastic capillary tubes
- **Work practice controls:** ban bending, recapping, or removing contaminated needles and other sharps (unless there is no alternative available)
- **Offer these:** use of personal protective clothing and equipment; free hepatitis B immunization to workers with potential exposure to BBP; postexposure evaluation and follow-up, including postexposure prophylaxis when appropriate; training in appropriate engineering controls and work practices

In order to further reduce healthcare workers' exposure to BBP, the BBP standard was amended in 2000, pursuant to the 2000 Needlestick Safety and Prevention Act [48]. Additional requirements were imposed upon employers, whereby employers shall keep a sharp injury log. Employers' exposure control plan shall be reviewed annually to reflect improvement of technology by considering and implementing effective newer, safer, medical devices designed to reduce or eliminate exposure to BBP. Employers shall also solicit input from nonmanagerial employees providing direct patient care in the assessment and implementation of effective engineering and work practice controls.

Among surgical personnel, sharp-tip suture needles are responsible for the majority of percutaneous injuries, causing 51–77% of these exposures [6, 49, 50]. Suture needle injuries can occur at different stages of the surgery. Examples include, but are not limited to, when team members pass needles hand to hand; when a needle is loaded or repositioned into the needle holder; when the surgeon/assistant is sewing toward himself/herself while the other team member is holding back other tissue; when a needle is left on the operative field; when a needle is placed in overfilled sharp containers; and when a needle is placed in poorly located sharps containers [51].

Suturing muscle and fascia frequently results in exposure injuries [49]. Blunt-tip suture needles can be used to suture less dense tissue such as muscle and fascia and have been shown to significantly decrease the risk of percutaneous injuries to surgical personnel [5]. OSHA, National Institute for Occupational Safety and Health (NIOSH), and the American College of Surgeons (ACS) currently recommend their use when applicable [5, 52].

Other OR work practices that have been shown to decrease the risk of percutaneous injury include the use of double gloves. The ACS recommends the universal adoption of the double glove technique, unless it may compromise the safe conduct of the operation or the safety of the patient [52].

OSHA and the ACS also recommend the use of a neutral zone to transfer sharps (except in situations where it may compromise the safe conduct of the operation). A sharp neutral zone is defined as a towel or magnetic pad used for the pickup and release of surgical sharps. This technique does not allow direct handling of instruments between team members [52].

Conclusion

Exposure to blood-borne pathogens in healthcare settings is a potential serious risk to all healthcare workers, especially surgeons. Prevention lies in applying standard precautions including hand hygiene, use of protective barriers and safer equipment, and appropriate use and disposal of needles and other sharp instruments. In the case where an exposure incident occurs, prompt recognition is crucial to avoid unintended complications and costs. All healthcare institutions should have a system in place with protocols that ensure early reporting, initiation of testing, and appropriate postexposure prophylaxis. In addition, it is important to assert the importance of follow-up counseling, to recognize the anxiety resulting from the exposure incident, and to provide psychological counseling and stress management if needed. Finally, it is essential to promote a culture of safety in healthcare settings, which will provide optimal protection and care for all patients and healthcare workers.

References

1. Needlestick transmission of HTLV-III from a patient infected in Africa. Lancet. 1984;2(8416):1376–7.
2. U.S. Department of Labor Occupational Safety & Health Administration. Regulations (Standards - 29 CFR) bloodborne pathogens [Internet]. p. 1910.1030. https://www.osha.gov/laws-regs/regulations/standardnumber/1910/1910.1030
3. Occupational Safety and Health Administration. Bloodborne pathogens and needlestick prevention [Internet]. [cited 9 Jul 2019]. https://www.osha.gov/pls/oshaweb/owadisp.show_document?p_id=10051&p_table=STANDARDS
4. Elseviers MM, Arias-Guillén M, Gorke A, Arens HJ. Sharps injuries amongst healthcare workers: review of incidence, transmissions and costs. J Ren Care. 2014;40(3):150–6.
5. NIOSH. Use of blunt-tip suture needles to decrease percutaneous injuries to surgical personnel. Saf Heal Inf Bull; 2007. http://www.cdc.gov/niosh/docs/2008-101/pdfs/2008-101.pdf
6. Makary M, Al-Attar A, Holzmueller CG, Sexton B, Syin D, Gilson MM, et al. Needlestick injuries among surgeons in training. N Engl J Med. 2007;356(26):2693–9.
7. Mannocci A, De CG, Di BV, Saulle R, Unim B, Nicolotti N, et al. How much do needlestick injuries cost? A systematic review of the economic evaluations of needlestick and sharps injuries among healthcare personnel. Infect Control Hosp Epidemiol. 2016;37(6):536–646.
8. Cooke CE, Stephens JM. Clinical, economic, and humanistic burden of needlestick injuries in healthcare workers. Med Devices Evid Res. 2017;10:225–35.
9. Henry K, Campbell S, Jackson B, Balfour H, Rhame F, Sannerud K, et al. Long-term follow up of health care workers with work-site exposure to human immunodeficiency virus. JAMA. 1990;263(13):1765.
10. Armstrong K, Gorden R, Santorella G. Occupational exposure of healthcare workers (HCWs) to human immunodeficiency virus (HIV): stress reactions and counseling interventions. Soc Work Health Care. 1995;21(3):61–80.
11. Worthington MG, Ross JJ, Bergeron EK. Posttraumatic stress disorder after occupational HIV exposure: two cases and a literature review. Infect Control Hosp Epidemiol. 2014;27(2):215–7.
12. United States Public Health Service. Updated U.S. Public Health Service guidelines for the management of occupational exposures to HBV, HCV, and HIV and recommendations for postexposure prophylaxis. Morb Mortal Wkly Rep [Internet]. 2001;50(RR11):1–42. https://www.cdc.gov/mmwr/preview/mmwrhtml/rr5011a1.htm
13. Tarantola A, Abiteboul D, Rachline A. Infection risks following accidental exposure to blood or body fluids in health care workers: a review of pathogens transmitted in published cases. Am J Infect Control. 2005;34(6):367–75.
14. Beltrami EM, Williams IT, Shapiro CN, Chamberland ME. Risk and management of blood-borne infections in health care workers. Clin Microbiol Rev. 2000;13(3):385–407.
15. Kidd-Ljunggren K, Holmberg A, Bläckberg J, Lindqvist B. High levels of hepatitis B virus DNA in body fluids from chronic carriers. J Hosp Infect. 2006;64(4):352–7.
16. Scott RM, Snitbhan R, Bancroft WH, Alter HJ, Tingpalapong M. Experimental transmission of hepatitis B virus by semen and saliva. J Infect Dis. 1980;142(1):67–71.
17. Irwin GR, Allen AM, Bancroft WH, Karwacki JJ, Brown HL, Pinkerton RH, et al. Hepatitis B antigen in saliva, urine, and stool. Infect Immun. 1975;11(1):142–5.
18. Victor Feinman S, Berris B, Rebane A, Sinclair JC, Wilson S, Wrobel D. Failure to detect hepatitis b surface antigen (Hbsag) in feces of hbsag-positive persons. J Infect Dis. 1979;140(3):407–10.

19. Bond WW, Favero MS, Petersen NJ, Gravelle CR, Ebert JW, Maynard JE. Survival of hepatitis B virus after drying and storage for one week. Lancet. 1981;317(8219):550–1.
20. Centers for Disease Control and Prevention. Prevention of hepatitis B virus infection in the United States: recommendations of the Advisory Committee on Immunization. Morb Mortal Wkly Rep. 2018;67
21. Savasi V, Parrilla B, Ratti M, Oneta M, Clerici M, Ferrazzi E. Hepatitis C virus RNA detection in different semen fractions of HCV/HIV-1 co-infected men by nested PCR. Eur J Obstet Gynecol Reprod Biol. 2010;151(1):52–5.
22. Rey D, Fritsch S, Schmitt C, Meyer P, Lang JM, Stoll-Keller F. Quantitation of hepatitis C virus RNA in saliva and serum of patients coinfected with HCV and human immunodeficiency virus. J Med Virol. 2001;63(2):117–9.
23. Suzuki T, Omata K, Satoh T, Miyasaka T, Arai C, Maeda M, et al. Quantitative detection of hepatitis C virus (HCV) RNA in saliva and gingival crevicular fluid of HCV-infected patients. J Clin Microbiol. 2005;43(9):4413–7.
24. Pfaender S, Helfritz FA, Siddharta A, Todt D, Behrendt P, Heyden J, et al. Environmental stability and infectivity of hepatitis C virus (HCV) in different human body fluids. Front Microbiol. 2018;9(504):1–8.
25. Paintsil E, He H, Peters C, Lindenbach BD, Heimer R. Survival of Hepatitis C virus in syringes: implication for transmission among injection drug users. J Infect Dis. 2010;202(7):984–90.
26. Hosoglu S, Celen MK, Akalin S, Geyik MF, Soyoral Y, Kara IH. Transmission of hepatitis C by blood splash into conjunctiva in a nurse. Am J Infect Control. 2003;31(8):502–4.
27. Sartori M, La Terra G, Aglietta M, Manzin A, Navino C, Verzetti G. Transmission of hepatitis C via blood splash into conjunctiva. Scand J Infect Dis. 1993;25(2):270–1.
28. Henderson DK, Fahey BJ, Willy M, Schmitt JM, Carey K, Koziol DE, et al. Risk for occupational transmission of human immunodeficiency virus type 1 (HIV-1) associated with clinical exposures: a prospective evaluation. Ann Intern Med. 1990;113(10):740–6.
29. Cardo DM, Culver DH, Cieseielski CA, Srivastava PU, Marcus R, Abiteboul D, et al. A case-control study of HIV seroconversion in health care workers after percutaneous exposure. N Engl J Med. 1997;337(21):1485–90.
30. Kuhar DT, Henderson DK, Struble KA, Heneine W, Thomas V, Cheever LW, et al. Updated US Public Health Service guidelines for the management of occupational exposures to human immunodeficiency virus and recommendations for postexposure prophylaxis. Infect Control Hosp Epidemiol. 2013;34(9):875–92.
31. World Health Organization. Occupational risks and management of bloodborne pathogens. In: WHO best practices for injections and related procedures toolkit. Geneva; 2010. p. 29–38.
32. Centers for Disease Control and Prevention. CDC guidance for evaluating health-care personnel for hepatitis B virus protection and for administering postexposure management. Morb Mortal Wkly Rep [Internet]. 2013;62(10). http://www.cdc.gov/mmwr/cme/conted.html
33. Beasley RP, Hwang L-Y, Stevens CE, Lin C-C, Hsieh F-J, Wang K-Y, et al. Efficacy of hepatitis B immune globulin for prevention of perinatal transmission of the hepatitis B virus carrier state: final report of a randomized double-blind, placebo-controlled trial. Hepatology. 1983;3(2):135–41.
34. Stevens CE, Toy PT, Tong MJ, Taylor PE, Vyas GN, Nair PV, et al. Perinatal hepatitis B virus transmission in the United States: prevention by passive-active immunization. JAMA. 1985;253(12):1741745.
35. Naggie S, Holland DP, Sulkowski MS, Thomas DL. Hepatitis C virus postexposure prophylaxis in the healthcare worker: why direct-acting antivirals don't change a thing. Clin Infect Dis. 2016;64(1):92–9.
36. Krawczynski K, Alter MJ, Tankersley DL, Beach M, Robertson BH, Lambert S, et al. Effect of immune globulin on the prevention of experimental hepatitis C virus infection. J Infect Dis. 1996;173(April):822–8.
37. Haase AT. Targeting early infection to prevent HIV-1 mucosal transmission. Nature. 2010;464(7286):217–23.

38. Irvine C, Egan KJ, Shubber Z, Van Rompay KKA, Beanland RL, Ford N. Efficacy of HIV postexposure prophylaxis: systematic review and meta-analysis of nonhuman primate studies. Clin Infect Dis. 2015;60(Suppl 3):S165–9.
39. Otten RONA, Smith DK, Adams DR, Pullium JK, Jackson E, Kim CN, et al. Efficacy of post-exposure prophylaxis after intravaginal exposure of pig-tailed macaques to a human-derived retrovirus (human immunodeficiency virus type 2). J Virol. 2000;74(20):9771–5.
40. Tsai C, Emau P, Follis KE, Beck TW, Benveniste RE, Bischofberger N, et al. Effectiveness of postinoculation (R)-9-(2-Phosphonylmethoxypropyl) adenine treatment for prevention of persistent simian immunodeficiency virus SIVmne infection depends critically on timing of initiation and duration of treatment. J Virol. 1998;72(5):4265–73.
41. Shih C-C, Kaneshima H, Rabin L, Namikawa R, Sager P, McGowan J, et al. Postexposure prophylaxis with zidovudine suppresses human immunodeficiency virus type 1 infection in SCID-hu mice in a time-dependent manner. J Infect Dis. 1991;163(3):625–7.
42. Wiboonchutikul S, Thientong V, Suttha P, Kowadisaiburana B, Manosuthi W. Significant intolerability of efavirenz in HIV occupational postexposure prophylaxis. J Hosp Infect. 2016;92(4):372–7.
43. U.S. Food and Drug Administration. FDA Drug Safety Communication: FDA to evaluate potential risk of neural tube birth defects with HIV medicine dolutegravir (Juluca, Tivicay, Triumeq); 2018.
44. Zash R, Makhema J, Shapiro RL. Neural-tube defects with dolutegravir treatment from the time of conception. N Engl J Med. 2018;379(10):979–81.
45. Department of Health and Human Services (HHS) Antiretroviral Guidelines Panels. Recommendations regarding the use of dolutegravir in adults and adolescents with HIV who are pregnant or of child-bearing potential [Internet]; 2018. https://aidsinfo.nih.gov/news/2109/recommendations-regarding-the-use-of-dolutegravir-in-adults-and-adolescents-with-hiv-who-are-pregnant-or-of-child-bearing-potential
46. Wald J. The psychological consequences of occupational blood and body fluid exposure injuries. Disabil Rehabil. 2009;31(23):1963–9.
47. Sohn JW, Kim BG, Kim SH, Han C. Mental health of healthcare workers who experience needlestick and sharps injuries. J Occup Health. 2006;48(6):474–9.
48. H.R. 5178—106th Congress: Needlestick Safety and Prevention Act [Internet]. 2000 p. HR 3801. https://www.govinfo.gov/content/pkg/BILLS-106hr5178enr/pdf/BILLS-106hr5178enr.pdf
49. Berguer R, Heller PJ. Preventing sharps injuries in the operating room. J Am Coll Surg. 2004;199(3):462–7.
50. Jagger J, Bentley M, Tereskerz P. A study of patterns and prevention of blood exposures in OR personnel. AORN J. 1998;67(5):979–96.
51. Davis MS. Advanced precautions for today's O.R.: the operating room professional's handbook for the prevention of sharps injuries and bloodborne exposures. Atlanta: Sweinbinder Publications LLC; 1999.
52. American College of Surgeons. American College of Surgeons (ACS) statement [Internet]. https://www.facs.org/about-acs/statements/94-sharps-safety

“I’m Missing a Sponge!” New Techniques in the Prevention of Foreign Body Retention

22

Scott E. Regenbogen and Samantha J. Rivard

Retained surgical items (RSIs) can include any surgical equipment (i.e., sponge, instrument, needle) unintentionally left inside a patient after an operation. RSIs result in significant patient morbidity, possible mortality, and excess healthcare costs. Over time, many strategies have been utilized to prevent the retention of surgical items. Traditionally, manual surgical counts and intraoperative plain imaging have served this purpose. More recently, new technologies have emerged, including bar-coded sponges and radio-frequency technology. This chapter focuses on reviewing RSI epidemiology, risk factors, and prevention methods—both standard practices and new technology.

RSIs are considered by many regulatory organizations to be “never events,” serious reportable incidents thought to be universally preventable, as defined by the National Quality Forum [1]. Since June 2005, the Joint Commission has classified RSIs as sentinel events that require immediate reporting, investigation with subsequent root cause analysis, and coordinated institutional response [2]. The Centers for Medicare and Medicaid Services (CMS) have also included RSIs on its list of hospital-acquired conditions. Therefore, since 2008, medical care resulting from RSIs is not reimbursed by CMS [3]. Many state and private health insurers have also adopted policies to not reimburse care associated with an RSI.

Retained surgical items represent significant complications for a variety of reasons. They may result in serious, even fatal injuries, and infectious complications, which require additional medical care, frequently manifested as increased length of stay, readmissions, and reoperations. Additionally, retained surgical item cases frequently lead to litigation and negatively affect the reputation of clinicians and hospital systems. All of these contribute to substantial healthcare costs.

S. E. Regenbogen (✉) · S. J. Rivard
Department of Surgery, University of Michigan, Ann Arbor, MI, USA
e-mail: sregenbo@med.umich.edu

J. J. Hoballah et al. (eds.), *Principles of Perioperative Safety and Efficiency*,
https://doi.org/10.1007/978-3-031-41089-5_22

Unfortunately, despite increasing attention to the prevention of RSIs, they remain the most common sentinel event reported to the Joint Commission, with 124 reported in 2017 and 121 in 2018 [4, 5]. Therefore, an understanding of the natural history, risk factors, and strategies for prevention of RSIs is critical for patient safety and surgical quality. As a community, we must recognize that while certain patient- and operation-specific factors may predispose to RSIs, human, team, and system factors contribute considerably.

Of note, heterogeneity exists in the terminology used in the published literature, which complicates the study of RSIs. The following terminology has all been utilized: retained foreign bodies, retained foreign objects, retained surgical equipment, retained surgical items, and retained sponges and instruments. Gossypiboma specifically refers to surgical sponges unintentionally left inside a patient during a surgical procedure. Other terms include textiloma, gauzoma, and muslinoma [6]. For the remainder of this chapter, the abbreviation RSI will be used to encompass "retained surgical items," including any surgical equipment (sponge, instrument, needle), which was unintentionally left inside a patient.

Epidemiology

The true incidence of retained surgical items is unknown and difficult to determine based on the nature of existing literature, which mainly consists of voluntary incident reporting, insurance and malpractice claims data, and retrospective reviews. Additionally, postoperative patients are infrequently screened for retained surgical items, which may take many years to become clinically relevant [6]. This results in a likely underestimation of true RSI incidence.

A landmark study based on malpractice claims estimated an incidence of 1 in 8801 to 18,760 of all inpatient operations [7]. However, this was felt to be an underestimate, and more recent literature cites an incidence of 1 in 5500 operations [8]. When focused on abdominal operations, incidence estimates increase to 1 in 1000 to 1500 cases [9, 10]. Although the risk of RSI is higher in emergency surgery, most events occur among elective operations.

The most common RSI is cotton materials, specifically sponges (52–69%), followed by surgical instruments (3–43%), and needles (9%) [7, 8, 11, 12]. It is not surprising that surgical sponges constitute the majority of RSIs as they are small and commonly used and become camouflaged when blood-soaked. Interestingly, needles were found to be a major cause of near misses, but less frequently result in an RSI [8].

Retained surgical items have been discovered in patients of all ages, within all body cavities, and throughout all subspecialties. The majority of RSIs are found in the abdomen or pelvis (46–65%) followed by the thorax (7.4–23%), vagina (22%), extremities (8%), head/neck (2%), natural orifices (mouth, rectum, urinary tract), and elsewhere (17%; including spinal canal, face, brain) [6, 7, 11, 13, 14]. In one series, 27.5% of RSI cases involved uncomplicated vaginal deliveries [14].

RSIs can be discovered immediately or take many years until discovery [11]. Throughout the literature, the average time to discovery of an RSI was 6.9 years, ranging from under 3 months to over 40 years [6]. However, the median time to discovery was 2.2 years because of high likelihood complications that occur within the first 2 years after surgery. Abdominal and pelvic locations were associated with significantly longer intervals to retained item identification and removal [13].

Natural History

The majority of patients discovered to have RSI undergo reoperation (65–83%) for removal of the item to treat or prevent complications [7, 8, 11, 13]. The complications associated with RSIs include adhesions (31%), abscess (24%), fistula (20%), small bowel perforation or obstruction (3–22%), and sepsis (7%) [6, 7, 11, 13]. In some cases, RSIs result in erosion into the gastrointestinal or genitourinary tracts, or vasculature [15]. Readmissions and increased length of stay from RSIs have been reported in 30–59% of cases [7, 8, 11, 13]. Mortality estimates range from 0 to 6% [7, 12, 13].

Some RSIs are discovered incidentally during the postoperative period, while others are discovered due to clinical signs and symptoms, and others remain hidden for years [11]. The majority of RSIs are discovered on imaging (67%) followed by self-exam or physical exam (24–30%) [7]. The most common imaging detection methods are CT scans (61%), then radiographs (35–51%), and ultrasound (34%) [7, 13]. Other technologies utilized include MRI, endoscopy, barium enemas, PET-CT, and mammography [6]. Some (9%) retained surgical items are not found until reoperation for complications [7].

Only a minority of patients (19%) report symptoms that prompted retained surgical item discovery. Those presenting with signs and symptoms report pain/irritation (42%), palpable mass (27%), fever (12%), nausea, emesis, and diarrhea. Of note, 48% of symptomatic RSI patients reported more than one symptom at presentation [6, 13]. Abdominal and pelvic RSIs were more likely to have clinically significant presenting symptoms [13]. Other nonspecific symptomologies included systemic inflammatory response syndrome and lack of expected clinical progress [11]. Therefore, for any patient with nonspecific or unexplained symptoms after surgery, it is recommended to obtain plain imaging, followed by CT imaging if radiographs are inconclusive [13].

The natural history of RSIs differs according to the duration that the RSI has been present. RSIs that have been present for longer periods of time are more likely to exhibit an inflammatory pathological response. Foreign material triggers the body's inflammatory response, which eventually leads to a fibrotic response manifesting as adhesions, granulomas, and, eventually, encapsulation. Only 16% of RSIs removed within 24 h were found to have inflammatory findings on pathology, compared to 42% of RSIs discovered between 24 h and 1 week, and 68% of RSIs discovered more than 6 weeks after surgery [13]. Most items retrieved beyond 24 h had one or more abnormal pathology findings, most commonly exudative reaction, fibrosis, and purulence/abscess. Fibrosis was more common in patients whose RSIs were discovered more than 1 week after retention [13].

Similarly, the clinical presentation correlates with the length of time of item retention. The majority of RSIs that were discovered less than 24 h postoperatively were asymptomatic, but some were acutely symptomatic or discovered incidentally on imaging [13]. RSIs that were discovered between 24 h and 3 months after retention were more likely to have inflammatory signs and symptoms including fever, fluid collections, abscesses, abnormal wound drainage, and fistulas. In a subset of patients that remained largely asymptomatic for years, RSIs were more likely to be discovered incidentally on imaging obtained for other reasons, or with new unexplained masses that were mistaken for neoplasms. Chronic manifestations may also include granuloma formation, tissue erosion, mass, and fistula/sinus formation [13]. Thus, early recognition and removal of retained surgical items are recommended to prevent long-term complications.

Retained surgical items incur a variety of negative consequences beyond the clinical morbidity, including ligation, negative publicity, and provider distress [7, 14]. The average cost of a retained surgical item is estimated at $95,000, which includes about $14,701 for unreimbursed readmission and reoperation costs [16]. Legal fees vary widely between states and specific cases, with a range of $37,041 to $2,350,000, with an average of $52,581 per case [7, 16]. By understanding the risk factors associated with RSIs and the prevention strategies available, these monetary figures represent potential healthcare cost savings.

Risk Factors

Approaches to the prevention of RSI have begun with attempts to define important risk factors. Identification of key risk factors for RSIs could enable additional screening for the highest risk cases. A meta-analysis of three retrospective, case-control studies of RSI risk factors found seven risk factors to be significantly associated with increased RSI risk, listed in order of highest to lowest risk [17]:

1. Incorrect surgical count
2. Unexpected intraoperative factors
3. More than one surgical team
4. Surgical count not performed
5. More than one sub-procedure
6. Duration of operation
7. Estimated operative blood loss more than 500 mL

Specifically, incorrect final sponge counts were associated with a 20-fold increased RSI risk [12].

Other factors thought to be associated with an increased risk of RSI are changes in nursing staff, emergency surgery, BMI, and operations performed "after hours." In one study, the incidence of RSI was nine times greater in emergency surgery [7].

Some studies suggest that the presence of surgical trainees reduced the risk of RSI by as much as 70% [11, 12]

Prevention

Every member of the perioperative team shares the responsibility for patient safety, with the ultimate goal of eliminating patient adverse events. Observational studies have identified team or system errors in more than 90% of cases of RSI, whereas isolated human error was responsible in only a small minority [13]. This finding suggests that, rather than individual culpability, RSI prevention requires interventions focused on team training and highly reliable systems. Many different institutional policies exist with the goal of preventing the occurrence of retained foreign bodies. Institutional policies differ in their components of surgical team training, manual surgical counts, traditional wound sweeps, use of intraoperative radiology, and technological advances.

Manual Surgical Count

Manual surgical counting has been used for decades as the main defense against retained surgical items. It is truly a multidisciplinary endeavor, relying on multiple team members, including circulating nurse, scrub technician, and surgeons. This process is highly prone to human error as it is a "simple task" performed in a complex environment, with multiple distractions and competing tasks [8]. The more times a count is performed, the incidence of possible error increases exponentially [8].

For standardization of the process, the Association of periOperative Registered Nurses (AORN) first published surgical count guidelines in 1976, which have undergone multiple revisions, with the most recent update in 2015 with the "Guideline for Prevention of Retained Surgical Items." The AORN standard practices recommend counting sponges, sharps, instruments, and miscellaneous items on all procedures with the possibility that a foreign object could be retained. They recommend that all cotton sponges be radiopaque. Counting practices are required to be audible and performed by two individuals, including the circulating nurse. Surgical counts should occur before the procedure for a baseline, when new items are added to the field, before closure of a cavity within a cavity (e.g., bladder), when wound closure begins, when skin closure begins or at the end of the procedure, at the time of permanent relief of either the RN circulator or the scrub person, and any time a discrepancy is suspected.

AORN further recommends proper steps for resolving an incorrect count, which include the certified surgical technologist and/or circulator informing the surgeon of incorrect count, visual search of the surgical field, and the surgeon performing thorough exploration of operative cavity. If item is not found, it is recommended to obtain an intraoperative X-ray, read by a radiologist, before surgical wound is closed and patient leaves the OR. All sponge, sharp, and instrument counts, as well as any additional procedures taken during a miscount, should be documented in the intraoperative record and patient's chart [18].

While manual surgical counting has remained the mainstay of RSI prevention for decades, many call into question its reliability due to dependence on human consistency and accuracy in a complex environment plagued with interruptions, time pressures, and multitasking. In retrospective studies, 62–88% of retained surgical items occur in operations for which a final count was erroneously documented as correct [6–8, 11, 12, 14]. In one study evaluating the value of counting, the observed sensitivity of manual surgical counts was 77.27%, specificity was 99%, and positive predictive value was 1.6%, owing to the low incidence of RSIs [19]. The positive likelihood ratio of an incorrect count was 113.3, indicating that cases with incorrect counts were over 100 times more likely to result in an RSI [19]. While these statistics point to a higher value of counting then found in the literature, surgical teams should be careful to assume a correct surgical count as protective against a retained surgical item, as it can lead to a false sense of security [8].

Another criticism of manual surgical counting relates to the time it takes to perform counting activities, which divert the attention of ancillary staff from the activities of the surgeon. A mean of 16.6 counting episodes occur per operation, each requiring an average of 8.6 min to perform, consuming up to 14% of operative time [20]. In many institutions, this increased operative time correlates with increased healthcare expenditures.

While retained surgical items are rare, count discrepancies are more common, occurring in about 1 in 145 operations or 0.69% of surgical procedures [19]. Count discrepancies are defined as any event in which a subsequent count does not agree with a previous one, indicating that there is no accurate representation of the number of sponges, needles, and instruments [20]. A prospective observational field study by Greenberg et al. in 2008 found that 1 in 8 operations incurred an intraoperative count discrepancy. Unresolved count discrepancies require thorough manual wound exploration, intraoperative radiographs, or both, which increase the operative time and therefore cost. After a discrepancy occurs, an average of 13 min is required to reconcile the discrepancy [20].

The majority of count discrepancies involve sponges (45%), followed by instruments (34%) and needles (21%). Most (59%) result from misplaced items, which are eventually found in the body, on the surgical field, or elsewhere in the OR. Alternatively, 38% of discrepancies result from errors in the written record [12]. Cases with personnel change, specifically circulating nurse or surgical technician, are three times more likely to have a discrepancy [20].

Count discrepancies are associated with prolonged surgery time, increasing 2.7-fold for every additional 2 h of surgery, as well as with operations later in the day, as well as those with a higher number of nursing teams involved [19]. Count accuracy also depends on the complexity and urgency of the operation, as well as the surgical team's fatigue and workload [19]. Count discrepancies were most common in transplantation (10.2%), cardiothoracic surgery, and neurosurgery (2–3%) [19]. In coronary artery bypass graft (CABG) surgery, each count discrepancy was associated with $932 of excess cost, associated with diagnostic testing and increased time spent in the OR. Extrapolating these expenses, the national cost of count discrepancies in CABG alone would be $24 million annually [19].

Recognizing that the majority of count discrepancies represent actual misplaced items, all count discrepancies warrant a thorough search and reconciliation [20]. Despite the inability of manual counts to prevent all RSIs, the role for manual surgical counts still exists because standard counting detects 82% of possible RSIs [21]. If no counting was performed, the incidence of retained surgical sponges might be as high as 67 per 100,000 operations [21].

Radiographs

Guidelines for use of radiographic detection of RSI vary widely between institutions. Some hospitals require radiographs in every open surgical case, while others selectively require radiographs in high-risk cases or only in those with discrepant counts. Some hospitals do not have radiography policies at all [7, 8, 22].

Intraoperative or dedicated postoperative plain radiographs are not completely protective. Radiographs do not appear to be reliable enough to prevent RSI, as intraoperative radiographs may have sensitivity as low as 67% [6, 8]. Up to 48% of RSIs have been missed on initial intraoperative radiographs, which contributes to a false sense of security [12].

This is attributed to the poor imaging quality of intraoperative radiographs and variable appearance of surgical sponges on plain films. The radiopaque threads on sponges are likely to be distorted and have been mistaken as sternal sutures, monitor wires, valve rings, and even linear tube markers, such as nasogastric tubes [23]. Cases have also been reported when an RSI was out of radiograph's view, which indicates that multiple films may be necessary. Therefore, an intraoperative radiograph reported as negative for a retained surgical item when counts are incorrect should not be taken as a definitive test [8].

The literature suggests that sponges and instruments are much easier to detect on imaging than needles [8]. Overall mean accuracy of intraoperative radiographs for needles is 74% and specificity is 80% for plain radiographs in the detection of retained surgical needles. While the overall reported sensitivity of 69% for needle detection on intraoperative radiographs appears higher than the sensitivity for any RSI detection on intraoperative radiograph, this statistic is misleading because it is highly dependent on needle size. Sensitivity for needles 25 mm or more in length was 99% compared to needles of 11–24 mm, which was 84%, and needles ≤10 mm, which was 29%. For reference, the length of a CTX needle on a 0 suture is 48 mm in length, an SH needle on a 3-0 suture is 26 mm, and a BV needle on a 6-0 suture is 11 mm. Some suggest that radiographs for lost needles smaller than 13 mm pose unnecessary radiation risk for little or no gain, as the clinical significance is debatable [11, 24].

In one institution that requires high-resolution postoperative survey film prior to patients being brought to the recovery room, 59% of RSIs were discovered through routine use of these dedicated films, despite reportedly correct surgical counts [8]. However, mandatory, even selective, radiology policies may not be cost effective or viable on the institution level. In a cost-effective analysis, both mandatory and selective policies had a relative cost-effectiveness ratio of over $1,000,000 per retained surgical sponge prevented, as compared with manual surgical counting alone [21]. Another study showed that performing intraoperative X-rays for every CABG in the United States would cost $42.4 million per year [19]. Additionally, mandatory or selective radiographs expose patients and healthcare providers to unnecessary radiation. When compared to newer technologies, which tend to focus only on surgical sponges, radiographs offer an added benefit in that they can identify a broader range of RSIs, including instruments and needles.

Some have advocated for the use of routine intraoperative radiographs in emergency operations, especially those in which the surgical count was bypassed due to patient condition. Although these cases involve significantly higher risk of RSI, an estimated 300 radiographs would still be required to prevent one retained surgical sponge in these high-risk procedures, at a cost of approximately $700 per emergency case [7, 15]. Nevertheless, intraoperative radiography has been considered by some to be less costly than a traditional counting strategy because of the avoided institutional costs (OR time, readmissions) and litigation expenses associated with RSIs [15]. Strategies for decreasing false-negative intraoperative radiographs include having attending surgeons confirm that the radiograph includes the area of interest, and direct contact with the radiologists to alert them of the RSI concern [15].

Technological Adjuncts

The frequency of counting discrepancies, high percentage of falsely correct manual surgical counts, and low sensitivity of intraoperative radiographs have fueled interest in technological adjuncts to help eliminate the occurrence of retained surgical items. Because sponges represent the majority (48–69%) of retained surgical items, they have been the target of almost all of the new technologies introduced commercially [7, 8, 11]. Devices brought to market have included bar-coded sponges and radio-frequency technology incorporated into surgical sponges. It should be noted that none of the following advances have been advocated as replacements for standard manual counts recommended by AORN, but instead have been used as supplements to current practices. These technologies are prone to electronic interference, mechanical failure, and operator-dependent error [12, 25].

Bar-Coded Sponges

To supplement manual counting, bar codes have been placed on surgical sponges to allow for computer-assisted sponge counting. Each sponge contains a unique data matrix code that is scanned prior to being added to the sterile field and again as each sponge is removed [21, 22, 26].

In 2008, Greenberg et al. performed a randomized controlled trial of a bar-coded sponge system in elective surgery and evaluated the incidence of count discrepancies in cases using bar coding versus traditional counting alone. The bar-coded sponge system detected count discrepancies twice as often as manual counting protocols. The detection of misplaced and miscounted sponges was significantly increased with the bar-coded sponge system. The technology did increase time devoted to counting by 3 min per case and did not decrease the likelihood of obtaining an intraoperative radiograph. By the end of the study, the majority of providers found the system easy to use, felt confident in its performance to track sponges, and believed that it had a positive effect on the counting process [22]. This study concluded that there was a potential to decrease the risk of retained sponges.

The Mayo Clinic implemented a similar bar-coded sponge counting system, and its institutional impact was published after 18 months of experience. Cima and colleagues also reported an increase in time spent counting sponges per operation, but no overall increase in operative time. The learning curve was reported as short, averaging four cases. After 18 months, the bar-code system eliminated retained surgical sponges, which previously occurred about every 64 days on average [26]. Staff surveys revealed that many staff believed that the system decreased the stress involved in manual counts and recognized the improved accuracy. Additionally, the reported increased cost per case was only $11.63 [26].

Using these data in a decision-analytic simulation, the bar-coding system was estimated to prevent about 97.5% of retained surgical sponges as compared to manual counting alone [21]. There was an incremental additional cost of $95,000 per retained surgical sponge prevented [21]. While bar-coded systems add value by preventing RSI cases at a reasonable cost, its limitations include its focus on sponges, with no effect on retained instruments or needles. Additionally, bar-coded systems cannot give insight about where a missing sponge is located, whether it be inside a patient, within the surgical field, or in the trash. Instead, it serves as a technological backup to counting [26].

Radio-Frequency Technology

The U.S. Food and Drug Administration-approved radio-frequency detection systems (RFDS) include radio-frequency-tagged sponges, a console with power source and monitor, and a detection wand or mat [26]. The radio-frequency chip embedded into surgical sponges is small enough not to interfere with typical sponge functionality. A detection wand with sterile cover is connected via a wire to the detection console, which generates visual and audible alarms when a sponge is detected while being passed over a patient. A variation on this technology utilizes a surgical mat, which is placed on the operating room table prior to the patient's arrival. On completion of surgery, pressing a button on the console activates the mat to scan the patient for a retained sponge. The mat technology avoids the potential of human scanning error introduced by the wand, as scanning too far from the patient may lead to false-negative results. Unlike the mat, the wand will also detect sponges located in other areas of the operating suite, including the surgical drapes and trash.

The benefit of the RFDS over bar-coded sponges is that it can be used for in vivo detection of any radio-frequency-labeled item. It should be noted that RF energy at wavelengths used by this technology has not been shown to expose humans to any deleterious effects [26]. Several prospective trials have sought to evaluate the value of radio-frequency technology on reducing retained surgical sponges.

Steelman et al. utilized a prospective, crossover, observer-blinded study design at the Veterans Affairs Medical Center in Iowa City in 2011, in which surgical sponges were placed behind patients' torsos to evaluate RFDS technology. Sensitivity and specificity of sponge detection by the RFDS technology were both 100%, with no false negatives or false positives. This indicates a much higher sensitivity and specificity than typical surgical counts and intraoperative radiographs. The scanning process lasted under 3 min, with an alarm sounding in less than 30 s when a sponge was detected. RFDS can indicate the presence of a sponge but not its exact location, evidenced by alarms when a sponge was located on the contralateral side of the body. Therefore, an alarm should prompt a thorough exploration of the cavity and not a dedicated quadrant search. There were some technical errors within this study when the console would alarm with name badges, proximity access cards, and, occasionally, pagers. However, software has since been updated to eliminate technical interference. Importantly, various internal metal implants and jewelry did not falsely activate the alarm [25].

Another prospective, crossover, double-blinded study was performed to investigate the RFDS utilizing the radio-frequency detection mat system. Notably, the RF mat is narrower than the operating room table, and the patient's abdominal cavity may exceed this width, especially in patients with higher BMIs. In patients with morbid obesity, the sensitivity of the RF mat was 96.9%, which decreased overall sensitivity to 98.1%, while specificity remained 100%. The RF wand was reevaluated in the morbidly obese as well but maintained 100% sensitivity and specificity. Therefore, the RF wand is preferable to the use of RF mat in patients with high BMI due to the mat's narrow width compared to body habitus [27].

University of North Carolina hospitals performed another study to evaluate the RFDS system, which included 2285 patients. All surgical sponge miscounts, with a rate of 1.53%, were successfully resolved with the use of RFDS technology. Sponges were ultimately found in surgical site (31.4%), within operative suite, surgical drapes, and emergency protocol deviations. No retained surgical sponges were encountered during the study period, but one near miss was detected by the RFDS technology. An additional $13.54 of added cost was associated with the implementation of the RFDS technology. Operating room staff reported an overall positive response to the technology, with high confidence of its ability to prevent retained surgical sponges [28].

When implemented among high-risk open-cavity emergency operations in a large county hospital, radio-frequency technology was found to be effective at preventing retained surgical sponges. Each case underwent traditional standardized manual counting, RFDS wand scanning, and intraoperative radiographic evaluation for detection of retained sponges, regardless of the count status. RFDS detected retained sponges in 0.5% of cases prior to cavity closure. Eleven near-miss events (sponges identified by RFDS and successfully retrieved before closure) were detected by the RFDS technology; 63.6% of these near misses occurred in trauma cases, specifically in those with sternotomies and then laparotomies. Sponge counts were recorded as incorrect 36.4% of the time and not performed in 45.5% of the time. In 18.2% of near-miss events, counts were recorded as correct, but RFDS technology identified retained sponge. All subsequent intraoperative radiographs had no evidence of RSS, indicating that RFDS missed no retained sponges. The additional cost of RFDS disposables was calculated at $0.17 for a 4 × 18 laparotomy sponge and $0.46 for 10-pack of 12-ply, 4 × 8 [29].

A cost-benefit analysis of radio-frequency technology was performed in 2014. Overall, radio-frequency technology implementation was associated with a 93% reduction in the rate of reported RSI when compared to a 77% reduction in places without RF technology implemented. Total additional cost to transition from radiographic detection to RF technology was estimated at $191,352 annually or $17.09 per case [30]. Similarly, in 2017, the estimated cost increase of $13–$17 per case was associated with radio-frequency technology implementation [31]. Generally, savings from decreased operating room time, intraoperative radiographs, and medical and legal costs were believed to outweigh the expenses associated with radio-frequency implementation. Overall, it is estimated to lead to more than $400,000 in savings per year after a switch to RFDS [30].

Conclusion

Retained surgical items represent a preventable and devastating adverse event. For decades, policies have focused on manual surgical counting, with supplemental intraoperative radiographs in cases of count discrepancies. Surgical sponge innovations, specifically bar-coded sponges and radio-frequency technology, have shown promise in preventing RSIs and should be considered for clinical use. However, only about 20% of hospitals in the United States have implemented these new technologies in existing standard protocols [31]. When implementing any new technology, institutions must consider their priorities including ease of use, cost-to-benefit ratio, availability of technology, implementation learning curve, and experience and preference of OR and hospital leadership.

References

1. National Quality Forum. Serious reportable events in healthcare—2011 update: a consensus report [Internet]; 2011. www.qualityforum.org
2. The Joint Commission. Sentinel events (SE), comprehensive accreditation manual for hospitals; 2013.
3. The Centers for Medicare and Medicaid. Hospital-acquired conditions [Internet]. https://www.cms.gov/Medicare/Medicare-Fee-for-Service-Payment/HospitalAcqCond/Hospital-Acquired_Conditions.html
4. The Joint Commission. Most commonly reviewed sentinel event types [Internet]. https://www.jointcommission.org/resources/sentinel-event/sentinel-event-policy-and-procedures/
5. The Joint Commission. Summary Data of Sentinel Events [Internet]. https://www.jointcommission.org/resources/sentinel-event/sentinel-event-data-summary/
6. Wan W, Le T, Riskin L, Macario A. Improving safety in the operating room: a systematic literature review of retained surgical sponges. Curr Opin Anaesthesiol. 2009;22(2):207–14.
7. Gawande AA, Studdert DM, Orav EJ, Brennan TA, Zinner MJ. Risk factors for retained instruments and sponges after surgery. N Engl J Med. 2003;348(3):229–35.

8. Cima RR, Kollengode A, Garnatz J, Storsveen A, Weisbrod C, Deschamps C. Incidence and characteristics of potential and actual retained foreign object events in surgical patients. J Am Coll Surg. 2008;207(1):80–7.
9. Hyslop JW, Maull KI. Natural history of the retained surgical sponge. South Med J. 1982;75(6):657–60.
10. Rappaport W, Haynes K. The retained surgical sponge following intra-abdominal surgery: a continuing problem. Arch Surg. 1990;125(3):405–7.
11. Lincourt AE, Harrell A, Cristiano J, Sechrist C, Kercher K, Heniford BT. Retained foreign bodies after surgery. J Surg Res. 2007;138(2):170–4.
12. Stawicki SPA, Moffatt-Bruce SD, Ahmed HM, Anderson HL, Balija TM, Bernescu I, et al. Retained surgical items: a problem yet to be solved. J Am Coll Surg. 2013;216(1):15–22.
13. Stawicki SP, Cook CH, Anderson HL, Chowayou L, Cipolla J, Ahmed HM, et al. Natural history of retained surgical items supports the need for team training, early recognition, and prompt retrieval. Am J Surg. 2014;208(1):65–72.
14. Kaiser CW, Friedman S, Spurling KP, Slowick T, Kaiser HA. The retained surgical sponge. Ann Surg. 1996;224(1):79–84.
15. Dossett LA, Dittus RS, Speroff T, May AK, Cotton BA. Cost-effectiveness of routine radiographs after emergent open cavity operations. Surgery. 2008;144(2):317–21.
16. Stawicki SP, Evans DC, Cipolla J, Seamon MJ, Lukaszczyk JJ, Prosciak MP, et al. Retained surgical foreign bodies: a comprehensive review of risks and preventive strategies. Scand J Surg. 2009;98(1):8–17.
17. Moffatt-Bruce SD, Cook CH, Steinberg SM, Stawicki SP. Risk factors for retained surgical items: a meta-analysis and proposed risk stratification system. J Surg Res. 2014;190(2):429–36.
18. Guideline for prevention of retained surgical items. AORN J 2016;102: P11.
19. Egorova NN, Moskowitz A, Gelijns A, Weinberg A, Curty J, Rabin-Fastman B, et al. Managing the prevention of retained surgical instruments: what is the value of counting? Ann Surg. 2008;247(1):13–8.
20. Greenberg CC, Regenbogen SE, Lipsitz SR, Diaz-Flores R, Gawande AA. The frequency and significance of discrepancies in the surgical count. Ann Surg. 2008;248(2):337–41.
21. Regenbogen SE, Greenberg CC, Resch SC, Kollengode A, Cima RR, Zinner MJ, et al. Prevention of retained surgical sponges: a decision-analytic model predicting relative cost-effectiveness. Surgery. 2009;145(5):527–35.
22. Greenberg CC, Diaz-Flores R, Lipsitz SR, Regenbogen SE, Mulholland L, Mearn F, et al. Bar-coding surgical sponges to improve safety: a randomized controlled trial. Ann Surg. 2008;247(4):612–6.
23. Bardes JM, Inaba K. The use of radiofrequency detection to mitigate the risk of retained surgical sponges. Adv Surg. 2017;51(1):219–27.
24. Ponrartana S, Coakley FV, Yeh BM, Breiman RS, Qayyum A, Joe BN, et al. Accuracy of plain abdominal radiographs in the detection of retained surgical needles in the peritoneal cavity. Ann Surg. 2008;247(1):8–12.
25. Steelman VM. Sensitivity of detection of radiofrequency surgical sponges: a prospective, cross-over study. Am J Surg. 2011;201(2):233–7.
26. Cima RR, Kollengode A, Clark J, Pool S, Weisbrod C, Amstutz GJ, et al. Using a data-matrix-coded sponge counting system across a surgical practice: impact after 18 months. Jt Comm J Qual Patient Saf. 2011;37(2):51–8.
27. Steelman VM, Alasagheirin MH. Assessment of radiofrequency device sensitivity for the detection of retained surgical sponges in patients with morbid obesity. Arch Surg. 2012;147(10):955–60.
28. Rupp CC, Kagarise MJ, Nelson SM, Deal AM, Phillips S, Chadwick J, et al. Effectiveness of a radiofrequency detection system as an adjunct to manual counting protocols for tracking surgical sponges: a prospective trial of 2,285 patients. J Am Coll Surg. 2012;215(4):524–33.

29. Inaba K, Okoye O, Aksoy H, Skiada D, Ault G, Sener S, et al. The role of radio frequency detection system embedded surgical sponges in preventing retained surgical sponges: a prospective evaluation in patients undergoing emergency surgery. Ann Surg. 2016;264(4):599–604.
30. Williams TL, Tung DK, Steelman VM, Chang PK, Szekendi MK. Retained surgical sponges: findings from incident reports and a cost-benefit analysis of radiofrequency technology. J Am Coll Surg. 2014;219(3):354–64.
31. TechNation. ECRI update: retained surgical sponges are a top hazard, technology solutions can help; 20 March 2019. [Internet]. https://1technation.com/ecri-update-retained-surgical-sponges-are-a-top-hazard-technology-solutions-can-help/

Principles of Perioperative Safety and Quality on the Global Stage

23

Meena Nathan Cherian, Jyotsna Agarwal, Raymond R. Price, Janet Martin, Adrian W. Gelb, and Davy Cheng

Patient Safety

Once the patient is scheduled for any surgical intervention, it is of paramount importance that we ensure the safety of the patient in the entire journey from admission until discharge from the hospital. In the healthcare delivery, while we accept that "to err is human," to deliberately ignore or skip the safety standards is unacceptable.

This chapter focuses on what the entire perioperative team must know about anesthesia and surgery to ensure patient safety and healthcare quality. An interesting quote from the International Committee of the Red Cross (ICRC) Anaesthesia Guidelines emphasizes the important role of anesthesia services, even in austere

M. N. Cherian (✉)
Global Health New Challenge, Geneva Foundation for Medical Education and Research, Versoix, Switzerland

J. Agarwal
Department of Anesthesiology and Pain Medicine, Hamdard Institute of Medical Sciences and Research, New Delhi, India

R. R. Price
Center for Global Surgery, University of Utah, Salt Lake City, UT, USA

J. Martin
Department of Anesthesia & Perioperative Medicine, Epidemiology & Biostatistics, London Health Sciences Centre, London, ON, Canada

A. W. Gelb
Department of Anesthesia and Perioperative Care, University of California San Francisco, San Francisco, CA, USA

D. Cheng
Schulich School of Medicine & Dentistry, Western University, London, ON, Canada

J. J. Hoballah et al. (eds.), *Principles of Perioperative Safety and Efficiency*,
https://doi.org/10.1007/978-3-031-41089-5_23

environments. "Surgeons perform big operations and small operations. There is no such thing as a small anaesthesia. Every anaesthesia is potentially fatal. The limits of operational activity in the theatre are not those of the surgeon's expertise. They are determined far more by the level of competency and sophistication of the anaesthesia department. There is only one other limiting factor that is as important as anaesthesia, if not more so, in determining the level of sophistication of surgery to be performed: postoperative nursing care" [1].

Some practical approaches that can guide both policy makers and healthcare providers (doctors, nurses, technicians, and support staff) are elaborated toward evidence-based strategies at the global stage to ensure patient safety in the perioperative care. These approaches for all surgical interventions including childbirth and injuries are applicable even in resource-limited settings and humanitarian emergencies.

The existing international standards of the World Health Organization (WHO), World Federation of Societies of Anaesthesiologists (WFSA), and recommendations from ICRC and Médecins Sans Frontières (MSF)—known also as Doctors without Borders—will be discussed toward ensuring perioperative quality and safety.

Background

It is often presumed that high-quality care is a luxury in low- and middle-income countries (LMICs) and difficult to measure, particularly in limited-resource healthcare settings. Safe and quality care can be delivered across geographical regions and resource settings with seven measurable and desired health outcomes [2]:

1. Effectiveness
2. Safety
3. People-centeredness
4. Timeliness
5. Equity
6. Integration of care
7. Efficiency

Universal health coverage (UHC) means that all individuals and communities receive the health services they need without suffering financial hardship. It includes the full spectrum of essential, quality health services, from health promotion to prevention, treatment, rehabilitation, and palliative care [3].

Safe Surgical and Anesthesia Services: Critical Component of UHC

UHC includes ensuring that surgical and anesthesia services are available to all when needed, also promoting equity, social justice, and human rights [4].

The unanimous passing of the World Health Assembly 68.15 Resolution in May 2015 by all 194 World Health Organization (WHO) member states (countries) on "Strengthening emergency and essential surgical care and anesthesia as a component of UHC" was a landmark in the global public health stage. It highlighted the global burden of surgical diseases and requested actions from the WHO and the member countries for providing safe surgical and anesthesia services, particularly in primary health care and first referral hospitals. It emphasized policies to set cost-effective priorities and minimum standards for skilled health workforce, infrastructure, equipment, medicines, supplies, infection control, pain management, perioperative mortality data, monitoring, and evaluation as a critical element of ensuring quality and safety [5].

Considering the magnitude of the global burden of surgical conditions—in pregnancy-related complications, injuries, congenital anomalies, cancer, acute abdomen, non-acute surgical conditions, and humanitarian crisis—access to safe, timely, and affordable surgical care and anesthesia is a critical component of UHC. Successfully reaching the specific health-related targets of the Sustainable Development Goals (SDGs) requires high-quality surgical services that ensure patient safety [6].

The surgical care community needs to focus on the wider population in the UHC context. Global efforts can be streamlined to improve safe and timely access to simple procedures that are cost effective and appropriate to perform in first-level hospitals that could reduce a significant proportion of the burden of surgical disease in LMICs [7]. The G4 Alliance, a coalition of more than 75 civil society organizations, collectively established its unifying global target as "Safe Surgical and Anaesthesia Care for 80% of the World by 2030" [8].

Global Situation of Perioperative Care

Even if surgery is provided, unsafe anesthesia will add to death or disability [9]. To improve patient safety and outcomes, successful anesthesia initiatives must be developed or expanded, including airway management (maintain airway, breathing, oxygenation); management of cardiac disturbances; and comprehensive perioperative care (comorbidities, pain management). These anesthesia initiatives are critical issues in many LMICs due to lack of investments in training, procurement, and maintenance of anesthesia and monitoring equipment, oxygen, and medicines, including opioids [9].

In the last 50 years, there has been a steady decline in the perioperative mortality rate (POMR) and anesthetic-related mortality (ARM) rates, despite taking higher risk patients for anesthesia. The greatest decline in POMR was in high-income countries (HICs), but the POMR incidence was two to three times higher in LMICs. Over the years, the risk of mortality solely due to anesthesia decreased progressively from 357 per million (before the 1970s) to 34 per million (in the 1990s–2000s). This could be attributed to the efforts to improve patient safety in the perioperative period over the years and suggested that it could become an indicator for patient safety.

In order to reduce this inequity, global priority should be given to utilizing evidence-based interventions in the LMICs' context in reducing the POMR and ARM [10] (Fig. 23.1).

A recent study on the global burden of postoperative death suggests that at least 4.2 million people worldwide die within 30 days of surgery each year, and half of these deaths occur in LMICs. This number of postoperative deaths accounts for 7.7% of all deaths globally, making it the third greatest contributor to deaths, after ischemic heart disease and stroke (Fig. 23.2). More people die within 30 days of surgery annually than from all causes related to HIV, malaria, and tuberculosis combined (2.97 million deaths) [11].

The May 2019 Report by the WHO Director General on Implementation of the 2030 Agenda for Sustainable Development emphasized that access to safe, timely, and affordable emergency and essential surgical and anesthesia care is a critical component of UHC.

Globally, 5 billion people lack access to this; 1.7 billion are children under the age of 15 years. This report also highlighted that 830 women die each day from complications of childbirth (commonly caused by obstructed labor and postpartum hemorrhage). A total of 6.3 million children under 15 years old died in 2017; many

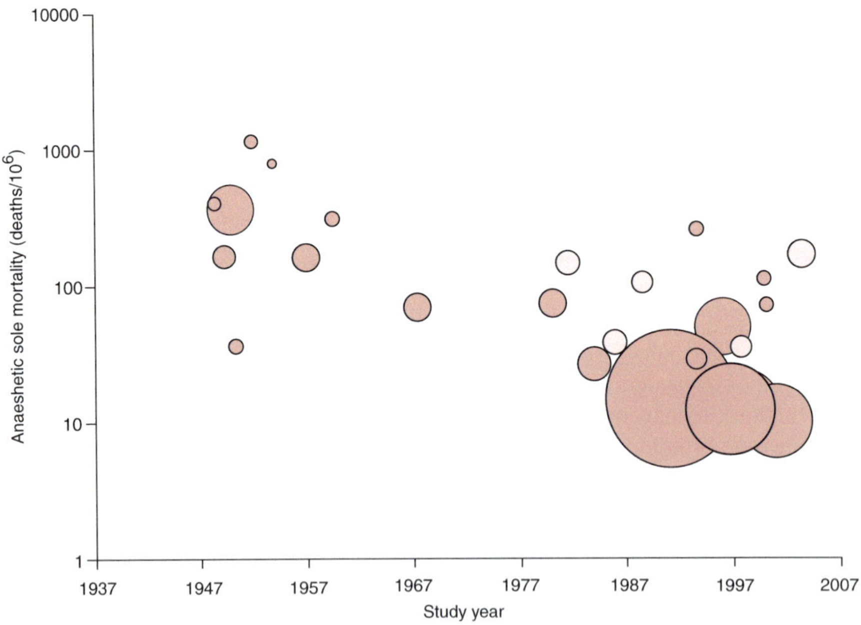

Fig. 23.1 Event rates for anaesthetic sole mortality by year. Every circle represents a study; the circle size is representative of the study's population size. The year represents the median year if the study reported a range of years. Low-income and middle-income countries are shown in light red (human development index [HDI]<0.8) and high income countries in dark red (HDI < 0.8). Reprinted from The Lancet, Vol. 380, Issue 9847, Bainbridge D, Martin J, Arango M, Cheng D; Evidence-based Peri-operative Clinical Outcomes Research (EPiCOR) Group, Perioperative and anaesthetic-related mortality in developed and developing countries: a systematic review and meta-analysis, 1075-81, Copyright (2012), with permission from Elsevier

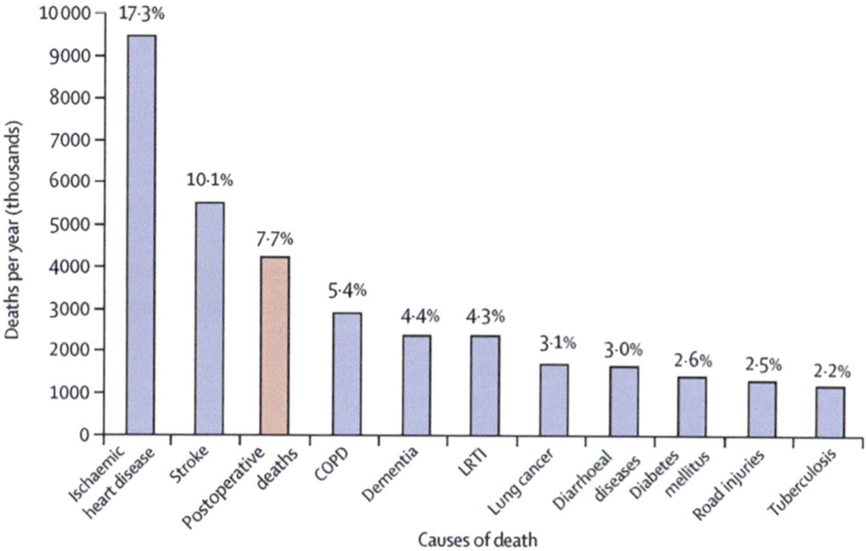

Fig. 23.2 Top ten global causes of death, 2016. Percentages are the proportion of total global deaths attributable to each cause. Data, except those on postoperative deaths, are from the Global Burden of Disease Study 2016. COPD- chronic obstructive pulmonary disease. LRTI- lower respiratory tract infections. Reprinted from The Lancet, Vol. 393, Issue 10170, Nepogodiev D, Martin J, Biccard B, Makupe A, Bhangu A; National Institute for Health Research Global Health Research Unit on Global Surgery, Global burden of postoperative death, Page 401, Copyright (2019), with permission from Elsevier

of these are caused by congenital malformations, violence and injury, and childhood neoplasms. Each year, 15 million people between the ages of 30 and 69 years die from a noncommunicable disease; about 85% of these deaths occur in LMICs and are a result of cardiovascular diseases (heart disease, stroke), cancer, and diabetes. Each year, 1.35 million die as a result of road traffic crashes, 93% of which occur in LMICs, and these are the leading cause of death for children and young adults aged 5–29 years. The majority of these conditions are most appropriately treated with surgical care [6]. There is a correlation between surgical access, anesthesia capacity, and patient safety on the one hand and mortality on the other hand [9].

Delivering Quality Perioperative Care

The World Health Assembly resolution 68.15 created an interest and better understanding in some players in the surgical global community, but more advocacy is needed in the global public health domain to improve surgical services on par with anesthesia services. Providing quality perioperative care requires a multi-sectoral approach, exploring financing mechanisms and appropriate resource allocation to improve training to meet local needs, in addition to monitoring and evaluation, and strengthening surgical care systems.

Safe and quality perioperative care takes into account the basic principles that the correct patient receives the correct procedure, performed on the correct site, at the correct time, while avoiding any harm.

Surgically correctable diseases constitute up to one-third of global burden of diseases, which implies universal and on-demand access to anesthesia and surgical care in all parts of the world, including remote areas. Maintenance of quality in these services is imperative, without which the core intent of improving patients' health will be defeated [12].

Surgical intervention should ensure patients' and healthcare providers' safety equally, at all levels of care (from tertiary to primary, elective and urgent, minor and major procedures, including in humanitarian crises) [13].

The first-level hospitals (rural, community hospital) receive referrals from health clinics and community centers that mostly require emergency surgical care. Often, these first-level hospitals lack trained anesthesia providers, which becomes a major barrier to providing essential emergency surgeries [7]. Therefore, priority should be given to improve the quality of perioperative care in these facilities through evaluation of minimum standards for infrastructure, equipment, medicines, supplies, data records, and skills of the surgical health workforce.

For a surgical intervention to be successful, strict measures are required during the entire perioperative period. Building an operating room is not enough for delivering safe and quality surgical services. It requires strengthening the entire surgical care system and investments in the implementation of a robust system, which, if ignored, has serious implication for the delivery of safe and quality perioperative care.

Perioperative care starts with a detailed preoperative check and continues with precise intraoperative and postoperative management until the discharge of the patient. Therefore, improvement in its safety and quality requires a multifactorial approach with safe infrastructure and maintenance of equipment, access to medicines, and a surgical workforce (anesthesia, nursing, technicians) trained and motivated to participate in quality measurement and improvement standards [14, 15].

"No single improvement in the care of surgical patients has had as profound an impact as the advancement of safe practices in anesthesia" [15].

With advancements in anesthesia and perioperative care, the ARM has reduced drastically from 2 per 10,000 to 1 in 200,000 in healthy patients. But it is not uniform globally. LMICs still have higher ARM rates, which can be as high as 1 in 300 [12].

This is due to absent or weak policies, lack of adherence to global standards, lack of development or consensus on national standards, and sometimes differing standards in hospitals within the same region. Even though anesthesia has advanced on par with surgical interventions, investments are not equally distributed in LMICs to enable high-quality anesthesia services to upgrade the equipment, medicines, skills of the anesthesia workforce, and continuing professional development.

Safe anesthesia for essential surgery is a basic human right [12]. Every patient must receive the highest standard of safe care possible, regardless of types of anesthesia and surgical procedure performed, or the patient's financial status. The recommended safety standards should not be ignored or compromised by the location, hierarchy, or resource availability of the healthcare delivery system [12].

Improving Safety and Quality of Perioperative Care

Anesthesia Safety

International Standards for a Safe Practice of Anesthesia were developed by the WFSA and the WHO, applicable globally both in HICs and in LMICs. This has been adapted by some countries in agreement with their national professional societies; however, these standards have not been implemented equally at all levels of care, resulting in "near misses" and perioperative morbidity and mortality. In addition, when these are reported (within the healthcare system or by media), it emphasizes the "blame factor" rather than investigating the implementation and adherence to national standards. The WFSA has set up recommendations in three categories: (i) highly recommended (minimum mandatory) standards, (ii) recommended standards, and (iii) suggested standards.

If the highly recommended minimum standards are implemented from the primary to the tertiary levels of health care that perform minor or major surgical interventions, it will assist countries toward meeting the 2018 Global Reference List of 100 Core Health Indicators (plus health-related SDGs), particularly the perioperative mortality rate (POMR) [16].

The Highly Recommended Standards are mandatory requirements that must be present in any setup providing general anesthesia, regional anesthesia, or moderate to deep sedation. Recommended and suggested standards should be followed as per resource availability.

Highly Recommended Standards include continuous presence of trained and vigilant anesthesia provider throughout anesthesia care, use of the surgical safety checklist, confirmation of endotracheal tube positioning by auscultation and end-tidal carbon dioxide, continuous monitoring of oxygenation and perfusion through clinical observation, noninvasive blood pressure (NIBP), and pulse oximetry.

Pre-anesthesia checkup includes formulation and documentation of anesthesia plan, written explained anesthesia consent, checking anesthesia equipment and medications prior to induction, clean labeling and date on medications, provision of supplemental oxygen to all patients undergoing general anesthesia or deep sedation, loud audible alarms for vital monitoring, and maintenance of detailed perioperative anesthesia records.

Postanesthesia care should be provided in recovery rooms with facilities of oxygen, suction, ventilation, and resuscitation capabilities. Continuous postoperative monitoring by a trained healthcare worker for airway, breathing, circulation, oxygenation, NIBP, and pulse oximetry, along with management of postoperative pain with adequate analgesics, is critical for safe postanesthesia care [12].

The WFSA recommends that anesthesiologists should have formal, documented training from the national accredited program and should be trained in proper and safe use of equipment [12].

Surgical Checklist

The WHO surgical checklist is a simple tool designed to improve the safety of surgical procedures by bringing together the entire operating team (surgeons, anesthesia providers, and nurses) to perform key safety checks during vital phases of perioperative care (Fig. 23.3) [15]:

(i) Prior to the induction of anesthesia
(ii) Prior to skin incision
(iii) Before the patient and team leave the operating room

A study in hospitals with a diverse clinical and economic environment in HICs and LMICs showed that the implementation of the WHO checklist decreased the rates of mortality and postoperative complications, thus improving the safety of surgical patients worldwide [17].

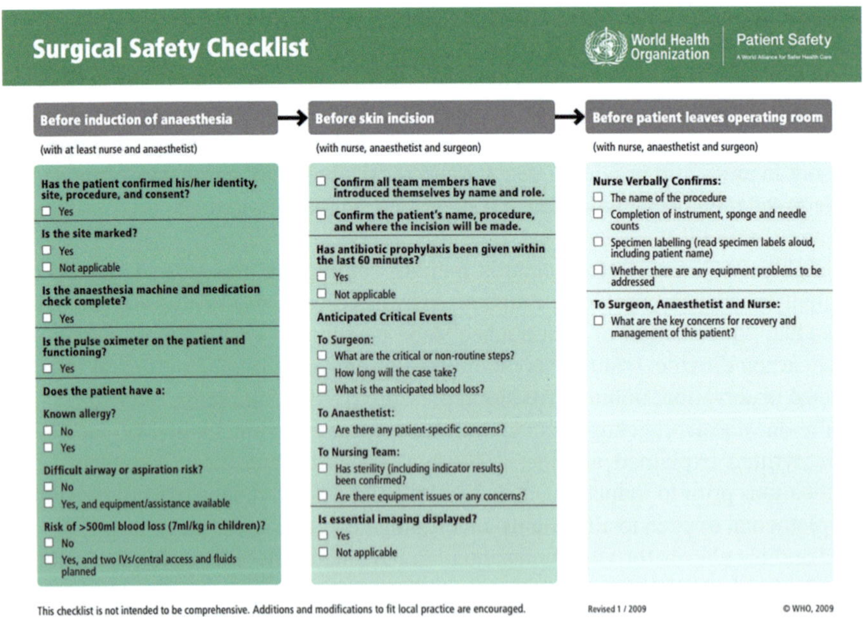
Surgical Safety Checklist

World Health Organization | Patient Safety

Before induction of anaesthesia
(with at least nurse and anaesthetist)

Has the patient confirmed his/her identity, site, procedure, and consent?
☐ Yes

Is the site marked?
☐ Yes
☐ Not applicable

Is the anaesthesia machine and medication check complete?
☐ Yes

Is the pulse oximeter on the patient and functioning?
☐ Yes

Does the patient have a:

Known allergy?
☐ No
☐ Yes

Difficult airway or aspiration risk?
☐ No
☐ Yes, and equipment/assistance available

Risk of >500ml blood loss (7ml/kg in children)?
☐ No
☐ Yes, and two IVs/central access and fluids planned

Before skin incision
(with nurse, anaesthetist and surgeon)

☐ **Confirm all team members have introduced themselves by name and role.**

☐ **Confirm the patient's name, procedure, and where the incision will be made.**

Has antibiotic prophylaxis been given within the last 60 minutes?
☐ Yes
☐ Not applicable

Anticipated Critical Events

To Surgeon:
☐ What are the critical or non-routine steps?
☐ How long will the case take?
☐ What is the anticipated blood loss?

To Anaesthetist:
☐ Are there any patient-specific concerns?

To Nursing Team:
☐ Has sterility (including indicator results) been confirmed?
☐ Are there equipment issues or any concerns?

Is essential imaging displayed?
☐ Yes
☐ Not applicable

Before patient leaves operating room
(with nurse, anaesthetist and surgeon)

Nurse Verbally Confirms:
☐ The name of the procedure
☐ Completion of instrument, sponge and needle counts
☐ Specimen labelling (read specimen labels aloud, including patient name)
☐ Whether there are any equipment problems to be addressed

To Surgeon, Anaesthetist and Nurse:
☐ What are the key concerns for recovery and management of this patient?

This checklist is not intended to be comprehensive. Additions and modifications to fit local practice are encouraged.

Revised 1 / 2009

© WHO, 2009

Fig. 23.3 WHO Surgical Safety Checklist. Reference WHO guidelines for safe surgery: 2009: safe surgery saves lives

Trauma Checklist

Trauma mortality rates have been reduced in many HICs, resulting from good planning and organization of trauma care services; more than 90% of injury deaths occur in LMICs [18]. The WHO trauma checklist emphasizes immediate steps (resuscitation and stabilization procedures) following the primary and secondary survey. It ensures recording the treatment given and next plans prior to handing over to the next team. The perioperative period in acute traumatic injury generally does not give enough time to arrange lifesaving items (chest tubes, resuscitation equipment, medicines, defibrillator, airway devices). These should be readily available, in adequate numbers, functioning with proper maintenance (like sterility, cold chain, charged battery, and expiry of unused items). Perioperative trauma care quality is influenced by overall patient care starting from the prehospital setting extending until rehabilitation (Fig. 23.4a, b).

Quality in trauma care aims at better monitoring of trauma care services, identification of problem areas, formulation and implementation of corrective strategies (such as protocols, education, communication, resource enhancement), monitoring their effectiveness, and ensuring achievement of intended results [18].

Strengthening of trauma quality improvement (QI) in LMICs aims at preventing deaths due to low-severity injuries. Trauma registry records all information such as the injury event, demographics, prehospital care, diagnosis, management, outcome of the patient, and cost of treatment. Quality in any service, including perioperative

Immediately after primary & secondary surveys:

Is further airway intervention needed? May be needed if: • GCS 8 or below • Hypoxaemia or hypercarbia • Face, neck, chest or any severe trauma	☐ Yes, done ☐ No
Is there a *tension* pneumo-haemothorax?	☐ Yes, chest drain placed ☐ No
Is the pulse oximeter placed and functioning?	☐ Yes ☐ Not available
Large-bore IV placed and fluids started?	☐ Yes ☐ Not indicated ☐ Not available
Full survey for (and control of) external bleeding, including:	☐ Scalp ☐ Perineum ☐ Back
Assessed for pelvic fracture by:	☐ Exam ☐ X-ray ☐ CT
Assessed for internal bleeding by:	☐ Exam ☐ Ultrasound ☐ CT ☐ Diagnostic peritoneal lavage
Is spinal immobilization needed?	☐ Yes, done ☐ Not indicated
Neurovascular status of all 4 limbs checked?	☐ Yes
Is the patient hypothermic?	☐ Yes, warming ☐ No
Does the patient need (if no contraindication):	☐ Urinary catheter ☐ Nasogastric tube ☐ Chest drain ☐ None indicated

Fig. 23.4 WHO Trauma Care checklist WHO 2016. WHO Trauma Care Checklist. WHO 2016; reference https://www.who.int/publications/i/item/trauma-care-checklist

LARGE-BORE IV PLACED AND FLUIDS STARTED?	☐ YES ☐ NOT INDICATED ☐ NOT AVAILABLE
FULL SURVEY FOR (AND CONTROL OF) EXTERNAL BLEEDING, INCLUDING:	☐ SCALP ☐ PERINEUM ☐ BACK
ASSESSED FOR PELVIC FRACTURE BY:	☐ EXAM ☐ X-RAY ☐ CT
ASSESSED FOR INTERNAL BLEEDING BY:	☐ EXAM ☐ ULTRASOUND ☐ CT ☐ DIAGNOSTIC PERITONEAL LAVAGE
IS SPINAL IMMOBILIZATION NEEDED?	☐ YES, DONE ☐ NOT INDICATED
NEUROVASCULAR STATUS OF ALL 4 LIMBS CHECKED?	☐ YES
IS THE PATIENT HYPOTHERMIC?	☐ YES, WARMING ☐ NO
DOES THE PATIENT NEED (IF NO CONTRAINDICATION):	☐ URINARY CATHETER ☐ NASOGASTRIC TUBE ☐ CHEST DRAIN ☐ NONE INDICATED

Before team leaves patient:

HAS THE PATIENT BEEN GIVEN:	☐ TETANUS VACCINE ☐ ANALGESICS ☐ ANTIBIOTICS ☐ NONE INDICATED
HAVE ALL TESTS AND IMAGING BEEN REVIEWED?	☐ YES ☐ NO, FOLLOW-UP PLAN IN PLACE
WHICH SERIAL EXAMINATIONS ARE NEEDED?	☐ NEUROLOGICAL ☐ ABDOMINAL ☐ VASCULAR ☐ NONE
PLAN OF CARE DISCUSSED WITH:	☐ PATIENT/FAMILY ☐ RECEIVING UNIT ☐ PRIMARY TEAM ☐ OTHER SPECIALISTS
RELEVANT TRAUMA CHART OR FORM COMPLETED?	☐ YES ☐ NOT AVAILABLE

Fig. 23.4 (continued)

trauma care, is a combined result of "human factors" and "system factors." System improvements make a large and long-lasting impact on quality improvement. Corrective strategies for individual provider performance include counseling and training. Some measures such as multidisciplinary morbidity and mortality conferences, recordkeeping, and computerized registries have consistently shown to improve trauma quality [18].

Safety and Quality Perioperative Care in Humanitarian Emergencies

Providing adequate perioperative safety should address workplace and health workers' safety, along with patient safety. Although any humanitarian crisis is challenging, it is still feasible to ensure safety and healthcare quality in an austere environment [19]. It is a common misconception that in an endeavor to provide medical care to a large number of patients, quality is inevitably compromised. However, it only requires adherence to context-adapted policies. Médecins Sans Frontières (MSF) recommendations for field anesthesia provide excellent guidelines to ensure perioperative safety, even in austere environments [20].

Specialty training of the entire team, along with flexibility and situational adaptability, is essential. Scarcity of workforce demands multitasking. An anesthesiologist may be required to double up as a pediatrician for newborn resuscitation, or as a circulatory nurse or a technical assistant. Preparedness for alternative plans (having plans A, B, and C) is useful. Patient privacy, dignity, and consent, in accordance with the local culture, should be respected. Basic principles of "first do no harm" and "best practice for most" are used. Simple and safe practices that are effective for the majority of patients allow maximum output with minimum dependence on sophisticated technology. Use of common, locally available, and affordable medicines and equipment enables a functional, sustainable medical unit, even after short-term projects conclude. Adherence to patient safety protocols in the perioperative period by the visiting surgical team, even if it is for short periods, can impact a behavioral change in the host health facility to continue following such practices. Recordkeeping and regular reviews are as important as any other surgical area to improve outcomes and maintain accountability, including in short surgical missions [21, 22].

The WHO Health Resources Availability Monitoring System (HERAM) allows the assessment and monitoring of the status of health facilities and the availability of health services and resources in areas affected by emergencies [23]. The WHO developed a global verification system for quality-assured emergency medical teams (EMTs) that meet the WHO EMT minimum standards for deployment in health emergencies [24].

Safe and Quality Perioperative Care in Childbirth

Fourteen million women globally suffer from postpartum hemorrhage, which is the largest direct cause of maternal mortality. The WHO Safe Childbirth Checklist targets major causes of maternal mortality, intrapartum-related stillbirths, and neonatal deaths. This checklist was developed with the goal to improve the quality of care during four points of childbirth in any level of healthcare facility (Fig. 23.5a, b) [25]:

1. At admission
2. Just before pushing or before C-section
3. Soon after birth
4. Before discharge

The WHO "global core indicators for assessing the quality of health care provided to mothers, newborns, and children in health facilities" include prenatal optimization, facilities for infection control, neonatal resuscitation, and availability of uninterrupted oxygen supply and essential lifesaving medicines, all of which enhance perioperative mother and child safety [26].

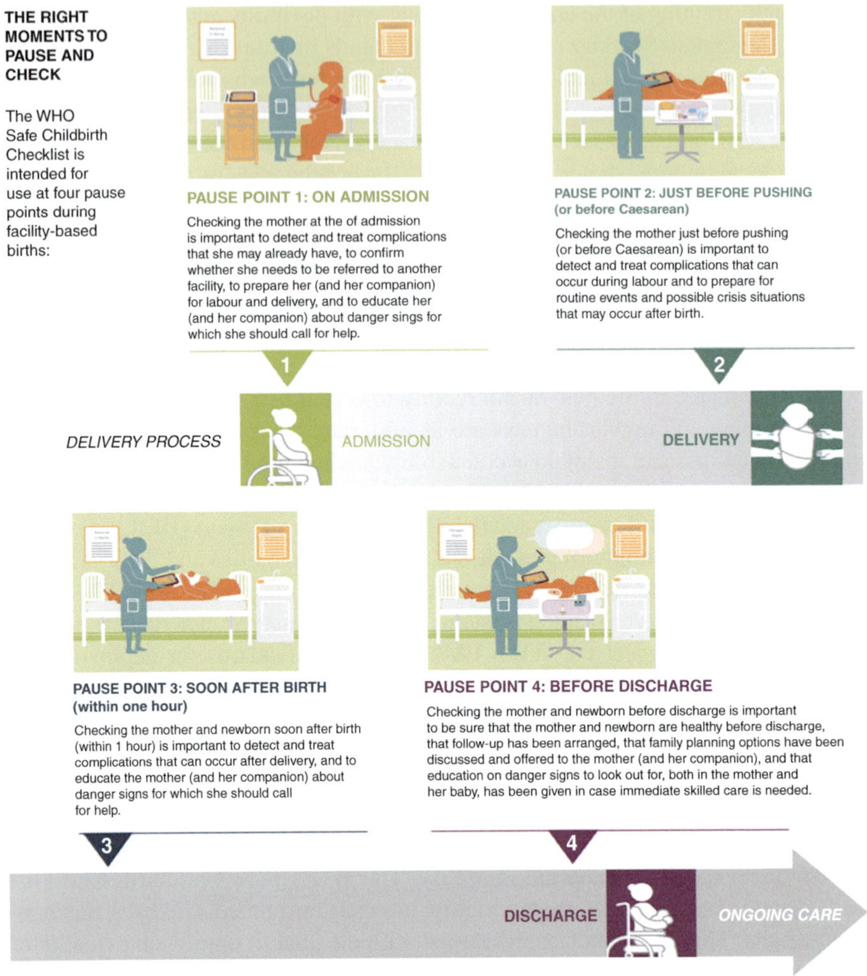

Fig. 23.5 The right moments to pause and check. WHO safe childbirth checklist is intended to use at four pause points during facility-based births. Reference WHO safe childbirth checklist implementation guide: Improving the quality of facility-based delivery for mothers and newborns. Geneva, WHO, 2015. https://apps.who.int/iris/bitstream/handle/10665/199177/9789241549455_eng.pdf ISBN 978 92 4 154945 5 (NLM classification: WQ 300)

Infection Control in Perioperative Care

Postoperative infections lead to prolonged hospital stays, more intensive care, and increased cost of care. Improving the quality of perioperative care infection control and antimicrobial resistance (AMR) plays a very important role globally at all levels of healthcare facilities, resulting in decreased health costs due to shorter hospital stay and less intensive care. The WHO standards and guidelines for perioperative infection control are:

(i) WHO standards on hand hygiene [27, 28]
(ii) WHO recommendations for prevention of surgical site infections and to combat AMR [29]

Pain Relief Is Essential for Quality Perioperative Care

Pain management is not just a "humanitarian" act; it is basic to the right to health [30–32].

It limits chronic pain, enables rehabilitation, and improves overall outcome. Inadequately treated pain can contribute to long-term disability, morbidity, and, rarely, mortality.

The "Reversed WHO Pain Management Ladder" is useful in the management of acute pain during a humanitarian crisis. It involves immediate pain relief with the use of strong opioids that are tapered gradually (Fig. 23.6) [33].

Often in LMICs at the district and subdistrict levels of care, optimum postoperative pain relief (particularly for children and women in labor) is not provided due to lack of medicines and a skilled health workforce.

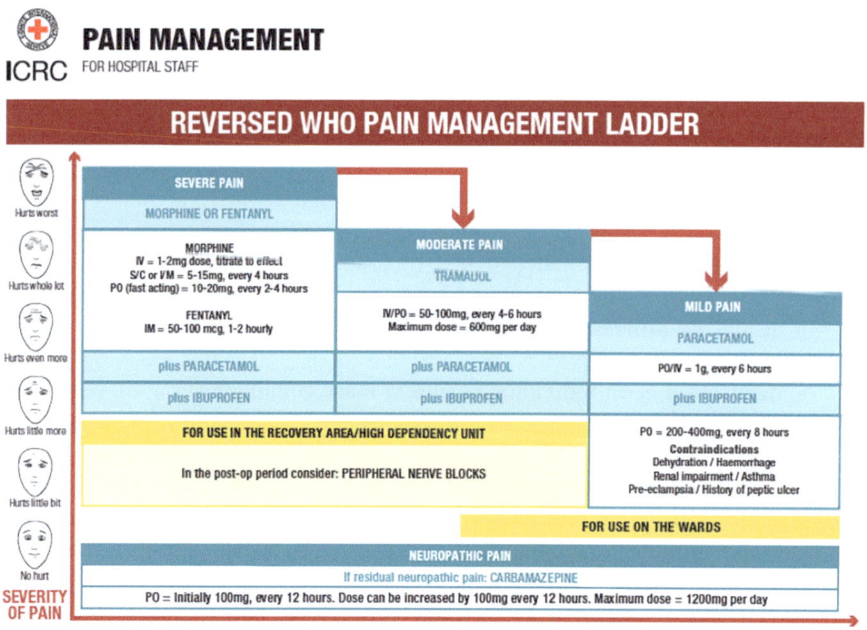

Fig. 23.6 Reversed WHO Pain Management Ladder. Reference Mahoney PF, Jeyanathan J, Wood P, Craven R. The ICRC Anaesthesia Handbook. Geneva: International Committee of the Red Cross, 2017: Annexure 3, Reversed WHO Pain Management Ladder; p 175

The WHO list of essential medicine includes effective and inexpensive analgesics, nonsteroidal anti-inflammatory medicines, and opioids, but they are frequently insufficient in supply. The postoperative surgical team is not allowed to administer these essential medicines or trained to administer safely, which may contribute to POMR [9]. The World Health Assembly resolution in 2015 (WHA 68.15) highlighted the limited access to opioids for perioperative pain relief in a large proportion of the global population and requested that member states take suitable action [5].

Effective regional anesthesia causes good analgesia, is opioid sparing, attenuates sympathetic stress response, and can sometimes avoid general anesthesia. Use of ultrasound has shown to improve efficacy and safety of regional anesthetic procedures.

Patient Safety in Perioperative Care

If investments are made into high-quality frontline health services, it will improve the quality and safety of patient care and resource utilization. This will generate a trust in health services in the community and therefore enhance local health security, which is a key to global health security [2].

Various WHO Global Patient Safety initiatives focus on improving perioperative safety. The first Global Patient Safety Challenge in 2005, "Clean care is safer care," aimed at reducing hospital-acquired infections (HAIs) with May fifth designated as Global Hand Hygiene Day [34].

The second Global Patient Safety challenge in 2009, "Safe surgery saves lives," focused directly on perioperative safety standards and led to the implementation of the evidence-based WHO Surgical Safety Checklist. The checklist aims at preventing errors from the preoperative until postoperative period and at improving communication amongst the team. Its use has been shown to reduce patient mortality by one-third (see Fig. 23.3) [15].

The third patient safety challenge in 2014, "Medication without harm," aimed at reducing avoidable medication-related harm and involves system improvements, role of healthcare professionals, and patient participation in ensuring medication safety [35].

Communication at an individual level and mass communication are both very important tools in ensuring the quality of trauma care and patient safety such as:

- Detailed patient monitoring charts and careful handing over at staff shift changes (Fig. 23.7)
- Clear and audible announcements by the team leader during surgery or resuscitation.

Announcement of codes like initiation of "massive transfusion protocol" or "disaster management" can activate all relevant departments simultaneously and reduce their response times (like early availability of blood from blood bank, preparation of operation theaters, readiness in intensive care units, resource mobilization, and enhanced patient care). Communication in patient safety has a very important role in reducing harm. In Australia, 11% of adverse events leading to permanent disability were found to be due to "communication issues" [36].

Lack of effective communication is an important factor in the majority of adverse events and is especially prominent in demanding situations like perioperative care. Patient handover (or handoff) communication starts from the receiving of the patient by healthcare providers, continues during handovers amongst caregiver teams, and finishes with handing over of patient to the family by a healthcare provider to maintain continuity of care. Communication strategies during patient handovers like SBAR (situation, background, assessment, recommendation) are designed to improve inter-professional collaboration and transfer of comprehensive information in an organized manner. It is considered a current best practice in communication that improves patient safety, especially in critical situations. "Repeat back" and "read back" steps, limiting communication during handover to that related to patient care, and trainings on effective communication and handover all help in minimizing errors during patient handover (see Fig. 23.7) [37].

Day care surgeries and ambulatory anesthesia involve early discharge of patients. Discharging the patient and handing over the patient to their family should

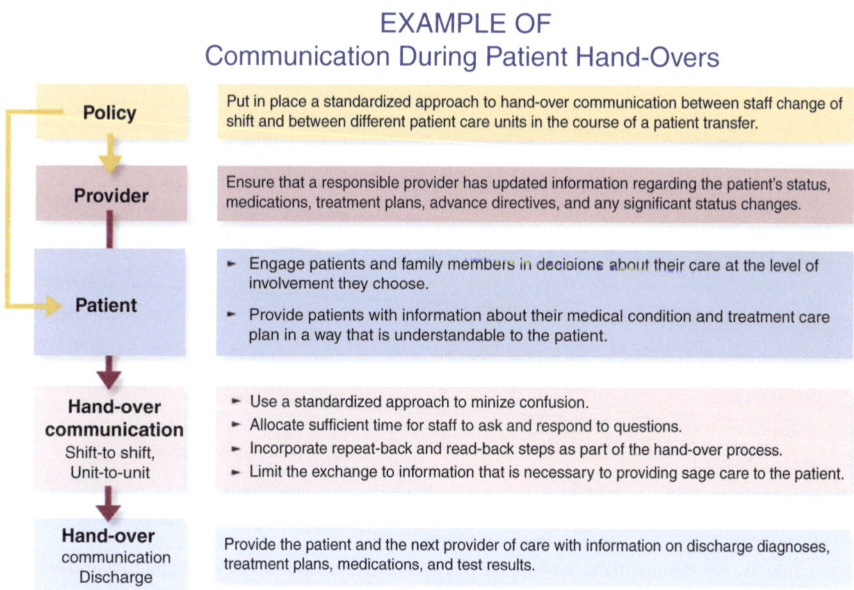

Fig. 23.7 Communication during patient hand-overs. Reference Communication during patient hand-overs. JCI WHO Collaboration Patient Safety Solutions | volume 1, solution 3 | May 2007

involve detailed communication with the patient and have the patient involved in their own care. The prescription, medications, and precautions should be explicitly told to the patient. When to contact and whom to contact in an emergency should be clearly written in the discharge paper. "Teach back" is a technique in which patients have to describe what they have understood about the medical advice given [37].

A 2004 WHO initiative "Patients for Patient Safety" was established to involve and engage patients in their own care. Patients should be communicated with in detail about their medical condition and the planned treatment and kept continuously involved in their management and decisions. Informed consent is also an integral part of patient safety. Patients should be encouraged to take ownership of their health, give relevant information to the healthcare provider before surgery, ask questions and clear their doubts regarding the perioperative period, follow medical advice, and try to familiarize themselves with medications and treatment, especially during home care. They should be actively involved rather than be a passive recipient of healthcare service. The WHO tool Patient Information for Surgical Safety engages and empowers the patient to ask key questions of the surgical care provider before and after any surgical intervention (Fig. 23.8) [38].

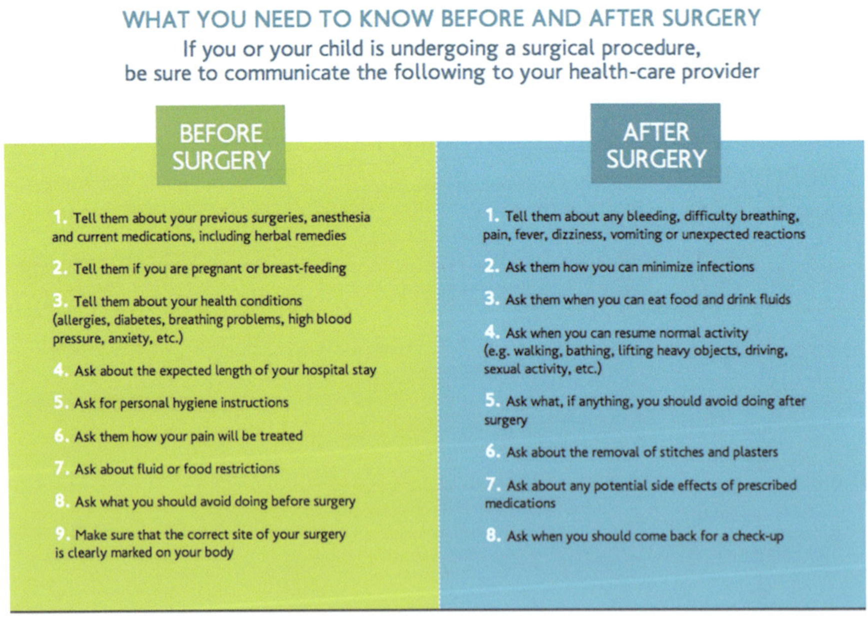

Fig. 23.8 WHO Patient information for surgical safety. Patient's Communication Tool for Surgical Safety. Who reference number: WHO/HIS/SDS/2015.18. Patient information for surgical safety: what you need to know before and after surgery (who.int) https://www.who.int/publications/i/item/WHO-HIS-SDS-2015.18. Reference https://www.who.int/surgery/publications/patients_communication_tool.pdf?ua=1. https://www.who.int/publications/i/item/integrated-management-for-emergency-and-surgical-care-(-imeesc)-toolkit

Strengthening Health Systems to Deliver Quality of Surgical Services Toward Achieving UHC

Improving quality and safety of surgical care services requires a "systems thinking" approach with locally adaptable interventions and strategies to reduce harm; data systems; professional development; and patient empowerment toward a sustainable environment. A recent study showed that UHC for SDG conditions could avert 8.6 million deaths per year, provided that investments are made for expanding health service coverage together with high-quality health systems [39].

Surgical (including anesthesia) services should not be seen in isolation in the tertiary level of care, but should be addressed from a perspective of strengthening health systems. Provision of safe and quality surgical care to a population requires a robust health system that has competent surgical personnel. In LMICs, a significant proportion of nonphysicians (clinical officers, surgical technicians, nurses) deliver surgical and anesthetic care with a wide variation of skills at the district and subdistrict healthcare facilities (Fig. 23.9) [40].

SDG3 indicators specifically emphasize quality and safety of essential health services; health workforce density distribution per 100,000 population; decrease in

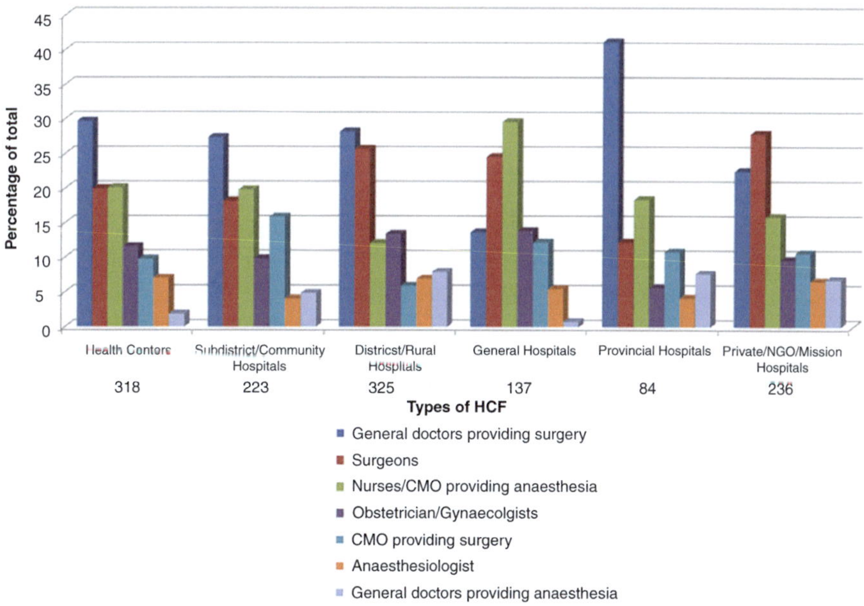

Fig. 23.9 Human resources according to types of healthcare facility. Reprinted from Sheik Ali S, Jaffry Z, Cherian MN, et al. Surgical human resources according to types of health care facility: an assessment in low- and middle-income countries. World J Surg. 2017; 41:2667. https://doi.org/10.1007/s00268-017-4078-4. Licensed under Creative Commons CC BY

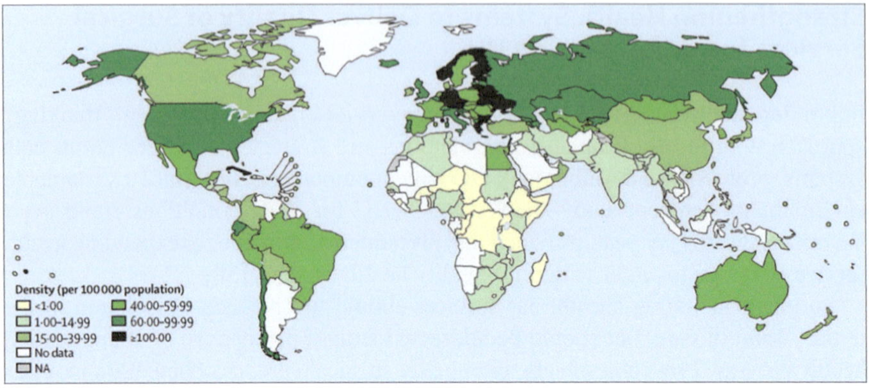

Fig. 23.10 Global distribution of surgeons, anaesthesiologists, and obstetricians, per 100,000 population. (NA = countries or territories that are not WHO members and thus excluded from our data). Reprinted from The Lancet Global Health, Vol. 3, Suppl. 2, Holmer H, Lantz A, Kunjumen T, Finlayson S, Hoyler M, Siyam A, Montenegro H, Kelley ET, Campbell J, Cherian MN, Hagander L, Global distribution of surgeons, anaesthesiologists, and obstetricians., Pages S9–11. Copyright (2015), with permission from Elsevier

perioperative morbidity and mortality including surgical procedures involving injuries and sexual and reproductive health; cancer and other surgical conditions; and abdominal and humanitarian emergencies (Fig. 23.10) [41, 42].

It is important to ensure that countries incorporate quality and safety of anesthesia and surgical care services. In their national health plans aligning with all the relevant programs such as maternal and child health, noncommunicable disease (injuries, cancer, aging, cardiovascular), neglected tropical disease, HIV, and humanitarian emergencies, capacity for essential surgery and anesthesia services is severely limited in LMICs due to shortfalls in physical infrastructure, human resources, and basic equipment and supplies, including continuous water, electricity, and oxygen [43–45].

Achieving post-2015 sustainable development goals, including universal healthcare, will require significant investment in surgery and anesthesia capacity [46].

Standard Tools Applicable Globally for Quality Surgical and Anesthesia Services

Several guidance tools, discussed below, have been developed by the WHO and the WFSA with professional bodies that could assist ministries of health and funders to make appropriate investments for improving the quality and safety of surgical and anesthesia services.

1. **WHO Situation Analysis Tool (SAT)**

   WHO SAT helps in assessing the gaps in emergency and essential surgical care at resource-limited settings and is used in several countries. The WHO

Integrated Management for Emergency and Essential Surgical Care toolkit contains guidance on improving safety and quality of surgical services [47, 48].

2. **WFSA Comprehensive Anesthesia Facility Assessment Tool (AFAT)**
   AFAT enables data collection and assessment of anesthesia practices, medicines, equipment, and workforce at the facility level, regional level, and national level. This data can help in the assessment of anesthesia capacity at the regional and national level, and resource management for the implementation of WHA resolution 68.15 [49].
3. **WFSA guidance on anesthesia machines**
   Because the supply of electricity and compressed gases varies from location to location, the WFSA has developed guidelines for those seeking to tender for and purchase anesthesia machines [50].
4. **Global standardization of medical gases**
   Guidelines on anesthetic gases' color coding and pin index system to ensure safe patient care globally have been developed by the International Organization for Standardization (ISO) and can be adopted by all countries [51, 52].
5. **WHO equipment donation**
   Donation of surplus medical equipment from high-resource settings to low-resource settings could help in bridging some gaps in healthcare service delivery. Effective donation requires proper execution. It involves understanding of recipients' context and providing support system and capacity-building programs for recipients. Guidelines and training modules on equipment donation have also been developed by the WHO [53].
6. **WHO Service Availability and Readiness Assessment (SARA)**
   WHO SARA is a tool for assessment and monitoring of health sector service availability and readiness and helps in health system planning and management. It contains indicators to assess readiness of surgical services and is used in several countries [54].

Improving Quality of Perioperative Care at the Global Stage

At the global stage, it requires understanding and commitments from all stakeholders (ministries of health and finance, professional and civil societies, nongovernment organizations, health providers, and managers) to invest in improving the quality and safety of perioperative care, which contributes to the SDG targets for maternal and child health, noncommunicable and neglected tropical diseases, and humanitarian emergencies.

In order to improve the delivery of safe and quality surgical and anesthesia services, it is important for both policy makers and health providers to adopt the following concrete improvement interventions/steps toward a robust health system:

1. Adapt existing global safety standards to develop national safety standards consistent with the local situation.
2. Sustainable investments to strengthen the implementation of safety standards to deliver quality care at all levels of healthcare facilities: The essential equipment

and medicines, and measures for infection control required to deliver safe perioperative care, should not be compromised in the district or primary level of healthcare facilities. It is often seen that anesthesia services in LMICs are compromised in terms of infrastructure and health workforce [43]. Performance-based assessment, implementation of safety protocols/checklists, and minimum safety standards in the healthcare facility will encourage financial investments.

3. Skilled surgical and anesthesia health workforce to meet the country's local needs: This will require both short-term and long-term training strategies (both midlevel health cadres and specialists), supervision, and ongoing evaluation of healthcare providers. These training programs should be licensed/accredited and approved at the national level by ministries of health, academia, and professional societies.

   Major deficiencies were found in specialist surgical workforce, especially surgeons, anesthesiologists, and obstetricians (SAO) in LMICs in a study by the Lancet Commission on Global Surgery and the WHO. It recommended SAO workforce of at least 20/100,000 to achieve SDG 3.8.1 by 2030. Globally, many countries are much below the target (see Fig. 23.10) [42].

   In LMICs at the district and subdistrict levels, much of the surgical (including anesthesia) care providers are nonphysicians (nurses, technicians). See Fig. 23.9 [40]. Quality of care provided by midlevel health workers has been studied in some LMICs such as Malawi, Mozambique, Cameroon, and Tanzania [55]. In some HICs, physician assistant/associate (USA, Ireland), surgical technicians, and other healthcare providers are trained to provide preoperative and postoperative care. Continuing professional development platforms for perioperative healthcare providers (doctors, nurses, technicians), e.g., online courses, training workshops, meetings, and conferences for recent updates, is essential.

4. Platform/forum for evaluation of implementation of quality and safety standards: For a sustainable quality anesthesia services at first referral level, rural and remote health facilities' policies need to be in place for the retention of trained anesthesia and surgical workforce. An appropriate environment has to be maintained (such as structured training and professional development, infrastructure, equipment, medicines, consistent financial remuneration, and established health posts) [56].
5. Using information technology (medical records, robust data system, patients' feedback) for choosing implementation of evidence-based interventions and evaluation, which will improve the quality of perioperative care in the local context

Three Practical Checkpoints Applicable Globally Toward the Patient's Safe Perioperative Journey

A prerequisite to quality perioperative care is a safe infrastructure with continuous water, electricity, oxygen supply, and a qualified trained surgical team. There are three checkpoints that guide the implementation of standard protocols and tools for the patient's safe perioperative journey that should be promoted globally.

First Checkpoint: Preoperative

- WHO Patient Information tool
- Preoperative anesthesia checkup (history, allergy, comorbidity, medications, labs, examination, consent, anesthesia and surgical plan, WHO Surgical Safety Checklist)
- Operating room checks prior to taking the patient into the OR:
  - Patient identification (correct patient, correct surgery, correct site)
  - Infection control (gloves, antibiotics, alcohol swabs, sterile instruments)
  - Equipment check (anesthesia, oxygen, suction, airway, operating room table, resuscitation, vital monitoring, pulse oximetry, end-tidal carbon dioxide monitoring)
  - Medicines (emergency, anesthetics, opioid)
  - Supplies (oxygen, intravenous fluids, disposable syringes with needles)
  - Trained staff (each member of the surgical team is trained/skilled in what they do: doctors/nurse/technician/assistants)
  - Intravenous access and blood requirements

Second Checkpoint: Intraoperative

- WHO Surgical Safety Checklist
- Critical surgical concerns
- Monitoring
- Maintaining record

Third Checkpoint: Postoperative/Recovery Room/Intensive Care/Ward

- Pain relief
- Monitoring (sometimes often the best successful surgical intervention performed in the OR can end up with a morbidity and mortality discovered much later in the postoperative period during transfer or in the ward)
- WHO Surgical Checklist: Discharge records are signed off before transfer to the next level of care
- Room check:
  - Infection control (surgical site infection, hand hygiene, etc.)
  - Equipment (oxygen, suction, monitoring vital signs, etc.)
  - Medicines
  - Supplies

Conclusion

The Sustainable Development Goals (SDGs) implementation agenda for 2030 calls for the global surgical community to act urgently in collaboration and partnership with local stakeholders to invest in improvements made specifically to the SDG core indicator targets relevant to emergency and essential surgical care and anesthesia.

These core indicators highlight the important areas required for coverage of quality essential health services that include service-specific availability and readiness; outpatient service utilization including inpatient admissions and surgical volume; perioperative mortality rate reduction in maternal, newborn, and children; noncommunicable diseases including injuries and cancer; interventions in neglected tropical diseases; and health system strengthening for quality and safety of care including access to medicines, health worker density and distribution, access to emergency surgery, output training institutions, and official development assistance to the medical research and basic health sectors [16].

Pursuing UHC through expanding coverage for health services alone is not enough. LMICs must strive to provide better quality of care (and improve surgical and anesthesia capacity); otherwise, deaths attributable to receiving poor-quality healthcare will not enable meeting SDG targets [39].

References

1. Giannou C, Baldan M. Anaesthesia and analgesia in war surgery. In: War surgery: working with limited resources in armed conflict and other situations of violence. Vol. 1. Geneva: International Committee of the Red Cross; 2009. p. 307.
2. World Health Organization, Organisation for economic co-operation and development, The World Bank. Delivering quality health services: a global imperative for universal health coverage. Geneva; 2018, p. 30. https://apps.who.int/iris/bitstream/handle/10665/272465/9789241513906-eng.pdf?sequence=1&isAllowed=y. Accessed 01 Aug 2019.
3. Universal health coverage. WHO Infographics. https://www.who.int/universal_health_coverage/infographics/en/
4. Debas HT, Donkor P, Gawande A, Jamison DT, Kruk ME, Mock CN, editors. Essential surgery, disease control priorities, vol. 1. 3rd ed. Washington, DC: World Bank; 2015. Preface; p xv.
5. World Health Assembly Resolution WHA68.15. Strengthening emergency and essential surgical care and anesthesia as a component of universal health coverage: addressing the public health gaps arising from lack of safe, affordable and accessible surgical and anesthetic Services. Geneva; 2015. http://apps.who.int/gb/ebwha/pdf_files/WHA68/A68_R15-en.pdf. Accessed 01 Aug 2019.
6. World Health Organization. EB144/11 Rev.1. Implementation of the 2030 Agenda for Sustainable Development: report by the director-general. Geneva; 2018. https://apps.who.int/gb/ebwha/pdf_files/WHA72/A72_11Rev1-en.pdf. Accessed 01 Aug 2019.
7. McCord C, Kruk ME, Mock CN, Cherian M, Schreeb JV, Russell S, English M. Organization of essential services and the role of first-level hospitals. In: Debas HT, Donkor P, Gawande A, Jamison DT, Kruk ME, Mock CN, editors. Essential surgery, disease control priorities, vol. 1. 3rd ed. Washington, DC: World Bank; 2015. p. 228.
8. Haider A, Scott JW, Gause CD, et al. Development of a unifying target and consensus indicators for global surgical systems strengthening: proposed by the global Alliance for surgery, obstetric, trauma, and anaesthesia care (the G4 Alliance). World J Surg. 2017;41:2426–34. https://doi.org/10.1007/s00268-017-4028-1.
9. McQueen K, Coonan T, Ottaway A, Dutton RP, Nuevo FR, Gathuya Z, Wilson IH. Anesthesia and perioperative care. In: Debas HT, Donkor P, Gawande A, Jamison DT, Kruk ME, Mock CN, editors. Essential surgery, disease control priorities, vol. 1. 3rd ed. Washington, DC: World Bank; 2015. p. 265–6.
10. Bainbridge D, Martin J, Arango M, Cheng D. Evidence-based perioperative clinical outcomes research (EPiCOR) group. Perioperative and anaesthetic-related mortality in developed and developing countries: a systematic review and meta-analysis. Lancet. 2012;380(9847):1075–81.

11. Nepogodiev D, Martin J, Biccard B, Makupe A, Bhangu A. Global burden of postoperative death. Lancet. 2019;393(10170):401.
12. Gelb AW, Morriss WW, Johnson W, Merry AF. International standards for a safe practice of anesthesia workgroup. World Health Organization-World Federation of Societies of Anaesthesiologists (WHO-WFSA) International Standards for a Safe Practice of Anesthesia. Can J Anesth. 2018;65:698–708.
13. Stewart B, Wong E, Papillon-Smith J, Trelles Centurion MA, Dominguez L, Ao S, et al. An analysis of Cesarean section and emergency hernia ratios as markers of surgical capacity in low-income countries affected by humanitarian emergencies from 2008–2014 at Médecins sans Frontières Operations Centre Brussels projects. PLoS Curr. 2015;7. https://www.ncbi.nlm.nih.gov/pmc/articles/PMC4395259/. Accessed 02 Aug 2019.
14. WHO Comprehensive Safe Hospital Framework, Geneva; 2015. https://hospitalsafetypromotionanddisasterpreparedness.files.wordpress.com/2018/03/comprehensive_safe_hospital_framework_2015_who.pdf. Accessed 02 Aug 2019.
15. WHO guidelines for safe surgery: safe surgery saves lives. World Health Organization. Geneva; 2009. https://www.who.int/patientsafety/safesurgery/tools_resources/9789241598552/en/. Accessed 02 Aug 2019.
16. World Health Organization. 2018 Global reference list of 100 core health indicators (plus health-related SDGs). Geneva; 2018. http://www.who.int/healthinfo/indicators/2018/en. Accessed on 02 Aug 2019.
17. Haynes AB, Weiser TG, Berry WR, et al. The safe surgery saves lives study group. A surgical safety checklist to reduce morbidity and mortality in a global population. N Engl J Med. 2009;360:491–9.
18. World Health Organization. Guidelines for trauma quality improvement programmes; 2009. https://apps.who.int/iris/bitstream/handle/10665/44061/9789241597746_eng.pdf?sequence=1. Accessed 02 Aug 2019.
19. Roth R, Frost EAM, Gevirtz C, editors; ; Atcheson CLH, assoc ed. The role of anesthesiology in global health: a comprehensive guide. Cham, Switzerland: Springer International Publishing; 2015.
20. Trelles Centurion M, Crestani R, Dominguez L, Caluwaerts A, Benedetti G. Surgery with limited resources in natural disasters: what is the minimum standard of care? Curr Trauma Rep. 2018;4(2):89–95.
21. Trelles M, Dominguez L, Stewart BT. Surgery in low-income countries during crisis: experience at Médecins Sans Frontières facilities in 20 countries between 2008 and 2014. Tropical Med Int Health. 2015;20(8):968–71.
22. Zitzman E, Berkley H, Jindal RM. Accountability in global surgery missions. BMJ Glob Health. 2018;3(6):e001025. https://www.ncbi.nlm.nih.gov/pmc/articles/PMC6326286/. Accessed 02 Aug 2019.
23. World Health Organization. HeRAMS Health resources availability mapping system. Geneva; 2009. http://www.who.int/hac/herams/en Accessed 03 Aug 2019.
24. World Health Organization. Emergency Medical Teams. Geneva; 2016. http://www.who.int/hac/techguidance/preparedness/emergency_medical_teams/en/ Accessed 03 Aug 2019.
25. World Health Organization. WHO Safe Childbirth Checklist. Geneva; 2015. https://www.who.int/patientsafety/implementation/checklists/childbirth/en/ Accessed 04 Aug 2019.
26. World Health Organization. Consultation on improving measurement of the quality of maternal, newborn and child care in health facilities. Geneva; 2014. http://apps.who.int/iris/bitstream/10665/128206/1/9789241507417_eng.pdf. Accessed 04 Aug 2019.
27. World Health Organization. WHO guidelines on hand hygiene in health care. Geneva; 2009. https://www.who.int/gpsc/5may/tools/9789241597906/en/. Accessed 04 Aug 2019.
28. World Health Organization. 10 facts on patient safety, updated Mar 2018. Geneva; 2018. https://wwwwhoint/features/factfiles/patient_safety/en/. Accessed 03 Aug 2019.
29. World Health Organization. WHO global guidelines for the prevention of surgical site infection. Geneva; 2016. https://www.who.int/gpsc/SSI-outline.pdf?ua=1. Accessed 03 Aug 2019.
30. Macintyre PE, Scott D, Schug SA, Visser EJ, Walker SM. Acute pain management: scientific evidence. 3rd ed. Melbourne: Australian and New Zealand College of Anaesthetists and Faculty of Pain Medicine; 2010.

31. Goucke R, MorrisseyW. Essential pain management: workshop manual. Wembley Downs: Roger Goucke & Wayne Morriss; 2011.
32. Size M, Soyannwo OA, Justins DM. Pain management in developing countries. Anaesthesia. 2007;62(Suppl 1):38–43.
33. Mahoney PF, Jeyanathan J, Wood P, Craven R. Anaesthesia handbook. Geneva: International Committee of the Red Cross; 2017.
34. World Health Organization. First global patient safety challenge: clean care is safer care. Geneva; 2005. https://www.who.int/gpsc/clean_care_is_safercare/en/. Accessed 03 Aug 2019.
35. World Health Organization. Third global patient safety challenge: medication without harm. Geneva; 2017. https://www.who.int/patientsafety/medication-safety/en/. Accessed 03 Aug 2019.
36. Zinn C. 14,000 preventable deaths in Australia. BMJ. 1995;310:1487.
37. Communication during Patient handovers. JCI WHO JCI WHO Collaboration Patient Safety Solutions, Vol.1, solution 3. May 2007.
38. World Health Organization. Patients for patient safety. Geneva; 2013. https://www.who.int/patientsafety/patients_for_patient/en/. Accessed 03 Aug 2109.
39. Kruk ME, Gage AD, Joseph NT, Danaei G, García-Saisó S, Salomon JA. Mortality due to low-quality health systems in the universal health coverage era: a systematic analysis of amenable deaths in 137 countries. Lancet. 2018;392(10160):2203–12.
40. Sheik Ali S, Jaffry Z, Cherian MN, Kunjumen T, Nkwowane AM, Leather AJM, et al. Surgical human resources according to types of health care facility: an assessment in low- and middle-income countries. World J Surg. 2017;41(11):2667–73.
41. United Nations. Transforming our world: the 2030 agenda for sustainable development. A/RES/70/1. Geneva; 2015. https://www.un.org/en/development/desa/population/migration/generalassembly/docs/globalcompact/A_RES_70_1_E.pdf. Accessed 03 Aug 2019.
42. Holmer H, Lantz A, Kunjumen T, Finlayson S, Hoyler M, Siyam A, et al. Global distribution of surgeons, anaesthesiologists, and obstetricians. Lancet Glob Health. 2015;3:S9–11.
43. Vo D, Cherian MN, Bianchi S, Noel L, Lundeg G, et al. Anesthesia capacity in 22 low and middle income countries. J Anesth Clin Res. 2012;3:207.
44. Belle J, Cohen H, Shindo N, Lim M, Velazquez-Berumen A, Ndihokubwayo JB, et al. Influenza preparedness in low-resource settings: a look at oxygen delivery in 12 African countries. J Infect Dev Ctries. 2010;4(7):419–24.
45. Kushner AL, Cherian MN, Noel L, Spiegel DA, Groth S, Etienne C. Addressing the millennium development goals from a surgical perspective. Essential surgery and anaesthesia in 8 low- and middle-income countries. Arch Surg. 2010;145(2):154–60.
46. Martin J, Tau G, Cherian MN, de Dios JV, Mills D, Fitzpatrik J, et al. Survey of the capacity for essential surgery and anaesthesia services in Papua New Guinea. BMJ Open 2015;5:e009841. Available at: https://bmjopen.bmj.com/content/5/12/e009841 Accessed 03 Aug 2019.
47. World Health Organization. Tool for situational analysis to assess emergency and essential surgical Care; 2007. https://www.who.int/surgery/publications/WHO_EESC_SituationAnalysisTool.pdf. Accessed 04 Aug 2019.
48. Osen H, Chang D, Choo S, Perry H, Hesse A, Abantanga F, et al. Validation of the World Health Organization tool for situational analysis to assess emergency and essential surgical care at district hospitals in Ghana. World J Surg. 2011;35(3):500–4.
49. World Federation of Societies of Anaesthesiologists. Anaesthesia facility assessment tool. https://www.wfsahq.org/resources/anaesthesia-facility-assessment-tool Accessed 04 Aug 2019.
50. World Federation of Societies of Anaesthesiologists. Safety and quality. Guidelines for tendering for anaesthesia machines. 2014. Available at: https://www.wfsahq.org/our-work/safety-quality. Accessed 04 Aug 2019.

51. International Organization for Standardization. Gas cylinders for medical use-marking for identification of content. ISO 32:1977. Geneva; 2017. https://www.iso.org/standard/3659.html. Accessed 04 Aug 2019.
52. International Organization for Standardization. Small medical gas cylinders—Pin index yoke type valve connectors. Geneva; 2004. https://www.sis.se/api/document/preview/905461/.
53. World Health Organization. Donation of medical equipment. Geneva; 2016. https://www.who.int/medical_devices/management_use/manage_donations/en/. Accessed 04 Aug 2019.
54. Spiegel DA, Droti B, Relan P, Hobson S, Cherian MN, O'Neill K, et al. Retrospective review of surgical availability and readiness in 8 African countries. BMJ Open. 2017;7(3):e014496.
55. Lassi ZS, Cometto G, Huicho L, Bhutta ZA. Quality of care provided by mid-level health workers: systematic review and meta-analysis. Bull World Health Organ. 2013;91(11):824–33. https://www.who.int/bulletin/volumes/91/11/BLT-13-118786-table-T5.html. Accessed 05 Aug 2019.
56. Cherian M, Choo S, Wilson I, Noel L, Sheikh M, Dayrit M, et al. Building and retaining the neglected anaesthesia health workforce: is it crucial for health systems strengthening through primary health care? Bull World Health Organ. 2010;88:637–9. https://apps.who.int/iris/handle/10665/270745. Accessed 05 Aug 2019.

The Role of the American College of Surgeons in Advancing Perioperative Safety and Efficiency

24

Julia R. Coleman and Patricia L. Turner

Introduction

Since its creation in 1913, the American College of Surgeons (ACS) has been a long-standing national leader in setting the standard of surgical practice and advocating for optimal patient care. With more than 82,000 members across 130 countries, the ACS has a global legacy of leadership with far-reaching effects on delivery of patient care and advocacy for surgical quality.

The four key principles of ACS, proposed by the organization's founders under the leadership of Franklin Martin, MD, FACS, are to (1) set standards, (2) build an appropriate infrastructure, (3) collect and analyze data, and (4) verify with outside experiences [1]. In the spirit of these four principles, in 1913, the ACS implemented professional and competency standards by establishing medical staff organizations in hospitals, exclusively acknowledging licensed practitioners in good standing, mandating regulations and policies regarding professional work, standardizing medical records, and requiring access to diagnostic and therapeutic resources [2]. Since then, ACS's mission and advocacy around perioperative safety and quality have expanded in a new era of rising health care costs and use of quality measure metrics (Fig. 24.1).

The College's commitment and leadership in this front have been in the form of standardized national databases for research focused on quality and safety, consensus statements and regulatory measures from collaborative multidisciplinary committees, and formalized educational programming for residents.

J. R. Coleman
Department of Surgery, University of Colorado–Denver, Aurora, CO, USA

P. L. Turner (✉)
American College of Surgeons, Chicago, IL, USA
e-mail: pturner@facs.org

J. J. Hoballah et al. (eds.), *Principles of Perioperative Safety and Efficiency*,
https://doi.org/10.1007/978-3-031-41089-5_24

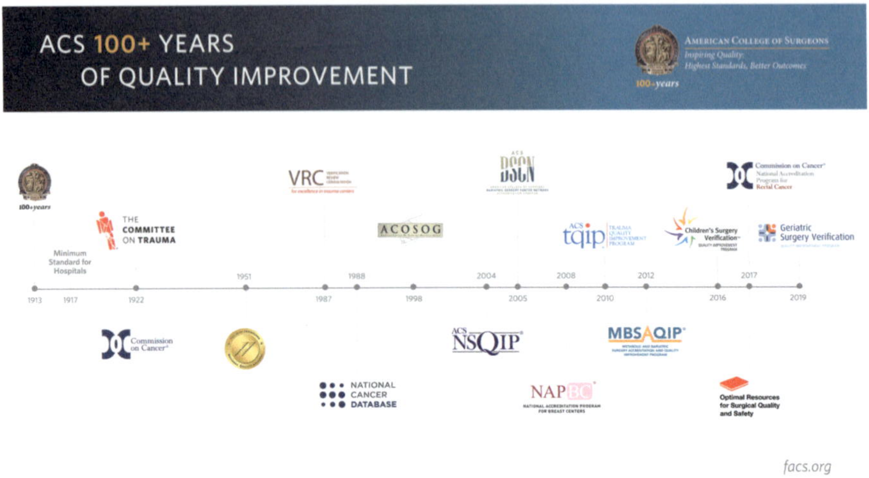

Fig. 24.1 A depiction of the 100+ year history of quality and safety programs put forth by the American College of Surgeons. Used with permission from the ACS

Perioperative Safety Through Promotion of Evidence-Based Practice: American College of Surgeons Databases

A core mission of the American College of Surgeons has been to collect, analyze, and disseminate data on perioperative patient care and outcomes to inform evidence-based practice guidelines and standards of care. This has led to the development of several quality improvement programs with nationwide databases, including the American College of Surgeons National Surgical Quality Improvement Program (ACS NSQIP); ACS NSQIP-Pediatrics, Trauma and Quality Improvement Program (TQIP); National Trauma Data Bank (NTDB); and National Cancer Database. The mission of promoting evidence-based practices has also spanned beyond the United States, with several international collaborative databases. These databases have had wide-ranging effects on various surgical specialties. Beyond promoting guidelines and standards of care, several courses have been created, including the Advanced Trauma Life Support (ATLS) course, which presents a concise approach to assessing and managing multiply injured patients.

ACS NSQIP, created by the Department of Veterans Affairs (VA) to compare risk-adjusted survival outcomes to the private sector and continued through ACS, is a national, validated, multispecialty outcome-reporting tool capable of assessing risk-adjusted outcomes, validating interventions, identifying areas for improvement, and promoting best practices and resource allocation [3]. When initially created, data from ACS NSQIP informed evidence-based care practice changes at the VA, which resulted in reduced morbidity and mortality rates at the VA by 43% and 47%, respectively, from 1991 to 2006 [3, 4]. With the motive to translate the ACS NSQIP to the civilian and private sector, the ACS and Agency for Health Care Research and Quality (AHRQ) awarded the Reporting System to Improve Patient

Safety in Surgery grant to 14 private sector hospitals and four community hospitals to examine risk-adjusted surgical outcomes. These data ultimately resulted in practice changes in reductions in postoperative morbidity, including surgical site infections and renal injury, leading to the ACS NSQIP becoming an open subscription program. Since its initial development in 1994, ACS NSQIP has expanded to now allow for predictive models for risk-adjusted 30-day morbidity and mortality in eight difference surgical specialties (general surgery, vascular surgery, noncardiac thoracic surgery, orthopedic surgery, urology, plastic surgery, otolaryngology, and neurosurgery). The culmination of the decades of ACS NSQIP data and the College's long tradition of developing successful quality programs for improving surgical care is *The Optimal Resources for Surgical Quality and Safety* manual (known as "The Red Book"). The publication, consisting of information on case review and peer review, credentialing and privileging, database and registries, and clinical practice guidelines, is the work of more than 100 contributing authors who are advocates of the health care quality movement. The Red Book now serves as a trusted resource for surgical leaders seeking to improve patient care in their institutions, departments, and practices.

One of the greatest impacts of ACS NSQIP has been identification of modifiable risk factors, leading to significant progress in evidence-based practice changes around perioperative safety in a population-, disease-, and phases of case-based approach. This has spanned various postoperative safety and quality outcomes around surgical site infections (SSIs) and sepsis [5–8] as well as urinary tract infections (UTIs) [6, 9, 10], venous thromboembolism [11], hospital length of stay [12–16], readmissions [17, 18], reoperation rates [11, 19], and mortality [6, 19–23]. The literature cited here is merely a small sample, with more than 2500 articles included in PubMed from analyses of ACS NSQIP data, which highlights the true impact and breadth of reach of ACS-driven education. The ACS NSQIP has become more developed and sophisticated over the decades, allowing it to more accurately identify hospital rates of outcomes, such as surgical site infections, as compared to the Centers for Disease Control and Prevention's National Healthcare Safety Network (NHSN) [24]. ACS NSQIP also led to the creation of a pediatric-based database, leading to research surrounding similar perioperative outcomes among neonatal and non-neonatal patients [25, 26]. This database includes nearly 100 hospitals and has promoted heightened awareness and data analysis around resource utilization, value-based metrics, and quality and safety measures [27], from evaluation of programs focused on reducing surgical site infection [28] to tools to predict perioperative morbidity risk factors [29, 30].

Adoption of ACS NSQIP into hospital performance standards and surgeon benchmarks has ultimately resulted in decreased morbidity and mortality of patients [31]. For example, Bliss et al. described adoption of surgical checklists for 73 surgeries and compared to 2079 historical control cases and 246 cases without checklist use; patient cases in which surgical checklists were employed perioperatively had significantly lower 30-day morbidity and safety-related events (in the form of surgical site infections and readmissions) [32]. Often, changes in health care delivery are prompted by the ACS NSQIP semiannual report. After having received the semiannual report with identification of their hospital as a high outlier for postoperative *Clostridium difficile* infections (CDIs), Turner et al. described employment of strategies to reduce CDIs in their hospital including antimicrobial stewardship optimization of preoperative order sets, modification of terminal cleaning practices, increased hand hygiene and personal protection equipment signage, improved antimicrobial stewardship, education through surgical grand rounds, and routine data feedback via ACS NSQIP. After implementation of these strategies, the observed rate of CDIs decreased significantly from 1.27% to 0.91% in 1 year alone [33]. In a similar success story of patient-centered, data-driven change, John et al. described response to ACS NSQIP semiannual report of higher SSI rates with audits of wound classification and SSIs, ultimately resulting in improved assessment, standardization, and prompt diagnosis of wound classification [34]. These stories highlight the significant translational impact of ACS NSQIP data.

Perioperative Safety Through Promotion of Collaborative Consensus Statement and National Recommendations

The American College of Surgeons has a long-standing precedent of establishing perioperative safety and quality improvement programs, beginning in 1917 with the creation of what would become the Joint Commission, a system for surveying institutions to determine whether hospitals were complying with College standards of care [1]. Programs focused on optimal patient care and perioperative safety comprise a myriad of collaborative efforts including, but not limited to, the Commission on Cancer (CoC), the Committee on Trauma (COT), the American College of Surgeons Oncology Group, the National Accreditation Program for Breast Centers (NAPBC), the American College of Surgeons Program for the Accredited Education Institutes, and the Metabolic and Bariatric Surgery Accreditation and Quality Improvement Programs.

Developed in the same spirit of ACS NSQIP, the Safety Program for Improving Surgical Care and Recovery (ISCR) was established in 2019, under the leadership of the Agency for Healthcare Research and Quality, the American College of Surgeons, and the Johns Hopkins Medicine Armstrong Institute for Patient Safety and Quality [35]. This collaborative effort aims to disseminate best practices in perioperative care to more than 750 hospitals across multiple procedures, from topics spanning postsurgical, specialty-specific pathways to perioperative safety outcome prophylaxis [35]. These best practices have been informed by decades of research on core surgical components of perioperative safety and quality, including patient education, bowel preparation, elimination of nasogastric tubes, minimization of surgical drains, early postoperative mobilization and feeding, conservative fluid management, prompt removal of urinary catheters, use of laxative and chewing gum, surgical site infection reduction bundles, glucose management, and venous thromboembolism [36–38]. These practice guidelines will ultimately allow for future evidence-based best practices and benchmarking of institutions across the nation and across surgical specialties.

In addition to the interdisciplinary, collaborative efforts of ISCR, the ACS has released several statements focused on perioperative safety to promote quality and benchmarking in surgery. In 1996, the ACS Board of Regents released the "Statement on Principles Underlying Perioperative Responsibility," which outlined the core responsibilities of the surgeon to ensure optimal patient care and perioperative safety in the form of diagnosis confirmation, review of appropriate management strategies, informed consent, proper preoperative preparation, safe operations, standardized postoperative care, and appropriate follow-up [39].

Beyond the expected conduct of the individual surgeon, the Board of Governors Surgical Care Delivery Workgroup and the Board of Governors Committee on Surgical Practice in Hospitals and Ambulatory Settings have issued several official statements on surgical patient safety focused on teamwork [40]. At the core of these statements, the ACS encourages health care organizations and hospitals to develop guidelines to ensure optimal perioperative safety. In 2018, the ACS issued a revised "Statement on Patient Safety in the Operating Room: Team Care," in which a team approach to communication and conduct in the operating room is encouraged [40]. In their "Statement on Surgical Patient Safety," the ACS also promotes adoption of a standardized curriculum developed by the Department of Defense focused on leadership, situation monitoring, mutual support, and communication: the Team Strategies and Tools to Enhance Performance and Patient Safety (TeamSTEPPS™) [41].

The focus on teamwork as an essential component of optimal perioperative and operative care was inspired by the formation of the Committee on Perioperative Care (CPC) in 2002 and the Council on Surgical and Perioperative Safety (CSPS) in 2004. CPC, a result of integration of the Committee on Operating Room Environment (CORE) and the Pre- and Post-Operative Care Committee (PPOC), works collaboratively with several organizations, including the American Society of Anesthesiologists and the American Association of Surgical Physician Assistants, to serve as the primary resource to the College on topics concerning perioperative care. Specifically, the committee develops and presents information and recommendations related to education, technology, standards of care, clinical and facilities management, and assessment of outcomes [42]. Similarly, CSPS includes representatives from the ACS, the American Society of Anesthesiologists (ASA), the Association of Registered Nurses (AORN), the American Society of Nurse Anesthetists (ANA), the American Society of Physician Assistants (AAPA), the American Society of Perianesthesia Nurses (ASPAN), and the Association of Surgical Technologists (AST) [43]. With the goal of collaborating on standards and guidelines for safe practice and patient safety, the CSPS has released several statements including "Statement on Health Care Industry Representatives in the Operating Room," "Statement of Blunt Suture Needles," and "Statement on the Prevention of Retained Foreign Bodies After Surgery" to promote standardized practices around perioperative safety and quality. CPC and CSPS are only a couple of exemplary demonstrations of ACS collaboratives, with other ACS partnering with the American Association for the Surgery of Trauma, the American Society of Breast Surgeons, the American Society of Transplant Surgeons, the Association of Women Surgeons, the Association for Academic Surgery, the Association for Surgical Education, and Eastern Association for the Surgery of Trauma, among others.

These interdisciplinary, collaborative groups for adult care led to the development of the ACS Task Force for Children's Surgical Care, a group composed of leaders in pediatric perioperative medicine, in 2012 [44]. Under the direction of the ACS and Children's Hospital Association (CHD), this task force has established benchmarks and recommendations around perioperative resource utilization and access and quality improvement and safety, as well as created the Children's Surgery Verification and Quality Improvement Program (ACS CSG) in 2017. ACS CSG now includes more than 125 pediatric surgical programs meeting specific requirements for leadership and resource availability and continues to expand [44].

Perioperative Safety Through Promotion of Resident Education and Collaboration with ACGME

While the American College of Surgeons has centralized its focus around patient safety, it also recognizes that an integral component of this is through education of future patient providers, surgical residents. In conjunction with the Accreditation Council for Graduate Medical Education (ACGME), the ACS has led the movement toward incorporation of perioperative safety into the curriculum of resident education. The ACGME and the American Board of Medical Specialties (ABMS) have defined six core competencies for all residents, all of which are essential for patient safety: (1) medical knowledge, (2) patient care, (3) interpersonal and communication skills, (4) professionalism, (5) practice-based learning and improvement, and (6) system-based practice [45]. Innovative curriculum design and promotion have been led by the ACS around these core competences to promote patient safety. In 2005, the ACS and Association for Surgical Education jointly co-sponsored a conference focused on national educational efforts relating to patient safety in surgery [46]. This conference led to a description of a comprehensive safety-centered curriculum focused on institutional culture, clinical teaching and learning, team training, simulation exercises, transitions in care, and handling of adverse events and errors.

Aligned with the mission of educating residents about standards of surgical care and implementation of quality-driven care, the ACS is part of a consortium led by the American Board of Surgery entitled the Surgical Council on Resident Education (SCORE). Formed in 2006, this nonprofit consortium of leaders in the US surgical education has a mission of improving the education of residents in general surgery and related specialties through development of a national curriculum. The SCORE portal, available to all residents across the country, delivers educational content across the six clinical competencies mentioned above and spans across patient quality and safety.

ACS recognizes that a core component of resident professional development is encouraging engagement in the College and nurturing leadership in the realm of patient quality and safety. The Resident and Associate Society of the American College of Surgeons (RAS-ACS) is an organization for surgical trainees and young surgeons within ACS, which provides an avenue for participation in ACS affairs, fosters development and use of leadership skills in organized surgery, and provides opportunities for opinions and concerns of young surgeons and trainees to be heard by ACS leadership. RAS-ACS activities, from journal clubs and hangouts to *ACS Bulletin* compositions and advocacy efforts, have focused on quality and safety, instilling a deep sense of commitment and value for patient quality and safety in the delivery of surgical care among resident trainees.

In addition to promoting education around perioperative safety in surgical resident curricula, the ACS has also been a leading voice in advocacy for resident involvement in patient care. Research from the ACS NSQIP database on resident involvement in patient care indicates longer operative times, but no difference in perioperative safety outcomes and morbidity and mortality rates, debunking myths and concerns about patient safety when residents are involved in patient care [47–50]. For example, in an evaluation of all orchiectomies for testicular cancer in ACS NSQIP from 2006 to 2013, resident involvement in patient care was associated with longer operative time, but no difference in length of stay, complications, or mortality [49]. In a study of all thyroid surgeries in 2011 from ACS NSQIP, those with resident involvement were associated with slightly longer operative time (119 min versus 102 min, $p < 0.001$), but unplanned reoperation rate was significantly *lower* in cases with residents, with no difference in overall postoperative complications [47]. Similarly, in a study of all patients undergoing microsurgical procedures from 2005 to 2012 in ACS NSQIP, resident involvement was not a significant risk factor for complications, flap failure, bleeding, and unexpected reoperation rates [51]. These studies highlight that resident involvement in patient care is not only safe, but also beneficial to patients. This emphasizes the importance of training residents with patient-centered, safety-focused curricula.

Conclusion

The American College of Surgeons will continue to be a leader in advocating for optimal patient care and focus on perioperative safety. This mission involves supporting ongoing database and risk calculator tools likes ACS NSQIP, fostering collaborative, multidisciplinary committees and task forces—in addition to timely and evidence-based practice recommendations—and promoting resident training centered on perioperative safety and quality. The American College of Surgeons has a history embedded in the mission of optimal patient care and will continue to lead the future in patient care quality and safety through standards and performance benchmarks, data-driven optimization in health care delivery, and excellence in training.

References

1. Hoyt DB, Schneidman DS. 100 years of inspiring quality at the ACS: how did we get here? J Pediatr Surg. 2014;49(1):25–8.
2. Wright JR Jr. The American College of Surgeons, minimum standards for hospitals, and the provision of high-quality laboratory services. Arch Pathol Lab Med. 2017;141(5):704–17.

3. Ingraham AM, Richards KE, Hall BL, Ko CY. Quality improvement in surgery: the American College of Surgeons National Surgical Quality Improvement Program approach. Adv Surg. 2010;44:251–67.
4. Khuri SF. The ACS-NSQIP: a new frontier in surgery. Surgery. 2005;138(5):837–43.
5. Ramly EP, Alami RS, Tamim H, Kantar R, Elias E, Safadi BY. Concomitant removal of gastric band and sleeve gastrectomy: analysis of outcomes and complications from the ACS-NSQIP database. Surg Obes Relat Dis. 2016;12(5):984–8.
6. deFreitas DJ, Kasirajan K, Ricotta JJ 2nd, Veeraswamy RK, Corriere MA. Preoperative inpatient hospitalization and risk of perioperative infection following elective vascular procedures. Ann Vasc Surg. 2012;26(1):46–54.
7. Shah DK, Vitonis AF, Missmer SA. Association of body mass index and morbidity after abdominal, vaginal, and laparoscopic hysterectomy. Obstet Gynecol. 2015;125(3):589–98.
8. Sutton E, Miyagaki H, Bellini G, Shantha Kumara HM, Yan X, Howe B, et al. Risk factors for superficial surgical site infection after elective rectal cancer resection: a multivariate analysis of 8880 patients from the American College of Surgeons National Surgical Quality Improvement Program database. J Surg Res. 2017;207:205–14.
9. Aminian A, Shoar S, Khorgami Z, Augustin T, Schauer PR, Brethauer SA. Safety of one-step conversion of gastric band to sleeve: a comparative analysis of ACS-ACS-NSQIP data. Surg Obes Relat Dis. 2015;11(2):386–91.
10. Sadeghi M, Leis JA, Laflamme C, Sparkes D, Ditrani W, Watamaniuk A, et al. Standardisation of perioperative urinary catheter use to reduce postsurgical urinary tract infection: an interrupted time series study. BMJ Qual Saf. 2019;28(1):32–8.
11. Nelson JA, Fischer JP, Wink JD, Kovach SJ 3rd. A population-level analysis of abdominal wall reconstruction by component separation in the morbidly obese patient: can it be performed safely? J Plast Surg Hand Surge. 2014;48(5):305–11.
12. Torabi SJ, Chouairi F, Dinis J, Alperovich M. Impact of advanced age on microvascular reconstruction of the lower facial third: an American College of Surgeons ACS-NSQIP study. Microsurgery. 2019;
13. Paredes AZ, Guzman-Pruneda FA, Abdel-Misih S, Hays J, Dillhoff ME, Pawlik TM, et al. Perioperative morbidity of gastrectomy during CRS-HIPEC: an ACS-ACS-NSQIP analysis. J Surg Res. 2019;241:31–9.
14. Schilling PL, Hallstrom BR, Birkmeyer JD, Carpenter JE. Prioritizing perioperative quality improvement in orthopaedic surgery. J Bone Joint Surg Am. 2010;92(9):1884–9.
15. Bovonratwet P, Ondeck NT, Nelson SJ, Cui JJ, Webb ML, Grauer JN. Comparison of outpatient vs inpatient total knee arthroplasty: an ACS-ACS-NSQIP analysis. J Arthroplast. 2017;32(6):1773–8.
16. Bovonratwet P, Tyagi V, Ottesen TD, Ondeck NT, Rubin LE, Grauer JN. Revision total knee arthroplasty in octogenarians: an analysis of 957 cases. J Arthroplast. 2018;33(1):178–84.
17. Hu K, Zhang T, Hutter M, Xu W, Williams Z. Thirty-day perioperative adverse outcomes after peripheral nerve surgery: an analysis of 2351 patients in the American College of Surgeons National Surgical Quality Improvement Program database. World Neurosurg. 2016;94:409–17.
18. Cloyd JM, Abdel-Misih S, Hays J, Dillhoff ME, Pawlik TM, Schmidt C. Impact of synchronous liver resection on the perioperative outcomes of patients undergoing CRS-HIPEC. J Gastrointest Surg. 2018;22(9):1576–84.
19. Weinberg D, Qeadan F, McKee R, Rogers RG, Komesu YM. Safety of laparoscopic sacrocolpopexy with concurrent rectopexy: peri-operative morbidity in a nationwide cohort. Int Urogynecol J. 2019;30(3):385–92.
20. Foster JM, Sleightholm R, Patel A, Shostrom V, Hall B, Neilsen B, et al. Morbidity and mortality rates following cytoreductive surgery combined with hyperthermic intraperitoneal chemotherapy compared with other high-risk surgical oncology procedures. JAMA Netw Open. 2019;2(1):e186847.
21. Rock AK, Opalak CF, Workman KG, Broaddus WC. Safety outcomes following spine and cranial neurosurgery: evidence from the National Surgical Quality Improvement Program. J Neurosurg Anesthesiol. 2018;30(4):328–36.

22. Haskins IN, Nowacki AS, Khorgami Z, Schulz K, Heinberg LJ, Schauer PR, et al. Should recent smoking be a contraindication for sleeve gastrectomy? Surg for Obes Relat Dis. 2017;13(7):1130–5.
23. Cramer JD, Patel UA, Samant S, Yang A, Smith SS. Liver disease in patients undergoing head and neck surgery: incidence and risk for postoperative complications. Laryngoscope. 2017;127(1):102–9.
24. Ju MH, Ko CY, Hall BL, Bosk CL, Bilimoria KY, Wick EC. A comparison of 2 surgical site infection monitoring systems. JAMA Surg. 2015;150(1):51–7.
25. Kim Y, Patel VA, Isildak H, Carr MM. An analysis of safety and adverse events following cochlear implantation in children under 12 months of age. Otol Neurotol. 2017;38(10):1426–32.
26. Raval MV, Dillon PW, Bruny JL, Ko CY, Hall BL, Moss RL, et al. American College of Surgeons National Surgical Quality Improvement Program Pediatric: a phase 1 report. J Am Coll Surg. 2011;212(1):1–11.
27. Cameron DB, Rangel SJ. Quality improvement in pediatric surgery. Curr Opin Pediatr. 2016;28(3):348–55.
28. Fawley J, Chelius TH, Anderson Y, Cassidy LD, Arca MJ. Relationship between perioperative blood transfusion and surgical site infections in the newborn population: an ACS-ACS-NSQIP-Pediatrics analysis. J Pediatr Surg. 2016;51(9):1397–404.
29. Valencia E, Staffa SJ, Faraoni D, DiNardo JA, Nasr VG. Prospective external validation of the Pediatric risk assessment Score in predicting perioperative mortality in children undergoing noncardiac surgery. Anesthand Analg. 2019;129(4):1014–20.
30. Basques BA, Lukasiewicz AM, Samuel AM, Webb ML, Bohl DD, Smith BG, et al. Which pediatric orthopaedic procedures have the greatest risk of adverse outcomes? J Pediatr Orthop. 2017;37(6):429–34.
31. Maggard-Gibbons M. The use of report cards and outcome measurements to improve the safety of surgical care: the American College of Surgeons National Surgical Quality Improvement Program. BMJ Qual Saf. 2014;23(7):589–99.
32. Bliss LA, Ross-Richardson CB, Sanzari LJ, Shapiro DS, Lukianoff AE, Bernstein BA, et al. Thirty-day outcomes support implementation of a surgical safety checklist. J Am Coll Surg. 2012;215(6):766–76.
33. Turner MC, Behrens SL, Webster W, Huslage K, Smith BA, Wrenn R, et al. Multidisciplinary approach to Clostridium difficile infection in adult surgical patients. J Am Coll Surg. 2019;228(4):570–80.
34. John H, Nimeri A, Ellahham S. Improved surgical site infection (SSI) rate through accurately assessed surgical wounds. BMJ Qual Improv Rep. 2015;4(1)
35. Ban KA, Gibbons MM, Ko CY, Wick EC, Cannesson M, Scott MJ, et al. Evidence review conducted for the Agency for Healthcare Research and Quality Safety Program for Improving Surgical Care and Recovery: focus on anesthesiology for colorectal surgery. Anesth Analg. 2019;128(5):879–89.
36. Kalogera E, Nelson G, Liu J, Hu QL, Ko CY, Wick E, et al. Surgical technical evidence review for gynecologic surgery conducted for the Agency for Healthcare Research and Quality Safety Program for Improving Surgical Care and Recovery. Am J Obstet Gynecol. 2018;219(6):563.e561–19.
37. Grant MC, Gibbons MM, Ko CY, Wick EC, Cannesson M, Scott MJ, et al. Evidence review conducted for the Agency for Healthcare Research and Quality Safety Program for Improving Surgical Care and Recovery: focus on anesthesiology for bariatric surgery. Anesth Analg. 2019;129(1):51–60.
38. Childers CP, Siletz AE, Singer ES, Faltermeier C, Hu QL, Ko CY, et al. Surgical technical evidence review for elective total joint replacement conducted for the AHRQ Safety Program for Improving Surgical Care and Recovery. Geriatr Orthop Surg Rehabil. 2018;9:2151458518754451.
39. American College of Surgeons. Statement on principles underlying perioperative responsibility. https://www.facs.org/about-acs/statements/25-perioperative. Accessed 14 Jul 2019.

40. American College of Surgeons. Statement on patient safety in the operating room: team care. https://www.facs.org/about-acs/statements/113-patient-safety. Accessed 14 Jul 2019.
41. Clancy CM, Tornberg DN. TeamSTEPPS: assuring optimal teamwork in clinical settings. Am J Med Qual. 2007;22(3):214–7.
42. American College of Surgeons. Committee on perioperative care. https://www.facs.org/about-acs/governance/acs-committees/committee-on-perioperative-care. Accessed 14 Jul 2019.
43. American College of Surgeons. Council on surgical and perioperative safety. https://www.ast.org/Aboutus/CSPS_Statements/. Accessed 14 Jul 2019.
44. Houck CS, Deshpande JK, Flick RP. The American College of Surgeons Children's Surgery Verification and Quality Improvement Program: implications for anesthesiologists. Curr Opin Anaesthesiol. 2017;30(3):376–82.
45. Sachdeva AK. Acquisition and maintenance of surgical competence. Sem Vasc Surg. 2002;15(3):182–90.
46. Sachdeva AK, Philibert I, Leach DC, Blair PG, Stewart LK, Rubinfeld IS, et al. Patient safety curriculum for surgical residency programs: results of a national consensus conference. Surgery. 2007;141(4):427–41.
47. Kshirsagar RS, Chandy Z, Mahboubi H, Verma SP. Does resident involvement in thyroid surgery lead to increased postoperative complications? Laryngoscope. 2017;127(5):1242–6.
48. Loppenberg B, Cheng PJ, Speed JM, Cole AP, Vetterlein MW, Kibel AS, et al. The effect of resident involvement on surgical outcomes for common urologic procedures: a case study of uni- and bilateral hydrocele repair. Urology. 2016;94:70–6.
49. Vetterlein MW, Seisen T, Loppenberg B, Hanna N, Cheng PJ, Fisch M, et al. Resident involvement in radical inguinal orchiectomy for testicular cancer does not adversely impact perioperative outcomes—a retrospective study. Urol Int. 2017;98(4):472–7.
50. Jubbal KT, Echo A, Spiegel AJ, Izaddoost SA. The impact of resident involvement in breast reconstruction surgery outcomes by modality: an analysis of 4,500 cases. Microsurgery. 2017;37(7):800–7.
51. Jubbal KT, Chang D, Izaddoost SA, Pederson W, Zavlin D, Echo A. Resident involvement in microsurgery: an American College of Surgeons National Surgical Quality Improvement Program analysis. J Surg Ed. 2017;74(6):1124–32.

Index

J. J. Hoballah et al. (eds.), *Principles of Perioperative Safety and Efficiency*,
https://doi.org/10.1007/978-3-031-41089-5

MIX
Papier aus verantwortungsvollen Quellen
Paper from responsible sources
FSC® C105338

If you have any concerns about our products,
you can contact us on
ProductSafety@springernature.com

In case Publisher is established outside the EU,
the EU authorized representative is:
Springer Nature Customer Service Center GmbH
Europaplatz 3, 69115 Heidelberg, Germany

Printed by Libri Plureos GmbH
in Hamburg, Germany